VITAMIN C AND CANCER:
MEDICINE OR POLITICS?

29 April 1985

To Arnold S. Relman, Editor
N E J M

Three months ago I wrote to each of the six Mayo Clinic authors of their paper published on 17 January 1985 in the New England Journal of Medicine, asking some questions about the paper. Not one of the six answered my letter.

I have now written them again, pointing out that this fact is evidence that they are involved in a conspiracy to suppress the truth.

Some time ago I wrote to you, asking for information about the process by which this fraudulent paper came to be accepted for publication in your journal. You have not answered my letter.

I hope that you will do me the courtesy of answering my letter. Your continued failure to do so would indicate that you also are involved in this conspiracy to suppress the truth.

I enclose a copy of my press release.

Yours truly,
Linus Pauling

The original draft of Linus Pauling's letter to Arnold Relman, editor of the *New England Journal of Medicine*, in the wake of the second Mayo Clinic trial of vitamin C. (Reproduced by kind permission of Linus Pauling)

Vitamin C and Cancer: Medicine or Politics?

Evelleen Richards

Science and Technology Studies Dept
University of Wollongong, Australia

St. Martin's Press
New York

First published in the United States of America in 1991

Printed in Hong Kong

ISBN 0–312–05242–1

Library of Congress Cataloging-in-Publication Data

Richards, Evelleen,
Vitamin C and cancer: medicine or politics? / Evelleen Richards
p.   cm.
Includes bibliographical reference and index.
ISBN 0–312–05242–1
1. Vitamin C — Therapeutic use — Political aspects.   2. Cancer —
Alternative treatment — Political aspects.   3. Vitamin therapy —
Political aspects.   4. Medicine — Research — Political aspects.
I. Title
RC271.A78R53 1991   90–8795
362.1'96994 — dc20   CIP

To Warwick,
whose idea this was

Contents

Acknowledgements

I owe debts of gratitude to a great many people who contributed to the making of this book.

My greatest debts must be to Linus Pauling and Ewan Cameron, who first welcomed me to the Linus Pauling Institute of Science and Medicine in 1983. With courage and generosity they gave me unrestricted access to their personal correspondence, manuscripts and referees' reports. Over the years, Ewan Cameron in particular, they unstintingly provided me with supplementary material, and responded patiently and graciously to my many questions and demands for information. Without them, in more senses than the obvious one of their centrality to the vitamin C and cancer dispute, this book could not have been written. Although they have not always agreed with my interpretation of their material, they have scrupulously refrained from any intervention in my project. They have given generously their permission for the many quotations from their private correspondence that I have used in my reconstruction of the controversy. I have great pleasure in thanking them both.

Emile Zuckerkandl, Director of the Linus Pauling Institute, was unfailingly courteous and hospitable, and provided some crucial material and information. I thank him for these and for our enjoyable debates on the social construction of science. Other Institute members I would like to thank include Mrs. Dorothy Monro, for her unflagging assistance in finding relevant correspondence and material in the vast, and as yet uncatalogued, Pauling Archives; Richard Hicks, Executive Vice-President, who patiently answered my questions on Institute funding and resources; and Steve Burbeck, Zelek Herman, Raxit Jariwalla, Rick Marcuson, Ruth Reynolds, Fred Stitt, Constance Tsao, and Dick Willoughby, for discussion of their research and Institute matters. I should also like to thank Dr. Robert Paradowski, Rochester Institute of Technology, who is working on the official Pauling biography, for his generous sharing of some valuable material.

For interviews or correspondence by mail, I would like to thank Dr. Robert E. Wittes and other personnel at the National Cancer Institute; Dr. Charles Moertel, Dr. Edward Creagan and Robert Horton of the Mayo Clinic; and Professor Kenneth J. Carpenter of the Department of Nutritional Sciences at the University of California, Berkeley.

I would also like to thank the investigative journalists, Peter Chowka and Ralph Moss, for their valuable information on the American alternative health network; and Ian Anderson, West Coast correspondent for

New Scientist, who gave generous access to his press clippings and files.

I owe much to Elizabeth Newland, who worked as research assistant in the initial phases of the project, and who is now waging her own brave struggle against cancer. Brian Martin gave encouragement, valuable advice, and ungrudgingly read and commented on each of the chapters of the book. Jerry Markle and Edward Yoxen kindly reviewed the manuscript at very short notice and offered stimulating and supportive comments. Other friends and colleagues who read chapters or gave intellectual encouragement or support include Ditta Bartels, Harry Collins, Louise Crossley, Anni Dugdale, David Edge, Richard Gillispie, Ron Johnston, Charles Kerr, Everett Mendelsohn, Harry Paul, Stewart Russell, Steven Shapin, John Schuster, David Turnbull, and Evan Willis. Anni Dugdale and David Selden gave research support in the final stages of manuscript preparation. I also wish to thank the students in my course on the 'Politics of Medicine and Health' at the University of Wollongong, who, over the years, were a responsive sounding board for many of the ideas contained in this book.

This research was aided by grants from the Australian Research Grants Scheme from 1981 to 1983, and from the University of Wollongong in 1983 and 1989.

I am grateful to Sage Publications for permission to use materials from: Evelleen Richards, 'The Politics of Therapeutic Evaluation: The Vitamin C and Cancer Controversy', *Social Studies of Science*, 18 (1988): 653–701. 1988 by Sage Publications, London, Newbury Park and New Delhi.

We must become the masters of medicine, not its servants. Let there be no misunderstanding: in the politics of medicine, it is we who must have the power, we who must set the policies.

Ian Kennedy, *The Unmasking of Medicine* (Kennedy, 1980)

The next thing [the judge] is going to say to me is, 'Look, I am an educated man and I wouldn't presume to decide between Linus Pauling and the Mayo Clinic. Here is a Nobel prize winning biochemist and here are fifteen doctors from the world's leading something and one tells me yes and the other tells me no, and how the hell am I going to decide? I don't know anything about biochemistry.' So he will say, 'Look Mr. [Attorney], you make a very interesting and persuasive argument, but on the other hand Mr.—— over here makes a very persuasive argument and I mean isn't this a question for scientists to decide? The history of science for a thousand years is that someone comes up with an idea, the establishment ridicules him, then fifty years later they find he was right and he becomes a saint. That's just life, and Pauling is in the great tradition of outcasts.' That's if I had a good judge. The worst is if I had a bad judge. He'd say, 'Look, Pauling is not a doctor – these guys are doctors; that's enough for me.' That could happen.

An Attorney's Advice to Linus Pauling at the height of the vitamin C and cancer controversy (Linus Pauling Institute, 1985c)

Introduction

In January 1985, the *New England Journal of Medicine* published the second negative study by Mayo Clinic researchers of the effectiveness of vitamin C as a cancer treatment. Once again, the media descended on the beleaguered Linus Pauling Institute of Science and Medicine. Three months later, Dr Linus Pauling dispatched a registered letter to the editor of the *Journal*, accusing him of publishing a 'fraudulent' paper and of being involved in a 'conspiracy to suppress the truth'.

What provoked these extraordinary allegations by America's most famous living scientist against the editor of its most powerful and prestigious medical journal? Five years down the track, what are we to make of the failure of the *New England Journal of Medicine* to publish Pauling's criticisms of the second Mayo study? The Mayo Clinic researchers will not respond to Pauling's letters. Why not? They have refused to share the raw data of the trial with him. Have they conclusively disproved Pauling's claims of the efficacy of vitamin C against malignant disease? Has Pauling, as they allege, violated the ethical code of science with his public denunciations of his adversaries and threats of litigation? Or is it, as Pauling asserts, that the ethical transgressors are his opponents – who have not refuted his claims but misrepresented them, who will not give him access to the data he needs, who have denied him a professional platform for his criticisms, and have forced him to go public in his efforts to make his own views heard? Who is right? What are cancer patients to do? How are we to understand this extended and acrimonious dispute? This is the cue for *Vitamin C and Cancer: Medicine or Politics?*

The vitamin C and cancer controversy has now continued for almost twenty years amidst mounting hostility and increasingly vehement charges and counter-charges of 'bias', 'fraud', and 'misrepresentation'. The dispute has been punctuated by running battles over publication and funding, by personal attacks on the scientific and ethical credibility of the disputants, and by media and political interventions. It has produced an avalanche of correspondence, manuscripts, publications, and newspaper reports. Its ramifications extend to the 'cancer establishment' and its institutions, various influential medical and scientific journals, the medical profession as a whole, nutritionists, the holistic health movement, the health food industry, the pharmaceutical industry, and to the many tens of thousands of cancer patients who currently take large doses of vitamin C. This story, as they say in the trade, has everything: the heroic confrontation of big business by little people over life and death issues;

1

allegations of scandal in high places; the central plot of a little-known surgeon from an obscure Scottish hospital locked in conflict with eminent researchers from one of the world's biggest and best-known medical clinics; and, of course, well upstage, the controversial and dominating presence of Linus Pauling – Nobel laureate and world-famous advocate of peace and vitamin C. This book, however, is less interested in exploiting the dramatic possibilities of the vitamin C and cancer story than in coming to grips with its implications.

Vitamin C and Cancer is about angry, dissident medicine. But it is also about bettering our understanding of the ways in which medical knowledge of disease and its treatment is produced, accepted, and applied. As a case study, the vitamin C and cancer controversy offers some valuable insights into the processes by which medical therapies are evaluated and put into practice. For this reason its history is relevant to all who wish to have a better understanding of, and, if possible, some input into the assessment and choice of available medical treatments.

Medical controversies are not new. As long as medicine and its practitioners have existed there have been disputes over the correct diagnosis and treatment of illness. Nor are protracted, rancorous and unresolved negotiations new to such disputes. The clinical epidemiologist, Alvan Feinstein, in discussing one such dispute over the interpretation of the randomized clinical study of certain agents for diabetic conditions, which was begun in the early 1960s and has still not been resolved, described it in the following terms:

> At the peak of the battle, the assaults from both sides contained emotional accusations, self-righteous fervour, and hyperbolic invective of a degree that has probably not occurred clinically since Pierre Louis more than a century earlier used statistical data to impugn the therapeutic value of blood-letting. (Feinstein, 1985)

What is comparatively new is the expectation by medical professionals, analysts, and critics alike, that such bitter conflicts may be resolved by the application of the scientific method to medicine in the form of the rigorously designed and properly applied controlled clinical trial (McKinlay, 1981; Doyle, 1983; Doyal and Doyal, 1984; Wallis, 1985; Silverman, 1985). According to what I shall term this standard view, science, in the form of the clinical trial, determines the 'correct' side of the debate, and it may then be safely assumed that the claims of the 'incorrect' side were somehow 'biased' by non-scientific factors, such as their own belief in the efficacy of their treatment, or their patients' expectations of improvement, or even economic or political considerations.

The standard view of medical controversies has its basis in the scientific status accorded to medicine and its practitioners, whereby medicine has been understood in its own terms as a body of objective knowledge about illness and its treatment. According to this viewpoint, medical knowledge is generated and practised by a group of experts, selected by achievement rather than social criteria such as class or gender, trained in scientific, rational, neutral processes, and regulated by an ethical code. But in recent years, coincident with the growth industry of medical criticism, this assumption has been questioned and revised. Modern medicine, its critics have argued, is replete with situations where remedies of questionable efficacy are routinely practised and prescribed, and ethically defended (Cochrane, 1972; McKeown, 1979; Kennedy, 1981; Inglis, 1983). Many modern medical techniques and therapies are viewed by their critics as not only ineffective but also harmful, and they have cautioned against the unbridled expansion of medical technology. The critics of medicine range from those within medicine itself who wish to instigate a measure of reform within the system, to those such as Ivan Illich, who adopts the extreme position that, on balance, medicine does more harm than good, and we would all be better off without it (Illich, 1977). This current dissatisfaction with modern medicine and its practitioners is not confined to such critics and the rapidly expanding literature which embodies their by now familiar critiques, but is more broadly diffused throughout western society. Every media story of some new medical breakthrough or wonder drug is counterbalanced by reports of adverse side effects, unnecessary surgery, over-investigation, and so on. The perceived deficiencies of western medicine are becoming a matter of major public concern and a particularly pressing concern to an increasingly defensive and embattled medical profession.

More particularly, because of the growing number of medical controversies that have become issues of public dispute, there is a growing public awareness that medical experts can and do disagree, that they are not infallible by virtue of their specialist access to some rigorous scientific testing process, that their 'objectivity' is not guaranteed by application of this method, and that non-technical and political assumptions influence their advice and decisions (Nelkin, 1979; Engelhardt and Caplan, 1987; Martin, 1988). Whether the confrontation is over the fluoridation of public water supplies, or about the side effects of the contraceptive pill, or over the implications of the consumption of a high-fibre or high-fat diet, we expect the experts to become involved, not just as consultants or providers of expertise, but as committed defenders or opponents of one side or the other. The well-documented decline of public trust in the infallibility and neutrality of expertise is consistent with a new approach to the interpretation of scientific knowledge that has recently engaged the attention of sociologists and historians of science.

It is now more than a quarter of a century since Thomas Kuhn published his classic *Structure of Scientific Revolutions* (Kuhn, 1962). This work made widely-known a conception of 'normal' science as a highly skilled activity which is routinely carried out by scientists within a shared or collectively established research tradition or 'paradigm'. A paradigm provides the framework of methodological assumptions, routine procedures, observational and experimental standards, criteria of interpretative judgements and so on, within which its adherents structure their work. According to Kuhn, a paradigm is established and maintained by a social collectivity or consensus. Scientists working in different paradigms are, in effect, living in different worlds. It follows from this that what counts as a true or false belief depends upon which paradigm a scientist works within. And, as each paradigm has its own unique and self-contained conceptual fabric and associated mode of practice, there are no independent scientific criteria or methodological procedures for judging whether one paradigm is preferable to another. This interpretation of Kuhn's work, therefore, offers a means of explaining disputes over 'true' or 'false' beliefs: disputing scientists may be seen to be arguing from the perspective of different paradigms (Pinch, 1986).

Recent work in the history and sociology of science has deepened this interpretation. In the process, it has presented a major revision of the conventional view of the objectivity and value-neutrality of scientific knowledge. Its most important implication for the purposes of this book is that it does not support the standard view that disputes over 'facts' and their interpretation can be resolved by the impersonal or 'objective' rules of experimental procedure. A large and growing number of sociological and historical studies have indicated that experimental design cannot be dissociated from the commitments of those who frame and evaluate the experiments. According to this revised view of scientific knowledge, where closure of a controversy has been achieved, it has resulted not from disinterested testing, but from the pressures and constraints exerted by the adjudicating community. These pressures and constraints include not only the accepted knowledge, evaluative standards, and practices of the community (the elements of its paradigm), but also the vested interests and social objectives that they embody. Together they shape the processes by which knowledge claims are accepted or rejected by the adjudicating community. Thus, within the terms of this 'constructivist' approach, scientific knowledge is not directly determined by the natural world as the standard view would have it; rather, knowledge is socially created or constructed. In other words, the 'truth' or 'falsity' of scientific claims is to be considered as residing in the interpretations, actions and practices of scientists rather than in nature. Scientific knowledge is actively constructed and endorsed by scientists, not passively given and ratified by nature (Bloor, 1976; Barnes, 1977; Mulkay, 1979; Knorr-Cetina, 1981; Shapin, 1982; Barnes and Edge, 1982; Albury, 1983; Collins, 1981,

1983, 1985; Pinch, 1986). This does not mean that anything goes, or that nature or reality does not constrain scientific conclusions. But it does mean that scientific knowledge is *not* value-free and politically and socially neutral as has generally been assumed. It means, further, that an understanding of the socially derived perspectives (the professional vested interests and so on) of the 'knowers' and their purposes is essential for the critical assessment of their knowledge and advice.

This is not just some abstruse piece of theorizing about science that may safely be left to armchair philosophers and sociologists. It has profound implications for medicine and its practitioners, for patients and their families, and for those concerned with the social implementation of medical therapies and techniques. If, as the new understanding of scientific knowledge suggests, social, professional, and economic interests play a significant part in the shaping of medical theories, practices, and treatments, then it follows that it can no longer be assumed that medical therapies and techniques can somehow be evaluated independently of those interests. According to the constructivist view, the idea of their neutral appraisal is a myth. Therapeutic evaluation must be seen as inherently a social and political process. We must expect that clinical trials, no matter how rigorously they are conducted, will inevitably embody the values or commitments of the assessors. They will not, as they are claimed to do, eliminate 'bias' from the evaluation of treatments. They cannot, therefore, provide definitive answers about the effectiveness of treatments. Nor will they be able definitively to resolve disputes over contentious treatments. This perspective calls into question the heavy investment of medical expertise in ever more tightly organized and rigorously controlled clinical trials, and the professional and public reliance on the supposed objectivity of the results of such trials. This in turn presents problems for regulators and policy makers – for those charged with the responsibility of ensuring that the public is not exposed to ineffective or dangerous treatments, and that the medical dollar is efficiently and effectively spent. On the positive side, it may be argued that the recognition of the inherent limitations of clinical trials in resolving questions of effectiveness and safety implies a greater reliance on social values and needs in the evaluation and choice of available treatments. It also implies a more prominent role for non-experts, for patients and the public at large, in the processes of assessment and decision making (Richards, 1988).

To date, there have been few attempts to analyse the production and evaluation of contemporary medical knowledge within the terms of this significant new approach. But such an analysis is well overdue (Wright and Treacher, 1982; Bury, 1986; Nicolson and McLaughlin, 1987). Moreover, as I have indicated, it would mesh with an incipient public perception of the contradictions and fallibility of much of contemporary medical opinion and practice. Together, they open the way for a more realistic interpretation of the medical expert's role in society – one which recognizes that the value of expert advice depends upon the professional vested interests and the larger social and economic objectives that it embodies.

This book is an attempt to examine and explain the dispute over the evaluation of vitamin C as a cancer treatment in the light of this new understanding of scientific experiment and scientific knowledge. The vitamin C controversy offers an exemplary instance of the contention that the conventional ideal of impartial assessment of therapies via the rigorously conducted clinical trial is unrealizable in practice. By looking in detail at this case I hope to demonstrate that the process of therapeutic evaluation may be better understood as inherently a political process, and to examine some of the implications of this claim.

WHY THE VITAMIN C AND CANCER CONTROVERSY?

Controversies represent one of the most rewarding sites for carrying out empirical research in the sociology of scientific knowledge (Collins, 1981, 1983; Pinch, 1986). In controversies a particular claim to knowledge about the natural world is under dispute, and the competing views of scientists about nature (and often a good deal else besides) are confronted and made overt. It is by looking at such areas of open conflict that the implicit professional and economic interests that shape the selection and interpretation of scientific evidence and evaluative procedures may be most easily identified and analysed. So during the course of controversies we may learn most about these critical processes which ordinarily are not visible to us.

Another important reason for the preference of many sociologists for controversy studies is that controversies most readily allow the analyst to treat the conflicting claims of the disputants symmetrically. This symmetrical viewpoint is the most important principle of the social constructivist approach to the study of science. It states that the sociologist or historian must attempt to explain adherence to all beliefs about the natural world, whether they be perceived to be true or false, in an equivalent or symmetrical way (Pinch, 1986). No set of beliefs or their advocates may be privileged over another. Studies of unresolved controversies permit the sociologist to study science that is still in the making. Retrospective judgements about the truth or falsity of the conflicting interpretations of nature may be avoided and the principle of symmetry is directly applied. By following the course of the controversy through to closure, the analyst is able to recover the sociological factors which explain how some beliefs become true and others false. To borrow the

apt metaphor of Harry Collins, we are then able to follow and understand the series of manipulations by which the 'ship in a bottle' of
any established scientific conclusion is constructed and inserted into the
bottle. Without this sociological appreciation of the processes by which
statements of fact are accredited or rejected, it is not easy to accept that
the 'ship' was ever just a bundle of sticks. It is as if we are living in a
world in which all 'ships' are already in bottles with the glue dried and
the strings cut (Collins, 1975).

For a number of reasons, the vitamin C and cancer controversy is a
particularly rewarding site for such sociological and historical analysis.
To begin with, it is a well-developed controversy. Positions are well
polarized and the 'core set' of disputants is well delineated (Collins,
1981). On the one hand are the deviants or vitamin C 'believers' who
charge their opponents with bias and prejudice, if not downright fraud,
and who claim that economic and political considerations are obscuring
not only an important scientific issue, but also their humanitarian
endeavour to bring relief to cancer patients. They are opposed by the
orthodox or 'non-believers', who assert that a valid scientific case has not
been presented either theoretically or experimentally for the efficacy of
vitamin C as a cancer treatment, that it has, in fact, been experimentally
disproved, and that megadoses of vitamin C are not only worthless but
dangerous for cancer patients who might forego effective conventional
treatment. The dispute has engendered a large scientific and medical
literature and has spilled over into the popular press. It readily suggests
conflicting areas of professional and economic interest.

More importantly for my purposes, from the outset the controversy
challenges the conventional medical wisdom that such disputes may be
objectively settled through rigorously conducted clinical trials. It presents the immediate problem of why, after two decades of negotiation
and recrimination and *two* trials by leading cancer researchers at one of
the most prestigious medical research institutes in the United States, the
question of the efficacy of vitamin C as a cancer treatment has still not
been definitively resolved. The history of this dispute has become almost
a paradigmatic instance of the limitations of the clinical trial in resolving
issues of medical controversy. As I have indicated in the introduction,
this is a crucial issue and is central to my analysis.

The vitamin C controversy has the further advantage as a case study
of the process of therapeutic evaluation, in that its history may be readily
and instructively compared with those of two other cancer treatments:
5-fluorouracil and interferon. Some revealing contrasts may thus be drawn
between the differing responses of the medical profession and research
bodies to these three putative anti-cancer drugs.

I have chosen 5-fluorouracil for comparative purposes because it is
typical of the powerful cytotoxic (literally cell-poisoning) drugs conven-

tionally employed in cancer treatment, and so allows the comparison of vitamin C with a cancer treatment which conforms with the established theoretical framework and clinical practices. Unlike vitamin C, which may be self-administered, 5-fluorouracil is a highly toxic drug that is administered in hospitals or clinics by cancer specialists. Although its use as a standard adjuvant treatment for gastro-intestinal cancer has been criticized in the literature for about the last fifteen years on the grounds of its ineffectiveness and toxicity, it is still in routine use.

Interferon, the much-touted and costly magic bullet against cancer which failed to live up to clinical expectations, but which, nevertheless, has recently been adopted into conventional cancer therapy, is especially amenable to comparative analysis with vitamin C. Its supposed mode of action is directly comparable with that which is claimed for vitamin C. One of the reasons why interferon supposedly attracted so much medical attention in the first instance was because it offered a 'unique therapeutic approach' in that it did not act as a toxin directly on the tumour cells, but through the immune system, and it was hoped that it would be free of the deleterious side effects of the conventional cytotoxic drugs. Exactly the same claim was made for the inexpensive and non-patentable vitamin C, but as we shall see, it provoked a very different response from funding bodies and the medical profession.

This contrast between the research and funding patterns and clinical assessments of vitamin C and interferon is particularly valuable to my analysis, in making explicit the larger socio-economic and political structuring of professional judgements about the efficacy of these putative cancer treatments.

The vitamin C controversy has added value as a case study because it is possible to offer a rich and uniquely detailed reconstruction of the course of the controversy. Over the ten-year period from late 1971 to the end of 1981, some 250 letters passed back and forth between Ewan Cameron, then Senior Consulting Surgeon to the Vale of Leven Hospital in Scotland, and Linus Pauling. During this time, except for a one-year interval from late 1978 to 1979 which Cameron spent in residence at the Linus Pauling Institute in California, he and Pauling met briefly on only a few occasions and they made only exceptional use of expensive trans-Atlantic telephone calls. These lengthy letters, usually ten or more closely typed pages in Cameron's case, document their long-term collaboration from its inception in November 1971, when the Scottish surgeon first wrote to Pauling, seeking his help in establishing Cameron's recently formulated ideas about the role of vitamin C in cancer therapy on a 'sound scientific basis'.

Their correspondence not only details their attempts to piece together a comprehensive theoretical argument for the therapeutic use of vitamin C and Cameron's efforts to find and present the clinical evidence to support their hypothesis, but also records their failures and setbacks, their publication and fund-raising problems, and the tactics they adopted for presenting and defending their controversial claims. The contents of these letters have been fleshed out in a number of separate interviews with Cameron and Pauling, and used in turn to cross check their independent recollections of events. As well, their correspondence with their leading professional opponents in the dispute, with editors, research and funding bodies, and their manuscripts and referees' reports, have all been utilized in this reconstruction of the controversy.

Linus Pauling's centrality to the conflict is beyond dispute. Without Pauling, there would be no controversy over vitamin C. Throughout, he has been and remains an indefatigable and prolific letter writer in pursuing his vitamin C claims, and his far-flung and carefully preserved correspondence has been an invaluable aid in the location of the theoretical arguments and clinical findings in their larger institutional and social contexts. It has also provided a major means of following the course of the controversy since 1982, when Cameron relocated to California to take up the position of Medical Director of the Linus Pauling Institute. This marks the point when the Pauling–Cameron correspondence, save for the occasional memo, necessarily terminates.

This wealth of source material has been supplemented with official documentation, newspaper and journal reports, and, where possible, interviews with some of the other participants in the dispute. It is this unusually rich endowment of source materials in the form of the Pauling-Cameron correspondence and supplementary documentation that makes the vitamin C and cancer controversy such an exceptionally favourable case for historical reconstruction. They allow the story to tell itself.

But, of course, no story tells itself. There is always a story teller. The same story could be told from a number of different viewpoints (within the constraints of the documentary and other evidence) by different story tellers. It becomes necessary to offer some further explanation of my approach to the reconstruction and analysis of this particular episode in the history of medicine.

TELLING IT LIKE IT IS

My preference for the documentary evidence of the Pauling correspondence over the sociologist's preferred evidence of the 'in-depth' interview stems primarily from my own historical training. This has accustomed me to working my way through some very large archival and published collections of letters, notebooks, and manuscripts, such as those of the nineteenth century naturalists, Charles Darwin, Richard Owen, and

Thomas Henry Huxley (Richards, 1983, 1987, 1989a, b). By and large, I have followed these same historical techniques of the selection and inter-pretation of the documentary evidence in piecing together the sequence of events in the contemporary vitamin C and cancer controversy. Where any contradiction with the recollections of the participants has occurred, the documents have been given priority. I agree with other historians of science that the recollections of scientists are notoriously faulty and unreliable, and that the historian is on much safer ground if able to refer to documentary material that is strictly contemporaneous with the events being reconstructed and analyzed. This is not to say that scientists are dishonest or have bad memories. Rather, this approach takes account of the inevitable retrospective changes in meanings and interpretations in ever-changing historical contexts (Rudwick, 1985).

My aim is to provide a fine-grained chronological reconstruction of the events which avoids such retrospective judgements. In this way I hope to recover as much as possible of what sociologists have termed the 'interpretative flexibility' of scientists' findings and the processes of consensus formation (Collins, 1985; Pinch, 1986). The historian's goal of telling the story like it really happened is here subserving the sociologi-cal purpose of telling what science and scientists are really like. Part II of this book comprises an attempt to write the story of the vitamin C and cancer controversy in this manner, in a style that does justice to the messiness and muddle of real science and real medicine. For this same reason, the analysis of the controversy is kept separate from the narrative, and is the subject matter of part three of this book.

As previously emphasized, this analysis is not confined to the vita-min C and cancer controversy, but is a comparative analysis of the medical evaluations of vitamin C and two accepted cancer treatments. This comparative analysis serves a number of purposes, some of which have already been touched upon. One of its as yet undiscussed purposes is that it is intended to counteract a systematic bias in the documentation of the controversy, in that the fullest records are those of the vitamin C '[246]believers'. This documentary bias, which is the inevitable outcome of Pauling's centrality to the dispute, has several implications for the reconstruction and analysis of the controversy – implications which are not necessarily to the advantage of the 'believers'. Perhaps the most sig-nificant is that it lays open to the closest scrutiny the expressed actions, beliefs and motivations of one side, while leaving those of their oppo-nents undeclared except in so far as they are willing to represent them to the other side or to the analyst and in published accounts of their work. The main danger of this situation is that the claims of those most closely scrutinized may be perceived to be 'biased' by the revelation of the supposedly 'non-scientific' factors which have fed into their assump-tions, procedures, and the presentation of their work, while those of their opponents remain relatively unscrutinized and, perhaps, are presumed freer of such contaminating influences. The other side of this coin is that the charges of non-scientific doings by the best documented side against their opponents are more thoroughly aired than the counterclaims and charges of their opponents, and may carry more weight. In this case, by extending the analysis beyond a single case study, I hope simultaneously to defuse these dangers and to carry out the explanatory goal of going beyond findings of bias or conspiracy by one side or the other to a better understanding of the social processes that shape both the making and breaking of medical claims about disease and its treatment.

I must refer also to a major, but little acknowledged, difficulty in the task of historical reconstruction and analysis of contemporary scientific events: the historian is not dealing with the musty archives of forgotten disputes on which the dust of history has safely settled, but with science in the making, with what has been very well described as the 'fierce fight to construct reality' (Latour and Woolgar, 1979). The historian is at the front lines of the battle, and may easily be caught in the cross-fire. Socio-logical studies of contemporary controversies are potential resources in social struggles over scientific or technical knowledge claims. The combatants have a good deal at stake in the historian's interpretation and presentation of news from the war zone. Their perceptions of what the historian is up to, or rather, of what the historian *should* be up to, inevitably enter into the reconstruction of the story. Both sides to the dispute have opposing and unshakeable convictions as to who are the heroes and the villains involved, and where truth and justice lie. If they do not welcome the historian's attempt to deal symmetrically with the claims of their opponents, they may withdraw their cooperation from the project or actively hinder the study. Alternatively, one side may react more sympathetically to the analysis, and attempt to win the analyst to their cause (Collins and Pinch, 1979, 1982; Mulkay *et al.*, 1983). Another problem is that the intervention by the analyst may disturb the dispute, and this may make it more difficult for this or other researchers to obtain access to participants and documents. I shall not detail my own experiences here except to note, lest their omission from the list of acknowledgements should invite adverse comment on the sources relied upon in this study, that I was unable to achieve interviews or correspondence with two leading disputants, Dr. Vincent DeVita of the National Cancer Institute and Dr. Arnold Relman, editor of the *New England Journal of Medicine*. Nor did Dr. Charles Moertel of the Mayo Clinic respond to my invitation to offer critical comment on the final manuscript.

The response to my attempts at a symmetrical analysis of the vita-min C and cancer controversy must be interpreted in the context of the novelty of social constructivist accounts of contemporary disputes over medical therapies. In the case of disputes involving alternative or marginal therapies, analysts generally have uncritically adopted the orthodox 'scientific' medical position. They focus almost exclusively on the 'unscientific', 'irrational' or 'unproven' claims of the alternatives, and perceive their analytical task in terms of explaining the popular 'mistaken' or 'credulous' adherence to such scientifically unproven or unjustifiable therapies. The most partisan of these analysts are committed to the exposure of 'quacks' and 'charlatans', and their studies have been incorporated into the anti-quackery crusades of orthodox organizations such as the American Medical Association and the American Cancer Society (Young, 1967, 1972; Holland, 1982). Within this context, a symmetrical analysis that does not privilege orthodox knowledge claims, but attempts to deal evenhandedly with the claims of orthodox oncologists and marginal therapists, is flying in the face of all tradition. As I have found, it invites the suspicion and hostility of orthodoxy and the equally problematic embraces of the unorthodox. In spite of my own best efforts to steer a prudent path through the minefield of contemporary controversy analysis, I now have reason to believe that the goal of neutral social analysis is as mythical in actual practice as the scientist's goal of neutral evaluation of competing therapies (Scott *et al.*, 1990).

As my whole analysis is directed at undercutting the conventional view that an objective scientific assessment of contentious therapeutic claims is possible, it would be disingenuous of me, to say the least, to claim that I can offer an objective interpretation of events. What I hope I offer are insights into the social and political processes of therapeutic evaluation as instanced by the comparative analysis of the vitamin C and cancer controversy. It is not my intention to advocate vitamin C or anything else as a treatment for cancer. Rather it is my intention that readers should draw their own conclusions, but that they should do so from the point of view of this revised definition of medical knowledge which treats these conflicts as essentially political issues where there are *no* impartial experts.

Nor is this book in any way intended as an exercise in 'doctor bashing'. Rather it is an attempt to go beyond such sterile criticisms to a better understanding of the inherent limitations of medical theory and practice. It is offered on the assumption that medicine and its practitioners and consumers have much to gain from attempting to come to grips with these phenomena as necessarily, and inevitably, *social* processes.

Much of what I have to say will come as no surprise to those who daily confront the contradictions and uncertainties of therapeutic evaluation and the unpredictability of treatment outcome. Many doctors, I think, would agree that medical knowledge of disease and its treatment is fallible; that it is not susceptible to conclusive and final validation; that it is open to professional and wider socio-economic influences; and that it must be handled with care and circumspection. But to convert these tacit understandings of the day-to-day reality of medicine into the specificities of the critical appraisal of the formal processes of treatment evaluation and, moreover, to accept in full the cognitive and social implications of such an appraisal, is to ask a great deal more of the medical professional. It requires that the professional must step outside the boundaries of professional knowledge and professional self-interest, and consider them as an outsider might. The difficulty of this for the fully-fledged professional might be equated with the difficulty that would be encountered in appraising our own every-day knowledge and customs from the point of view of Barry Barnes' visiting extra-terrestrial (Barnes, 1985). The medical reader of these pages accordingly is invited to the demanding but rewarding task of suspending professional judgements and values for the purposes of this discussion – in effect, to adopt the role of the visiting Martian.

By the same token, the non-medical reader who is cast in the role of de facto extra-terrestrial, is cautioned against the invocation of easy prejudices and generalizations. From a Martian point of view, the mythical beliefs, ritual practices and protective taboos of the earthlings under scrutiny may be inconsistent and irrational; they may be sustained not directly by experience, as the earthlings claim, but by collective belief and for the interested ends of certain dominant tribes and elites. But Martians are invited to consider whether, had they been adopted by and brought up as earthlings, they too might not have succumbed to similar delusions; and further, to reflect upon whether their own taken-for-granted Martian beliefs and customs are as rational, experientially-based, and free from self-interest as they assume.

The book is organized in three main parts. Part I sets the scene for the reconstruction of the controversy. It sketches the social and intellectual setting of the conflict, introduces the interested parties and briefly explains their social and institutional affiliations. Part II is necessarily the longest section of the book. It may be read together with part one as a complete story in itself by those readers who are interested in the history of the controversy but who do not wish to engage with its theoretical and practical implications. It reconstructs the original sequence of events from late 1971 to the present, with as little interpretative commentary as is consistent with the clear presentation and understanding of an inevitably shortened and tightened history of those events. Generous quotations have been included with the aim of letting the participants tell as much of the story as possible, and of recapturing the complexity, confusion, and essentially *social* aspects of the making and breaking of medical knowledge. The rhetoric, invective and scandal are of interest not for their own sake, but because they and the general tone of the participants' exchanges are integral to the course of the controversy.

Part III offers a comparative analysis of the controversy in its institutional and social contexts. The implications of the study for a more adequate understanding of the processes of therapeutic evaluation are explored. The roles of professional power and broader social influences, such as consumer choice or market forces, in the constitution of medical knowledge are assessed. Finally, some suggestions for the practical applications of this analysis are offered.

Part I

Interested Parties and the Background to the Controversy

Medicines are a focus of powerful economic, social, and emotional forces.

> Jasper Woodcock, 'Medicines – The Interested Parties'
> (Woodcock, 1981)

I asked Professor Thomas Jukes, a nutrition expert at the University of California at Berkeley, how he feels about the claims made for vitamin C. Jukes scurries over to a bookcase and fishes out Pauling's *Vitamin C and the Common Cold*. In case you haven't read Professor Pauling's book, you should know that he gives a great deal of credit to a Dr Irwin Stone, a chemist, for putting him on the trail of vitamin C. . . . Jukes, bristling with rising indignation, struggling to control the fury in his voice, his angry eyes darting over the page, reads the appropriate passage. 'This man Stone is a brewing chemist. He worked for Wallenstein out on Long Island.'

Jukes slams shut the heavy reference book. 'He writes Pauling and says, "Dear Dr Pauling, I hope you live forever". Remember the salutation the king used to get, "O King, live forever"? So Pauling thinks, say, this is great. So he went on this vitamin C kick. I heard recently that he couldn't attend a meeting of the AMA because he was home with a cold. Did you hear that?'

> John Fried, *Vitamin Politics* (Fried, 1984)

Dear Friend,

Did you know that safe nutritional treatments have been discovered that can help control and even cure cancer?

It's true!

But because of government red tape and the questionable efforts of the medical and pharmaceutical industries – over *1,200 Americans will die of cancer today without even knowing about these cancer treatments!*. . . .

Why, you ask? Why is such a promising area of cancer research and treatment given only token support by the medical establishment?

I'll tell you why!

From the doctors who treat cancer patients – to the pharmaceutical companies which make chemotherapy drugs – cancer is a multi-billion dollar a year industry.

But cancer control through nutrition doesn't make money.

'Project CURE' Mailout Leaflet, 1985.

1 Charting The Terrain

What this country needs is a good five-cent pill! – some 'magic', easy-to-swallow little pellet that can slow aging, minimize heart disease, aid recovery from dozens of infectious and degenerative ailments, and inoculate us against countless health problems that stem from emotional stress and environmental pollutants.

THE GOOD NEWS
Happily, such a thing exists – in pill form, as supplemental powders, and, of course, in a number of foods . . . We are speaking of vitamin C . . .

THE BAD NEWS
More often than not, all the good news about all the things that vitamin C can do gets drowned in a sea of confusion. The real truth gets held hostage while a philosophic tug-of-war rages between adherents of two extreme positions: those who claim vitamin C can do everything and those who claim it does nothing. While this unfortunate slugging match takes place, a vast middle ground of solid scientific information is overlooked. . . .

Dr Emanuel Cheraskin *et al.*, *The Vitamin C Connection*
(Cheraskin *et al.*, 1983)

1.1 INTRODUCING VITAMIN C

Vitamin C (ascorbic acid or ascorbate) is essential for human health. It cannot be synthesized by humans, and must be obtained from dietary sources, primarily vegetables and fresh fruits. In human beings deprived of vitamin C, the life-threatening nutritional deficiency disease scurvy develops. That ascorbic acid is the essential nutrient for the prevention and treatment of scurvy has been accepted medical wisdom since the 1930s, when Albert Szent-Gyorgyi was awarded the Nobel Prize for its discovery and isolation. But very little else about this contentious substance has achieved such unanimity of medical opinion.

Fundamental to the vitamin C controversy is the concept of 'optimum' dietary levels of ascorbic acid. The debate over its therapeutic or preventative role hinges on whether the amount of ascorbate necessary to prevent scurvy is similar to the amount necessary for optimal health. No international consensus has ever been reached on the officially recommended daily allowance (RDA) or intake of vitamin C, which varies from country to country around the world. In the United States, the Food and Nutrition Board of the National Research Council (a subdivision of the National Academy of Sciences) is charged with the responsibility of determining the RDAs of vitamin C and other essential nutrients and minerals. It is a responsibility that carries with it wide socio-economic implications. RDAs are used in planning menus in schools, hospitals, and the armed forces, in government food assistance programmes, as the basis for nutrition labelling on food packages, and for the regulation and control of vitamin manufacturing and marketing. Down the years, they have generated vehement and costly scientific and medical controversy, political interventions, marketing manipulations, congressional hearings and litigation. The RDA of vitamin C (for males) has oscillated from 75mg in 1941, to 60mg in 1968, then to 45mg in 1974, and back to 60mg in 1980 (Carpenter, 1986).

In 1985, the Committee on Dietary Allowances of the Food and Nutrition Board, which reportedly had become increasingly concerned about the 'growing public obsession' with vitamins and the potential dangers of vitamin overdose, again revised and reduced the RDAs for a number of vitamins and minerals. Their draft report (which recommended an RDA for vitamin C of 40mg) became the subject of intense and unresolved dissension within the National Academy of Sciences. The chairman finally announced that no report would be issued, owing to an 'impasse resulting from honest differences of scientific opinion' (Marshall, 1985; Dale, 1987).

This definitional impasse reflects the deep, and apparently irreconcilable, differences of opinion that have arisen over the physiological, and above all, the putative therapeutic role of vitamin C. The latter, especially in the form of megavitamin therapy, has become the centre of the bitterest and most intractable of these conflicts.

Megadoses (one or more grams per day) of vitamin C are now widely promoted and used as treatment or supportive treatment for a wide range of conditions: the common cold, cancer, schizophrenia, drug addiction, improved wound repair, and atherosclerosis (Lewin, 1976; Basu and Schorah, 1982; Cheraskin *et al.*, 1983; Pauling, 1986; Carpenter, 1986; Levine, 1986; Burns *et al.*, 1987). As the literature enumerating its medical benefits has grown, so has the literature opposing such claims. The controversy has become particularly intense over long-term megavitamin C therapy in cold prevention and in cancer treatment.

While the vitamin C and cancer controversy cannot be considered in isolation from the common cold debate, my focus is on the area of cancer treatment.

Vitamin C has been connected with the treatment of cancer since the early 1930s, when it was first isolated by Szent-Gyorgyi. Most of the early experimental subjects were animals and only low dosages of vitamin C were tested – from about 25 to 50mg. This seems to have been initially because vitamin C was relatively scarce and expensive. But the trend continued after the late 1930s, when the large-scale production of synthetic vitamin C made it more accessible and cheaper. By this time the first estimates of the human requirement for vitamin C had been made at between 15 to 30mg per day (Carpenter, 1986), and it has been suggested that these early low estimates consolidated the low-dose trend in cancer research (Stone, 1972). It was not until the 1970s and the advent of megavitamin therapy, that megadoses were used in the treatment of cancer.

Earlier research had emphasized a relationship between vitamin C deficiency and cancer, and was concerned with the association of vitamin C with tissue growth and physiological activity and the relative importance of the vitamin to the growth and maintenance of neoplastic (cancer) cells. It is important to note that this early work on vitamin C, while equivocal in its interpretation of the effectiveness of vitamin C in cancer treatment, was not regarded as controversial or unorthodox, being published in such mainstream journals as *Cancer Research* and the *British Journal of Cancer* (Richards, 1988). But neither did it engender much interest in the medical world, primarily because it coincided with, and was overtaken by, the rapid development and promotion of the powerful cytotoxic drugs which have dominated cancer chemotherapy ever since. Vitamin C was allegedly excluded from the official ongoing screening programme for cancer-killing drugs because it was deemed to be too non-toxic for consideration. In 1969, a dissenting team of National Cancer Institute researchers criticized this trend, arguing that in their view it was precisely this property of vitamin C which made it of such potential value in cancer treatment:

the future of effective cancer treatment will not rest on the use of host-toxic compounds now so widely employed, but upon virtually host-nontoxic compounds that are lethal to cancer cells, of which ascorbate ... represents an excellent prototype example. (Benade *et al.*, 1969)

Their opinion was not shared by most mainstream cancer researchers. When, a few years later, Linus Pauling and Ewan Cameron began their collaborative research of vitamin C and cancer, they had to confront the almost total lack of interest in or dismissal of their work by a powerful amalgam of conservative institutional and professional interests – those I term the orthodox or 'unbelievers'. In their turn, in order to secure a hearing for their views and promote their orthodox evaluation and acknowledgement, they have invoked the support of an alternative array of backers and sponsoring interests – those I refer to as the alternatives or vitamin C 'believers'.

Before I proceed to identify these interested parties and map the complexities of their affiliations and interactions in Chapters 2 and 3 it is necessary to carry out a brief survey of the site of the dispute, the battlefield as it were, and to indicate some of the more important aspects of the conventional evaluation of cancer treatments.

1.2   THE BATTLEFIELD: THE TREATMENT OF CANCER

In the western world, about one in every three people contracts cancer, and one in five dies from it. In the United States, cancer is the second leading cause of death (after heart disease), accounting for approximately one in five deaths each year. In 1985 an officially estimated 462,000 deaths occurred from cancer, and 910,000 serious new malignancies were diagnosed. If we add to these the less serious cases of skin cancers (400,000) and carcinoma in situ (limited to one small site of the cervix or breast, 50,000), then over a million new cases of cancer are treated each year (NCI, 1985a; Page and Asire, 1985). Even according to official figures, the survival rates for the major cancers (lung, breast and bowel) have improved little over the last thirty-five years. According to some prominent epidemiologists and biostatisticians, the odds of dying from cancer have increased rather than diminished during that time (Bailar and Smith, 1986). A 1987 commissioned report on these contentious cancer survival rates by the U.S. General Accounting Office concluded that for the majority of cancers examined, actual improvements had been 'slight', and that the extent of improvement for specific cancers 'is often not as great as that reported' (United States General Accounting Office, 1987). Not only are cancer statistics the centre of a great deal of controversy in the medical literature, but there is little unanimity over the very definition and interpretation of cancer, and another major controversy surrounds its causes and prevention (Epstein, 1979; Doll and Peto, 1981; Cairns, 1978, 1985).

Against this background of grim statistics, doubt and uncertainty, 'cancerphobia' has become deeply entrenched in western culture. At the popular cultural level, by contrast with the more optimistic pronouncements of those connected with its funding, research and treatment, cancer more often evokes fear, distrust, and desperation.

Cancer is the 'dread disease', characterized by its mysterious onset and its insidious and relentless progression. In America, in particular, the history of cancer over the last hundred years is the history of the tensions between a more confident, affluent, and science-oriented, orthodox 'anti-cancer alliance' and a cancer 'counterculture'. This cancer counterculture has been traditionally perceived as more pessimistic, less affluent, popular-based, and, above all, sceptical of the dominant orthodox explanations and treatments of the disease and of the claims to expertise by 'establishment' cancer practitioners (Patterson, 1987). It was the dominant anti-cancer alliance which built up the pressure during the late 1960s in the U.S. for a federal 'war on cancer'. Their intensive political campaign culminated in the National Cancer Act which was signed into law by President Nixon towards the end of 1971. The National Cancer Act committed billions of dollars to the war on cancer and, almost from its inception, it has been at the centre of a divisive public conflict over the spending of the cancer dollar. Also, as the gap between the promises and the reality of the much-heralded but ever-elusive cancer cure has widened, the ideological differences between the orthodox anti-cancer alliance and the cancer counterculture have become more overt.

The dominant model of disease in the western world is that of scientific medicine. This model, often termed the 'biomedical model', is technical and reductionist in its emphasis. It provides the framework within which cancer is conventionally treated by surgery, radiation therapy and/or chemotherapy. It is the latter kind of treatment, chemotherapy, with which this study is primarily concerned.

Cancer chemotherapy owes its origin to the great period of laboratory medicine of the late nineteenth century, when the theory of specific aetiology (the idea that particular diseases have particular causes or pathogens) led to the notion of specific therapy – the so-called 'magic bullets', chemical weapons which would home in on the target pathogens and injure nothing else (Diesendorf, 1976; Dixon, 1978). The first of these, a synthetic arsenic compound called Salvarsan (a byproduct of the chemical dye industry, forerunner of the modern pharmaceutical industry) was developed in 1909 as both active and specific agent against the syphilis germ. The chemotherapeutic revolution in medicine culminated in the antibiotics and the synthetic antimicrobial drugs of the twentieth century, 'wonder drugs' which produced near-miraculous cures of a wide range of previously intractable and dreaded infectious diseases. Their spectacular successes not only legitimated the theory of specific aetiology, but also generated the extremely profitable and powerful modern pharmaceutical industry.

The concept of specific aetiology was part of a larger development in scientific medicine – what medical sociologists and historians have called the 'reconstitution of illness as disease' which occurred in the early nineteenth century with the growth of hospital medicine. Medical attention then shifted from the sick person to the disease, and doctors became preoccupied with the disease entity rather than the patient (Foucault, 1973; Figlio, 1977). The limitations of this approach, which ignores the social and psychological dimensions of illness, have become the subject of a well-developed critique of the biomedical model (Engel, 1977; Doyal and Doyal, 1984). It has been argued that the dramatic decline in mortality rates from infectious diseases in the western world was due less to the triumphs of twentieth century specific drug therapy than to the late nineteenth century improvements in water supply, sanitation, nutrition and housing. These public health improvements had little to do with nineteenth century medicine or its practitioners. Furthermore, it is argued, social and environmental factors remain the major determinants of health and illness. For these reasons modern medicine, dominated by the biomedical model, has been able to make little headway with the cure or control of the twentieth century epidemic of degenerative diseases such as cancer (McKeown, 1979; Kennedy, 1981; Inglis, 1983).

Nevertheless, the curative reputation of modern scientific medicine rests largely upon the generally perceived success of the chemotherapeutic revolution. It was this that inspired the extensive programmes to synthesize and test chemicals to deploy as specific weapons against specific cancers, beginning with the trials of the cytotoxic properties of the mustard gases which began after the second world war. Most of this early work was carried out in the United States. In 1954, the National Cancer Institute was given $3 million by Congress to establish a Cancer Chemotherapy National Service Centre, and within a few years it had developed an intensive chemotherapy programme, absorbing almost half its budget, and testing thousands of chemicals a year. By 1970 the anti-cancer potential of some 400,000 drugs had been explored (Patterson, 1987).

The early trials of the cytotoxic drugs focused on the childhood leukaemias and lymphomas which were almost invariably rapidly fatal. In time, after a great deal of trial and error, some impressive cure rates were achieved by using the cytotoxic drugs at the highest tolerable levels and simultaneously in suitable combinations, with the aim of eliminating as many cancer cells as possible at the one time. These two principles of chemotherapy (maximum tolerable dosages and combination chemotherapy), established by their success in this area, have since been applied to most other cancers, but with far less effect. With the exception of the childhood leukaemias, Hodgkin's disease, and a few other rare cancers, the results of chemotherapy are problematic (Bush, 1984; Cairns, 1985).

Overall, British cancer specialists have been much more conservative in their approach to chemotherapy than their American counterparts who, it is estimated, currently treat more than a quarter of all cancer patients with some form of chemotherapy. The National Cancer Institute assesses the number of patients undergoing cancer chemotherapy at more than 200,000 each year. The cancer authority John Cairns, in reporting these numbers, commented:

> For a dangerous and technologically exacting form of treatment these are disturbing figures, particularly since the benefit for most categories of patients has yet to be established. (Cairns, 1985)

Oncology, the specialty concerned with the treatment of cancer, is a fast growing field. The number of certified clinical oncologists in the U.S. is currently around 6,000, of whom about 3,500 are medical oncologists specializing in the chemotherapeutic treatment of cancer. Collectively, under the scrutiny of the American Medical Association and the individual specialty boards, oncologists set the standards for the diagnosis and treatment of cancer within orthodox medicine in the United States. They currently employ more than fifty drugs to prevent cancer cells from growing, multiplying and spreading. These drugs are used alone or in groups (combination chemotherapy), and may be used in combination with surgery and/or radiation therapy (combined modality treatment), or after surgery or radiation treatment to destroy any remaining cancer cells (adjuvant chemotherapy) (NCI, 1984; 1985b).

The theoretical basis of cancer chemotherapy is that, since cancer cells grow and divide very quickly, the drugs used are those chemicals most likely to affect fast-growing cells. Ideally, cancer chemotherapy aims preferentially to destroy cancer cells without harming normal tissue, but, since a wide variety of normal cells, such as those of the skin, the lining of the gastrointestinal tract, the reproductive system, and the bone marrow, also divide very quickly, they too can be harmed by the highly toxic anti-cancer drugs. Individual tolerance of these cytotoxic drugs varies considerably, but most patients experience some side effects. Among the acute side effects are hair loss, mouth ulcers, nausea, vomiting, fatigue, anaemia, and lowered resistance to infections. The latter two effects are linked to the suppression of the bone marrow, which is responsible for the production of blood cells and the maintenance of the immune system. Longer-term or remote effects can include organ damage, sterility, and the development of secondary cancers (somewhere between five and ten per cent of surviving patients die of leukaemia in the first ten years after adjuvant chemotherapy for breast cancer) (Cairns, 1985).

Because they are so dangerous, in western countries the cytotoxic drugs are available only on prescription and must be administered under the close supervision of a registered medical practitioner, usually a specialist oncologist experienced in the use of the particular drug. Some drugs are administered by mouth, but most are injected or infused, and treatment usually takes place in the doctor's office, in hospital or a clinic (NCI, 1985b). During treatment the patient's response must be constantly monitored by a battery of diagnostic tests and clinical evaluations. 5-fluorouracil, for example, carries with it the following warning:

> It is recommended that FLUOROURACIL be given only by or under the supervision of a qualified physician who is experienced in cancer chemotherapy and who is well versed in the use of potent antimetabolites. Because of the possibility of severe toxic reactions, it is recommended that patients be hospitalised at least during the initial course of therapy.

The *Physicians' Desk Reference* goes on to state that 5-fluorouracil is a highly toxic drug with a narrow margin of safety. The ratio between effective and toxic dose is small and 'therapeutic response is unlikely to occur without some evidence of toxicity'. Even with 'meticulous selection of patients and careful adjustment of dosage', severe blood toxicity, gastrointestinal haemorrhage 'and even death' may result from the use of 5-fluorouracil. 'Adequate therapy' is usually followed by bone marrow suppression, mouth and oesophageal inflammation (which may lead to sloughing and ulceration), diarrhoea, anorexia, nausea and vomiting. Other possible side effects include hair loss, dermatitis, pigmentation, gastrointestinal ulceration and bleeding, generalized allergic reactions, ataxia, headache, disorientation, and fever. There have also been reports of chest pain, tachycardia (abnormally rapid heart rate), breathlessness, and other changes indicative of heart disorders (PDR, 1989).

The problem for cancer chemotherapists is to balance the cell-destroying effects of the drug against its toxicity, so that the patient is not destroyed along with the tumour. Accordingly, cytotoxic drugs are usually administered on an intermittent basis over a period of months, with short bursts or courses of administration, followed by drug-free periods during which the damaged normal cells recover and the unwanted side-effects subside.

The evaluation of the cytotoxic drugs, where efficacy has to be balanced against toxicity, presents well-recognized problems. A 'consensus statement' on adjuvant chemotherapy released by a committee of the U.S. National Institutes of Health Consensus Development Panel in 1980 stated that 'the basic measure of therapeutic benefit is therapeutic survival with an acceptable quality of life' (Inglis, 1983). However, as the Panel itself recognized, because the concept of an acceptable quality of life is itself so arbitrary and difficult to assess, in actual practice the efficacy of chemotherapy is assessed primarily by means of its more measurable effects on the growth and spread of the tumour and on the time the patient survives from diagnosis, or from start of treatment (survival time) (Buyse *et al.*, 1984). It is this elusive and difficult to measure concept of quality of life, which is understandably of crucial concern to patients and their families, which lies at the heart of much of the current criticism of cytotoxic therapy (Faulder, 1985).

For instance, the current five-year relative survival rate for cancer of the colon (one of the commonest cancers in the western world) is 53 per cent (NCI, 1985a), i.e., out of every 100 patients diagnosed as having cancer of the colon, only 53 can expect to be alive at the end of five years. (The number of real survivors is lower than this, as the relative survival rate is calculated after other potential causes of death are eliminated.) To put it another way, about one in every two patients with colon cancer will die within five years. Cancer of the colon is also acknowledged to be one of the cancers most resistant to chemotherapy. Yet in the United States it is routinely treated by adjuvant chemotherapy with 5-fluorouracil, either alone, or in combination with other cytotoxic drugs. This routine practice has been heavily criticized in the medical literature. For instance, a recent large-scale trial reported in the *New England Journal of Medicine* found that patients who had surgery alone and no chemotherapy survived slightly longer than those who had both surgery and chemotherapy. Apart from the short-term debilitating effects of such chemotherapy (which are hardly negligible, in view of the average length of time that patients survive with this condition), seven of the 284 patients given chemotherapy died of leukaemia, and one from the acute toxic effects of the treatment (Gastrointestinal Tumour Study Group, 1984; Cairns, 1985).

The medical uncertainty and controversy over the treatment of cancer extends beyond the cytotoxic drugs to radical surgery and radiation therapy. In this situation, there are increasing protests from cancer patients and the proliferating consumer and self-help and support groups that represent their interests, that the price they are called upon to pay for increasing their survival odds is too high – that the marginal gains they might make in survival times do not outweigh the deleterious effects of the treatments to which they are subjected (Inglis, 1983; Faulder, 1985; Patterson, 1987; Byrski, 1989). This debate has not been confined to the 'fringe' literature or to the public media, but has also featured in the professional literature and institutions. For example, a patient-advocate on the U.S. National Cancer Advisory Board and two officials of the National Cancer Institute recently contested the benefits of adjuvant chemotherapy for breast cancer and the medical definition of 'tolerable' or 'acceptable' side effects in the journal of the American Cancer Society:

> When doctors say the side effects are tolerable or acceptable, they are talking about life-threatening things like a drop in your white blood cells or vomiting to the point where you have to go into the hospital for intravenous nutrition. But if you just vomit so hard that you break the blood vessels in your eyes, or you have a sore mouth that can be treated by putting a paste of baking soda in your mouth at night, they don't consider that even mentionable. And they certainly don't care if you go bald. (Kushner, 1984)

Criticism of the emphasis of cancer research on cytotoxic chemotherapy and of the aggressive overuse of the cytotoxic drugs has also come from insiders within the National Cancer Institute itself. The official response to such criticism has been to concede that the risks and side effects are cause for concern, but to dispute the charge of the 'only marginal' benefits of chemotherapy, arguing rather that it has brought about substantial gains in the treatment of cancer (Patterson, 1987).

In spite of such official reassurances, the indications are that cancer research and treatment are perceived as contentious. As the burgeoning literature in the area attests, more and more cancer patients are rejecting the conventional methods of treatment and substituting (or supplementing them with) the 'alternative' or 'complementary' therapies (Cassileth *et al.*, 1984; Cassileth and Brown, 1988; Fink, 1988; Fulder, 1989). These are generally claimed by their proponents to be non-toxic and therefore free from the dangerous and distressing side effects of the cytotoxic drugs (Cameron and Pauling, 1979; Moss, 1980; Harrison, 1987).

Alternative cancer therapies have a long history of association, stretching back into the nineteenth century, with the heterogeneous American cancer counterculture (Patterson, 1987). For as long, they have been the target of orthodox institutional and professional attack and state anti-quackery legislation. This long submerged conflict came to a head in the late seventies with the stalling of the war on cancer and the cultural and social ferment of the aftermath of the Vietnam War and Watergate. An increasing number of vocal critics attacked the dominant anti-cancer alliance and its well-financed organizations and institutions along with organized medicine and the profession of medicine in general. While many of these critics advocated social or environmental solutions to the cancer problem, others promoted self-reliance and deprofessionalization and confronted the orthodox biomedical model with their support for holistic interpretations of health and disease (see section 2.6). Within this climate of iconoclasm and outspoken criticism of orthodoxy and its professional practices and expertise, alternative approaches to cancer (particularly those which could be linked with holism and the emphasis on self-help) flourished as never before. The stereotype of the poor and uneducated as the major utilizers of alternative cancer therapies is not supported by more recent studies that have shown that those using unorthodox approaches tend to be better educated members of the middle classes (Cassileth *et al.*, 1984).

The medical profession, especially that segment whose specialty is the research and treatment of cancer – oncology – has reacted to this trend towards alternative approaches by invoking their own professional claims to scientific expertise and objectivity. In particular, they denigrate the theoretical and evidential bases of alternative treatments (which are accordingly designated 'unproven' by their orthodox critics), and persistently decry their lack of evaluation by accredited oncologists and by accredited methods of cancer treatment assessment (American Society of Clinical Oncology, 1983).

There are, however, formidable obstacles in the way of the orthodox evaluation of unconventional cancer treatments, and most have never been formally evaluated (see Chapter 3.5). Vitamin C is unique amongst marginal cancer therapies in having been evaluated by the canonical randomized controlled clinical trial (see section 1.4), and it took a Pauling to achieve it.

1.3   NATIONAL DIFFERENCES IN MEDICAL ORGANIZATION AND PRACTICE

In Scotland during the seventies, when Ewan Cameron carried out his clinical trials of vitamin C at the Vale of Leven Hospital, oncology was not a distinct specialty as in the United States and cancer was treated by general physicians and surgeons (Raven, 1990). The first Scottish Oncological Association was not formed until 1972, and was open to anyone interested in cancer treatment. It had an initial membership of around one hundred, including surgeons, physicians, pathologists, radiotherapists, researchers, and only a few of the new breed of medical oncologists. Cameron was a founding member and was elected to its governing council. Pauling was elected an Honorary Member at his suggestion. In the United States, in contrast to this informal situation, oncology was an established specialty and subject to rigid statutory controls and professional demarcations.

Again, in Scotland in the seventies, cancer was treated much more conservatively than in the United States. Surgery and radiotherapy were the standard treatments, and the cytotoxic drugs that were in routine use in the United States were seldom administered. These national differences in organization and practice are significant elements in the history of the vitamin C and cancer controversy.

Yet another set of important national differences relates to ethical practices in the two countries, and these will be brought out in the next section on cancer clinical trials.

1.4 CANCER CLINICAL TRIALS

Within the context of the uncertainties and controversies surrounding cancer treatments, cancer clinical trials have taken on an enhanced significance as the arbiters of what is and what is not an appropriate and effective treatment for cancer. In the U.S., more than a third of the total federal government allocation for the evaluation of all clinical procedures is devoted to the evaluation of cancer chemotherapy (Relman, 1983). In 1986, the National Cancer Institute officially listed some 1000 active cancer clinical trials across the country (NCI, 1986). Cancer clinical trials have become practically an industry in their own right, and have spawned a whole new specialty which is responsible for their methodological and statistical rigour and interpretation. Their design undergoes continual refining, and while there is considerable diversity of opinion about the appropriate methodology for the assessment of cancer treatments (as of all therapies), the randomized controlled clinical trial (RCT) has emerged as the leading method of assessment. On the grounds that it most effectively excludes both the bias of the investigators and any placebo effect or expectation of benefit for patients, it has been elevated by its advocates into the 'ultimate means of applying the scientific method to the practice of medicine' (Chalmers, 1981; Buyse *et al.*, 1984; Silverman, 1985). Cancer treatment decisions are ostensibly defended or endorsed primarily on the basis of this method. Unconventional treatments, if they are to achieve orthodox acceptance, must undergo evaluation via this professionally endorsed clinical method (Moertel, 1978a, 1986a).

Clinical evaluations of new cancer therapies are conventionally carried out in three phases (Sylvester, 1984):

Phase I The therapy is administered to a human being for the first time and screened for toxicity and maximim tolerated dose. Extensive prior animal screening has almost always been conducted.

Phase II The therapy is screened for potential anti-tumour activity in a limited number of patients with the same type of tumour and with advanced measurable disease. The purpose of a phase II study is to see whether the drug has sufficient activity at an acceptable level of toxicity to warrant further testing in a larger number of patients. Traditionally, phase II trials have been uncontrolled, although some critics have argued the necessity for their being RCTs (Chalmers, 1981).

Phase III If the phase II trial is positive, the relative efficacy of the drug is compared with either placebo or the best available conventional treatment, either alone on in combination with other drugs. As phase III trials are expensive and time-consuming, they are not usually undertaken without adequate preliminary Phase I and II trials.

It is now conventionally assumed that a Phase III trial must be a randomized controlled trial. However, RCTs are comparative latecomers to the research scene. As late as 1979, in an analysis of the types of controls used in therapeutic trials and reported in the *New England Journal of Medicine*, Chalmers found that only 57 per cent were randomized (Chalmers, 1981). In the area of cancer treatment, the majority of cytotoxic drugs, including 5-fluorouracil, have been applied widely in practice *without* prior evaluation by RCTs (Geehan and Freireich, 1974; McKinlay, 1981; Buyse *et al.*, 1984). Ewan Cameron's clinical trials of vitamin C were carried out primarily between 1972 and 1979, and were historically and concurrently controlled; that is, Cameron compared the survival times of patients given vitamin C with a matched set of randomly selected control cases (some concurrent, some not) from the same hospital who had not been given vitamin C. But his studies were rejected by the medical community on the grounds that they were not prospectively randomized, and therefore were open to the bias of the investigators. The two trials of vitamin C at the Mayo Clinic were designed to fulfil all the methodological criteria of the randomized, prospective, double-blind controlled clinical trial.

In the randomized prospective controlled trial, patients at a comparable stage and site of disease are randomly allocated (for example, by toss of a coin) to different treatments, one of which is the therapy in question, and the other of which may be the best available standard therapy or an inert placebo (a dummy pill made to look and taste like the substance under evaluation). The group receiving the standard therapy or placebo is the control group; the group receiving the therapy being tested is the experimental group. The efficacy of the experimental therapy is evaluated by a statistical comparison of the responses of the experimental and the control groups. Ideally, the trial is 'double-blinded', i.e., it is organized in such a way that neither the patients nor the experimenters are aware of the treatments allocated until the trial is concluded and the results are statistically analyzed. Thus the bias of the researchers and any placebo effects on the patients are supposedly excluded and the methodology is argued to ensure the objective evaluation of the efficacy of the therapy in question. However, such masking or blinding is rarely possible in cancer trials where the different drugs have distinctive side-effects (Buyse *et al.*, 1984).

The problems and pitfalls of the design and evaluation of controlled clinical trials have been exhaustively canvassed in the literature. Ethical considerations have proved the most contentious. Many critics (including many physicians) argue that RCTs are unethical on the grounds that randomization compromises the physicians' efforts to provide optimum individual care for their patients, and that RCTs require a control treatment in which patients are usually deprived of active medication. Defenders of the RCT have tended to dismiss such ethical objection by physicians as motivated by their self-interested avoidance of the experimental evaluation of the therapeutic effectiveness of their procedures and remedies (Finney, 1982). In countering this charge, it has been argued that recent advances in statistical theory and clinical epidemiology have rendered the use of historical or concurrent controls and other adjustment techniques in non-randomized cancer clinical trials as effective and reliable methods of evaluation as the RCT (Geehan and Freireich, 1974; Lortat-Jacob *et al.*, 1978; Feinstein, 1985; Schaffner, 1986).

Another set of ethical difficulties, of particular concern to cancer patients, surrounds the issue of 'informed consent'. Some medical researchers have argued that the full disclosure of risks and benefits to prospective entrants into an RCT would prejudice the outcome of the trial, and that the patient should not be involved in the decision making process (Kopelman, 1986). Richard Peto, the leading British cancer epidemiologist and biostatistician, has been particularly outspoken on this point. He calls informed consent 'a legalistic trick to devolve what should properly be the doctor's responsibility onto the patient. It may serve a useful purpose in warding off American lawyers, but in less litigious countries it is not necessary unless the doctor concerned feels it to be so' (Lortat-Jacob *et al.*, 1978). As Peto implied, the situation in Britain is that doctors are not legally obliged to disclose the risks of a proposed trial of an experimental medication to the patient, nor even to inform the patient of his or her participation in a clinical trial. Indeed, it is not standard practice for doctors to tell patients that they have cancer. Hence, following this customary practice, Ewan Cameron's patients were not directly informed that they were suffering from incurable terminal cancer, and their vitamin C was always described as a 'medication which might help a little' (Cameron and Campbell, 1974). By contrast, in the U.S., a 1978 Code of Federal Regulations made it mandatory for all researchers receiving federal government grant money to obtain informed consent from all patients included in clinical trials (Buyse *et al.*, 1984). So, in conformity with this Code, patients participating in the Mayo Clinic trials of vitamin C were fully informed of the nature of the experimental medication under investigation and of its possible risks and benefits. These distinctions also became a major source of contention in the vitamin C and cancer controversy.

In the U.K., following on the inquest in 1982 into the death of an eighty-three year old woman with bowel cancer (who had been entered into a randomized controlled clinical trial without her knowledge or consent and who died from the acute toxic effects of the experimental cytotoxic drug she was given), there has been increasing demand by cancer patients and those who represent their interests for their right to fully-informed consent for their participation in clinical trials. As well, the necessity for such trials has been questioned, and doubts have been cast on their scientific rigour. Above all, patients and their families have argued that such trials and assessments do not take sufficiently into account the patient's quality of life (Inglis, 1983; Faulder, 1985).

Similar methodological criticisms have been made by critics from within the profession, notably by the clinical epidemiologist Alvan Feinstein. He has criticized what he describes as the 'quasi-religious devotion' to randomized trials, and argued that clinical trials are notoriously faulty, value-laden, and beset with design and interpretative pitfalls (Feinstein, 1977, 1985). Feinstein also insists that the emphasis on quantification is dehumanizing and leads to the neglect of the socio-economic and psychological dimensions of disease in the evaluation of therapies:

> We shall advance the progress of neither science nor humanity by obsequious adherence to scientific doctrines that provide quantitative glitter and 'statistical significance', while dehumanising our data, confusing our sensibility, and diverting our attention from the people who are the only proper subjects for the study of mankind. (Feinstein, 1972)

In response to such criticism, defenders of the randomized controlled trial have recently made some efforts to include quality of life assessments in therapy evaluations, but there is as yet little unanimity on how such assessments are to be made and standardized. The consensus in a recent authoritative text on cancer clinical trials seems to be that without such standardization, 'quality of life or quality of survival should not be given decision making relevance' (Van Dam *et al.*, 1984).

But even quantitative measurements have their shortcomings. Amongst other problems, the quantitative assessment of a patient's response to treatment is subject to a non-negligible measurement error (Moertel and Hanley, 1976). For example, different physicians measuring the dimensions of a tumour in the same patient may make significantly different estimates of its size. For this and other reasons many specialists argue that survival times are the most important criteria of treatment success; but survival measurements also have many difficulties, one of them being the heterogeneity of starting points which can be chosen. This, as we shall see, became yet another point of contention in the vitamin C and cancer dispute. There is, in fact, as yet no standardization in the quantitative, let alone the qualitative, assessment of cancer therapies. 'The oncology literature', as one expert in the area has put it, writing in the same authoritative text on cancer clinical trials, 'is a jungle of free-enterprise approaches to clinical trial interpretation and data reporting. The reader must approach the literature with a *caveat emptor* philosophy' (Carter, 1984).

2 The Vitamin C 'Believers'

I am a scientist, a chemist, physicist, crystallographer, molecular biologist and medical researcher. Twenty years ago I became interested in the vitamins. I discovered that the science of nutrition had stopped developing. . . .

I thought that all I needed to do was to present the facts in a simple, straightforward, and logical way in order that physicians and people generally would accept them. I was right, in this expectation, about the people but wrong about the physicians, or perhaps not about the physicians as individuals but about organized medicine.

Linus Pauling, *How to Live Longer and Feel Better*
(Pauling, 1986)

Why has this information not been publicized? Why have the American people not been told of the helpful research done in the field of nutrition and cancer? Why are the physicians not listening? One young medical student told me why. He said that if physicians stray away from the dogma of surgery, radiation, and chemotherapy, their colleagues will think they are 'health food nuts' and they will be ridiculed and denied research grants! So what is the real reason for this cover up of nutrition information? Money!

Ruth Yale Long,
Crackdown on Cancer With Good Nutrition (Long, 1983)

The most prominent figures in the vitamin C and cancer dispute are indubitably Linus Pauling and Ewan Cameron. They have been jointly responsible for elaborating the theoretical rationale for the therapeutic use of vitamin C in cancer; Cameron's consistently encouraging clinical results have fuelled the controversy; and Pauling has brought his great prestige and consummate political and networking skills to the promotion and negotiation of their claims. Pauling has never hesitated to take what the medical profession regards as a strictly scientific issue into the wider social and political arena in order to obtain funding for his research and a wider hearing for his views, with the result (as his critics acknowledge) that vitamin C megadose has become one of the leading alternative treatments for cancer. It is the professional preserve of a growing number of orthomolecular practitioners, and is promoted by the popular holistic health movement and the booming health food industry. In his confrontation with orthodox medicine, Pauling can draw on the support of these allies with whom he maintains close ties.

2.1   LINUS PAULING

Linus Pauling (born 1901) is possibly the most eminent living scientist in the world, and one of the most controversial. As some measure of his public visibility and stature, a survey in the British journal *New Scientist* in the mid-1970s ranked him with Newton, Einstein and other legendary figures in a list of the twenty most important scientists of all time (Anon., 1975). But Pauling's detractors are almost as legion as his admirers. Over the long years of his professional career he has weathered many a political and scientific storm, while the barometer of public opinion has veered from 'genius' to 'fellow-traveller', from 'maverick' to 'national treasure'. Even in old age, Pauling remains a case-hardened and formidable adversary. Beneath his trade-mark, shabby black beret, he dominates interviews and public platforms, defying the criticisms that have rained down on his peace and vitamin C crusades. With a felt-tipped pen (his only concession to modern writing technology), remarkably few alterations, and an admirable clarity of style, he drafts his still-regular contributions to scientific journals; and, with single-minded determination, he pursues his paper war with his vitamin C opponents.

During the 1930s and 40s, Pauling made enormous contributions to the science of chemistry and to the development of molecular biology with his work on chemical bonding. His classic text, *The Nature of the Chemical Bond*, has become one of the most cited scientific works of this century (Huemer, 1986; Garfield, 1989). Pauling received his first Nobel Prize, for chemistry, in 1954. He has authored several other books and more than three hundred papers on the structure of crystals, quantum mechanics, the nature of the chemical bond, the structure and properties of proteins and antibodies, and molecular structure in relation to biology and medicine. He holds honorary doctoral degrees from about twenty-seven universities, including Yale, Harvard, Cambridge and Oxford, and membership of some sixty scientific societies. Besides the Nobel Prize, he has received many other prestigious scientific awards and honours, including the Davey Medal of the Royal Society in England, the Pasteur Medal in France, and the National Medal of Science in the United States.

Pauling's interests have always been more wide-ranging than chemistry and biology. His publications include more than a hundred papers and books on science and world affairs. In the 1950s and 60s he emerged as a leading anti-war activist when his campaign against the testing of nuclear weapons and his much-acclaimed book, *No More War!*, invoked a public controversy which led to the suspension of atmospheric testing in 1963, the year after Pauling was awarded the Nobel Peace Prize for his efforts in this area. During his campaign Pauling was subjected to the temporary lifting of his passport by the Department of State, to a gruelling appearance before an investigative congressional subcommittee in 1960, and to intense and often offensive media criticism which impugned his citizenship and alleged that he had pro-communist sympathies. In the mid-sixties, in an attempt to counter such allegations, Pauling initiated a series of law suits. One of these created a legal precedent when a badly-instructed jury found that the newspaper concerned could not injure the reputation of so eminent a man (Anon., 1966; Paradowski, 1986; Serafini, 1989). These experiences inured Pauling to public controversy and to the processes of litigation, and he has, over the years, acquired a very good understanding of the American law of libel which he has not been averse to invoking in his more recent confrontations with 'organized medicine'.

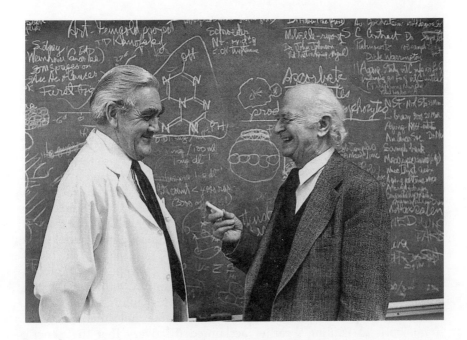

Ewan Cameron and Linus Pauling.

(Courtesy of the Linus Pauling Institute of Science and Medicine, Palo Alto, California)

Pauling's left-wing politics and alleged 'subversive' activities had made him a controversial enough figure in American science and public life, but this controversial image was exacerbated by his entry into the health debate in 1970 with the publication of his book *Vitamin C and the Common Cold*. He is now best known as the world's leading advocate of vitamin C megadose (one or more grams per day) for the maintenance of 'optimum health' and as treatment or supportive treatment for a wide range of conditions, including the common cold, schizophrenia, cancer, improved wound repair and cardio-vascular disease. His assumption of this new and increasingly contentious role has alienated some former admirers and, to a certain extent, undermined his professional standing and stature. As a journalist who interviewed him in 1978 perceived his situation:

> doors that had been open to him for almost half a century were suddenly slammed shut. People have accused him of suddenly entering his dotage. Others have lumped him together with the Mexican laetrile doctors, practitioners of holistic medicine and faith healers. (Collier, 1978)

Pauling's advocacy of vitamin C is often depicted in such terms, and he is usually identified (and has come to identify himself) with the alternative or holistic health movement. But underneath he is still very much the traditional reductionist and molecular biologist whose work paved the way to the development of molecular biology. It is essential to note that his work in orthomolecular medicine is compatible with the orthodox or biomedical model of disease, and may be best understood as a development of his earlier work in molecular biology. Indeed, in a number of respects, vitamin C as preventative or therapy for the common cold or cancer smacks of the medical 'magic bullet' so decried by holists. Pauling's advocacy of the human requirement of a daily megadose of vitamin C is predicated on the reductionist hypothesis that at some stage in their evolution, humans lost the ability to synthesize this essential nutrient through a mutation in their DNA and consequently suffer from a genetic disease, hypoascorbemia, or vitamin C deficiency of the blood (Pauling, 1970b). Pauling did not originate this concept but adapted it from an idea of the industrial chemist and vitamin C enthusiast, Irwin Stone, who first interested Pauling in vitamin C (Pauling, 1970a; Stone, 1972). The hypothesis is assimilable to the same molecular biological framework as Pauling's earlier acclaimed discovery that the genetic disease, sickle-cell anaemia, was caused by an inherited molecular defect (Pauling *et al.*, 1949). It was in connection with this work that Pauling invented the concept of 'molecular disease' and coined the term to describe it. In 1968, he went a step further and introduced the term 'orthomolecular' to describe the new approach to medicine and psychiatry that he and a few others were advocating. 'Orthomolecular' literally means 'right molecules', and Pauling defined orthomolecular medicine as:

> the achievement and preservation of good health and the prevention and treatment of disease by regulating the concentration of molecules that are normally present in the human body. Important orthomolecular substances are the vitamins, especially vitamin C. (Pauling, 1968, 1978)

However, Pauling's attempt to explain psychiatric states and diseases such as the common cold in these terms and, above all, the intrusion of this non-physician into therapeutics, found little favour with the medical profession. His ideas were almost immediately attacked by psychiatrists, physicians and nutritionists as 'unscientific' and unfounded (APA Task Force Report, 1973; Pauling, 1976; Marshall, 1986; Carpenter, 1986). Pauling's efforts to rebut such labels and defend his position embroiled him in controversy, which, as it became increasingly polarized, pushed him inexorably into the alternative camp and to alternative sources of funding for his orthomolecular research. His position at Stanford University, where he had been invited to set up a laboratory in 1969, became untenable when he was no longer able to obtain funding or laboratory space for what was viewed as increasingly contentious research. In 1973, with a former pupil and associate Dr Arthur B. Robinson, he set up an independent institute for orthomolecular research near Stanford, which subsequently became the Linus Pauling Institute of Science and Medicine (see section 2.3).

In spite of his medical marginalization, Pauling has always sought orthodox recognition and evaluation of his claims. He has persistently brought his considerable energy and well-developed political skills, along with his still powerful scientific and public prestige, to bear on these ends. Pauling has proved himself a consummate publicist. Although, as I shall document, his and Cameron's papers have been rejected by leading medical journals such as the *New England Journal of Medicine* and *Cancer*, and on one notorious occasion by the *Proceedings of the National Academy of Sciences*, Pauling has won some notable publishing and fund-raising battles. His prestige has even survived the continuing allegations by Arthur Robinson (co-founder with Pauling of the Linus Pauling Institute), that in an early experiment on the effect of vitamin C on skin cancer in mice, Pauling suppressed data that conflicted with his claims (see section 2.4). In spite of the adverse world-wide publicity engendered by Robinson's allegations, Pauling has pressed on undaunted with his campaign for official recognition and accreditation of his and Cameron's claims.

His greatest achievement was in convincing a reluctant and foot-dragging National Cancer Institute, through a personal diplomatic campaign that has been described as 'almost Kissingeresque', to sponsor a clinical trial of his and Cameron's claims at the Mayo Clinic, and when that proved negative, to successfully campaign for a retrial. When the results of that second trial were published at the beginning of 1985, they were again negative. Since that time, Pauling has been denied any mainstream establishment forum for his and Cameron's criticisms of this trial, and he has been reduced to a public slanging match with the Mayo Clinic team, whom he accuses of publishing a 'fraudulent' paper and issuing 'false and misleading' claims about the inefficacy of vitamin C in cancer treatment (Pauling, 1986). In spite of his belief that his claims about vitamin C have never been dealt with in an unbiased and objective fashion by the medical profession, Pauling's faith in scientific method as the supreme arbiter of truth remains undiminished, and he continues his campaign for yet another trial which will 'objectively' evaluate his and Cameron's claims.

2.2 EWAN CAMERON

A similar process of professional marginalization and exclusion has attended the medical career of Pauling's close collaborator of the past two decades, Ewan Cameron. Since his early retirement from the post of Senior Consulting Surgeon at the Vale of Leven hospital in 1982, Cameron has been Senior Research Professor and Medical Director of the Linus Pauling Institute. He describes his professional background as 'perfectly conventional, even conservative by many standards', and is uncomfortable with his current identification with alternative medicine. He ruefully concedes that his 'seemingly absurd conclusion' of late 1971 that such a simple, non-toxic and readily available substance as vitamin C might have some therapeutic value in such a 'bafflingly complex disease as cancer', and the reaction of the members of his profession to his and Pauling's attempts to theoretically elaborate and demonstrate this, have in effect marginalized him. He also concedes that without Pauling's backing and active intervention, he would never have been able to take his research on vitamin C as far as he has, nor have reached such a wide professional and lay audience.

Although he described himself as an 'obscure Scottish surgeon' in his first letter to Pauling (see Chapter 4), Cameron was quite well-known professionally in Scottish surgical and cancer circles and had established a reputation as offering some promising theoretical insights into the cancer process. His theoretical work had even received some recognition in the United States.

Cameron graduated in medicine from the University of Glasgow in 1944, and completed his postgraduate education in general surgery, being elected a fellow of the Royal Colleges of Surgeons of both Edinburgh and Glasgow. In 1956 he was appointed Consultant Surgeon to Vale of Leven District General Hospital and associated hospitals, Dunbartonshire, and from 1973 until 1982, he served as Chairman of the Hospital's Division of Surgery with responsibility for some 100 beds. He also served on various other district and Scottish medical committees and associations, and in 1975 was made Honorary Consultant in General Surgery to the Royal Navy in Scotland (an appointment which requires a high security clearance and offers some measure of his acceptance in conventional circles). His major interest has always been in the treatment of cancer, and at the time he first contacted Pauling he had a number of published papers in the area to his credit and was the author of a book *Hyaluronidase and Cancer*, published by Pergamon Press in 1966.

While his earlier theoretical approach to the understanding and treatment of cancer fell outside the mainstream approach to the disease, Cameron's work was certainly not viewed as unorthodox or controversial, and his book was fairly well reviewed. It received its best airing in the United States in Solomon Garb's influential book of 1968, *Cure for Cancer: A National Goal*, which helped pave the way to the National Cancer Act of 1971. Garb devoted a whole chapter to reviewing Cameron's approach to the control of cancer through inhibition of its invasiveness, and thought the approach promising enough to 'deserve intensive research'. As we shall see, Cameron's advocacy of vitamin C in cancer treatment was based on his assimilation of vitamin C into this framework, as a naturally occurring inhibitor of hyaluronidase, the enzyme he considered responsible for the invasiveness of cancer cells.

Both Cameron and Pauling, therefore, have orthodox backgrounds in their respective professions, and their advocacy of vitamin C in cancer treatment may be related in both cases to theoretical frameworks they have developed over the course of long professional careers. In Pauling's case, his work in this area had gained him a Nobel Prize, and Cameron had also received a degree of professional recognition for his. Yet as a result of their advocacy of vitamin C, both have been marginalized by their orthodox opponents. Nevertheless, like Pauling, the audience Cameron wants to convince is the professional medical one ('the body to which mentally I still belong'), although he is angered by what he perceives as their consistent hostility to his findings and their unwillingness to judge them impartially.

By insisting on orthodox acknowledgement and evaluation of their claims, Pauling and Cameron have made their own scientific integrity and credibility the central issue in the dispute. It is clearly in their interests to promote their credibility by demonstrating their adherence

to standard scientific and ethical procedures and practices; to justify their
theoretical arguments and experimental results by whatever means they
have at their disposal; and to allege, and if possible demonstrate, the bias
and prejudice of their detractors and opponents.

2.3　THE LINUS PAULING INSTITUTE

The Linus Pauling Institute has had a chequered career since its foundation as the Institute for Orthomolecular Medicine in 1973, with funding
being its major and continuing problem. It was founded as a tax-free non-
profit organization. Pauling and Robinson originally looked to traditional
sources of funding such as government grants, pharmaceutical companies and wealthy benefactors in order to finance their orthomolecular
research. When it became clear early in the piece that such sources
were not particularly interested in investing in increasingly controversial
research, the name of the foundation was changed to the Linus Pauling
Institute for Science and Medicine in the hope that the Pauling name
would prove more of a draw card for funding. However, Pauling's
ability to attract the large public and private grants to which he had
become accustomed in the heyday of his molecular biology research
was waning. By the mid-seventies the financial resources of the Institute
had reached such a low ebb that some alternative source of funding had
to be devised. It was just at this stage that the first published reports
of Cameron's preliminary Vale of Leven trials of vitamin C became
available, and the fund-raising activities of the Institute were largely
reorganized around their promising potential.

Cameron had been made a Non-resident Fellow of the Institute at
the beginning of 1974, and his vitamin C and cancer data were publicized in a campaign directed at the public, and particularly at the
burgeoning movement for self-help and alternative medicine. The campaign included the mailing of hundreds of thousands of form letters to
subscribers to the magazine *Prevention* and other publications of the alternative nutrition and holistic health movement. These letters described
Cameron's and Pauling's research and solicited donations for its continuance. As well, in an attempt to attract tax-exempt donations from
the well-to-do, eye-catching advertisements were placed prominently
in the *Wall Street Journal* and other likely financial publications, such
as:

　For Sale – One Thousand Mice With Malignant Cancer – $138 Each

　*Linus Pauling – Nobel Prize Chemistry 1954, Nobel Prize Peace 1963, Nobel
　Prize Vitamin C 19??*

Such blatant advertising raised establishment eyebrows, but the campaign met with an immediate and heavy response and the donations flooded in. Since that time, although it has managed to achieve some substantial government and private funding, the Institute has continued to draw the major part of its income from this source of some fifty to sixty thousand small donors who support its orthomolecular research. In return, they receive the Institute's *Newsletter* and (upon request) copies of its scientific publications which keep them in touch with its research activities. The continuing success of this direct mailing campaign depends on the ability of the Institute's research programme to fulfil the expectations it arouses that progress is being made in the nutritional conquest of cancer and other diseases. The outcome of the vitamin C and cancer controversy is therefore directly relevant to the economic viability of the Institute, and the *Newsletter* has been directed to maintaining the high profile of the Pauling–Cameron research, and to disputing the results of the two negative Mayo Clinic trials.

The Institute runs on a shoe-string budget of around \$3,000,000 per year. It currently employs around fifty people, not all of whom work full-time. About thirty-five of these are involved in active research. At times the Institute has been stretched to the limit in finding their salaries and the equipment for their research. Some researchers accept lower salaries than they might command elsewhere in order to work there and a few of the more elderly researchers draw no salaries at all. Of its senior personnel, only Pauling has a full-time secretary. Pauling, who holds the official position of Chairman of the Board of Trustees, now takes no part in the day-to-day running of the Institute and has very little contact with its personnel. Nevertheless, he is its inspiration and its members are determined that the Institute should continue as a 'monument' to Pauling.

But this intention points up the continuing dilemma of the Institute. Because of the inevitable association of orthomolecular research with unorthodox science and medicine, the Institute has had a hard struggle to attain scientific accreditation and recognition, and is sensitive to its categorization as 'unorthodox'. It is anxious to project itself 'not as a Vitamin C Institute' but as an 'organization working in the medical and basic biological sciences'. Under the direction of Dr Emile Zuckerkandl (the current president and director) the Institute has branched out into basic molecular biological and biochemical medical research, involving such conventional high technologies as gene cloning and DNA sequencing, and has received a degree of recognition in this area. It has forged some associations with researchers at near-by Stanford, and work performed at the Institute has received attention at major scientific meetings and recently attracted two substantial National Cancer Institute grants for basic research into the molecular mechanisms of the cancer process. Zuckerkandl himself, like Pauling with whom he formerly worked at the

California Institute of Technology, has a background in molecular biology and edits the *Journal of Molecular Evolution*. The connection between this reductionist, high-technology, basic molecular research and the 'applied' nutritional focus of the orthomolecular research at the Institute is much stressed by Zuckerkandl, but to a certain extent they sit uneasily side by side, a schism reflected in the funding strategies of the Institute. So long as orthomolecular research is viewed as unconventional and controversial, it cannot readily attract traditional funding. In order to survive, the Institute must either move more directly into conventional research at the risk of compromising its founding purpose of researching and promoting orthomolecular medicine, or it must remain largely dependent on alternative sources of funding with all their attendant problems of uncertainty, lack of continuity, and erosion of scientific status.

2.4   THE ROBINSON AFFAIR

The whole area of vitamin C and cancer research has been a sensitive issue at the Institute since 1978, when Arthur Robinson, who had been a founding trustee and President of the Institute since 1975, brought a reported $25.5 million lawsuit against the Institute for alleged breach of contract. Robinson followed this up by initiating twelve or so defamation suits against various individuals at the Institute, including Pauling and the executive vice president. In the attendant publicity it was alleged that there had been a falling out between Pauling and Robinson over the conduct of a series of experiments at the Institute concerning the relation between vitamin C ingestion and the incidence of skin cancer in mice.

Robinson continues with his allegations in any forum available to him. But since all other parties to the 'Robinson affair' are exceedingly reluctant to discuss the affair with outsiders, it is difficult to determine the exact course of events. It appears that Robinson introduced a new element into the mouse experiments, a diet of raw fruit and vegetables in which he had become interested through his working association with Eydie Mae Hunsberger, the wife of a wealthy company owner and author of a best-selling book, *How I Conquered Cancer Naturally* (Mae with Loeffler, 1975). According to Robinson, he fed the Hunsberger diet plus vitamin C in very high doses to one of the groups of mice in the experiment with spectacular results. This particular group showed a much lower incidence of cancerous skin lesions than any other group in the experiment. Moreover, the group fed the Hunsberger diet alone did as well as the group fed very high levels of vitamin C. By contrast, the group fed the mouse equivalent of the Pauling–Cameron recommended dose of 10 grams per day had, by Robinson's account, twice as many skin lesions as the controls who were fed a normal mouse diet (Robinson, 1979). Pauling apparently aroused Robinson's hostility by insisting that the experiments proceed with vitamin C alone and without the involvement of the Hunsbergers, whom he regarded as amateurs. Robinson resisted this directive and relations between the two deteriorated to the point where they could no longer work together. Robinson was dismissed from his post. After five years of litigation Robinson settled for a reported out-of-court settlement of $575,000 in 1983, and the whole affair was apparently over.

For several years, Pauling and the Institute found it extremely difficult to counteract the heavy financial costs and adverse world-wide publicity engendered by the affair, especially Robinson's sensational continuing allegation that Pauling suppressed the mouse data in relation to Robinson's experimental finding that vitamin C at the doses recommended by Pauling actually led to a twofold increase in the incidence of mouse skin cancer (Grant, 1979; Carroll, 1979; Grauerholz, 1984; Serafini, 1989). The real course of events is now impossible to determine, having disappeared in the welter of claim and counterclaim. But it is worthy of note that before his disagreement with Pauling, Robinson wrote a memo to Pauling explaining and dismissing this experimental result as possibly related to the fact that mice, unlike humans, synthesize their own vitamin C and might need fairly high doses of oral vitamin C in order to replace the potentially more effective internally produced vitamin. This suggests a fair degree of reinterpretation of this finding after Robinson had left the Institute. Moreover, contrary to Robinson's claim of suppression, Pauling has actually published the contentious data in a paper on these mouse experiments where they are explained away as having no statistical significance (Pauling *et al.*, 1982). Robinson has never formally published his own experimental findings and he now reportedly identifies a strong political component in his and Pauling's disagreement (Grauerholz, 1984; Serafini, 1989).

Senior personnel at the Institute explain the out-of-court settlement reached with Robinson as 'unmerited' but dictated by the crippling costs associated with the defence of the individuals concerned and the loss of research time while they were testifying. Even so, the decision not to proceed to trial and the vindication of their counter-claims has provided those opposed to Pauling's vitamin C claims with further ammunition, and the accusation of 'fraud' has been bandied about fairly freely among Pauling's leading medical opponents.

2.5 MEGAVITAMIN THERAPY AND ORTHOMOLECULAR MEDICINE

Megavitamin therapy is one aspect of orthomolecular medicine and involves the use of very large amounts of vitamins in the control and treatment of disease. The basis of megavitamin therapy is that the 'optimum' intake of vitamins in most cases is very much larger (ten to a hundred times) than the officially recommended daily intakes, and that this optimum intake varies widely from individual to individual. Its practitioners place much emphasis on the 'naturalness' and non-toxicity of their naturally-occurring therapies. This claim extends to terminology, so that Pauling, for instance, categorically rejects any comparison between vitamins and drugs, and is insistent that vitamins (even when taken in the very large amounts he advocates) are not drugs but *foods*:

> Drugs are dangerous, vitamins are safe. The vitamins are *foods* – essential foods, required by human beings for life and good health. They are safe, even when taken in large amounts. Side effects occur only infrequently and are rarely serious. Also vitamins are inexpensive, compared with most drugs. (Pauling, 1986)

Pauling accordingly contrasts the 'orthomolecular' medicine he promotes with the 'toximolecular' approach of drug-based conventional medicine. These terminological distinctions are as much ideologically as theoretically based, and are central to the vitamin C and cancer controversy.

Pauling remains its best-known advocate, but in recent years megavitamin therapy has become the professional preserve of a growing number of orthomolecular physicians who have secured a position on the periphery of conventional clinical medicine (Williams and Kalita, 1977; Hoffer and Walker, 1978; McMichael, 1981; Lesser, 1980). Over the years, the practitioners of orthomolecular medicine have grown in numbers and strength to the point where it is now recognized as one of the leading unorthodox or marginal therapeutic systems. There are now orthomolecular institutes and academies, and orthomolecular journals and societies, and it is possible to take orthomolecular diplomas and degrees. Its practitioners are seeking and taking on all the trappings of professionalism. Pauling, who coined the name and founded the first orthomolecular institute, is the intellectual inspiration and acknowledged patron of this emerging professional system. He is the founding Honorary President of the American Orthomolecular Association (founded in 1975), which claims approximately 500 physician members (Lesser, 1980; Pauling, 1986). Their heavy professional investment in the demarcation of vitamins from drugs underlies the vigorous opposition of orthomolecular physicians to the proposed regulation of high-dose vitamins as over-the-counter 'drugs' (see section 2.7).

According to Pauling, it is 'not easy' to be an orthomolecular physician, and he and the practitioners of orthomolecular medicine claim harassment from the medical establishment which, they say, is threatened by the purported benefits and low costs of megavitamin therapy. In 1984, Pauling testified on behalf of the current president of the Orthomolecular Medical Association, who had his California medical license revoked by the California Board of Medical Quality Assurance. One of the charges against him was that he was using an unproven method of cancer treatment. He was forced to move to another state in order to continue his practice of medicine (Pauling, 1986; Jukes, 1986).

Orthomolecular practitioners also claim that a double standard prevails in the orthodox criticism of megavitamin treatments: while the most rigorous proof of the efficacy of such treatments is demanded, the flimsiest of anecdotal evidence is produced in demonstration of their toxicity (Pauling, 1986). As well, it is alleged that double-blind randomized studies that have been carried out by orthomolecular physicians are resisted or disregarded by orthodox critics, and that establishment institutions are not interested in replicating such studies or instituting others (Hoffer and Osmond, 1960; Hoffer, 1980). Generally, megavitamin therapists have placed the onus for the disproof of their disputed therapies squarely on their orthodox critics. *They* in turn have demanded convincing preliminary evidence of the efficacy and safety of megavitamin therapy, and have alleged evasion of evaluation by orthomolecular practitioners (Yetiv, 1986).

2.6 THE HOLISTIC HEALTH MOVEMENT AND THE 'FREEDOM FIGHTERS' FOR ALTERNATIVE CANCER TREATMENTS

While it aspires to professional status and orthodox recognition, orthomolecular medicine keeps one foot firmly in the holistic health movement through its naturalistic basis and its emphasis on nutrition. The highly eclectic holistic health movement may be located in the context of the current broad dissatisfaction with the way that orthodox medicine is organized and practised (Berliner and Salmon, 1979a, 1980; Guttmacher, 1979; Salmon, 1984; Aakster, 1986; Fulder, 1989).

Largely an outgrowth of the counterculture and the human potential movement of the late sixties and early seventies, holism has been influenced by Chinese medical practice, Eastern philosophy, nineteenth century American health practices, and, more recently, the 'New Age' movement. Beyond drawing together the diverse practitioners who place themselves outside the mainstream of modern medicine, there are therefore problems in its definition, and these are compounded by the multitude of theories and therapies that have been linked to the movement by their advocates. Generally, holism rejects the reductionism and mechanism of scientific medicine, is highly critical of its technological and interventionist orientation, and aims at the integration of body, mind and spirit. Each individual is considered as a unique conjunction of these aspects and must be approached and treated as an integrated whole. The holistic emphasis is on prevention, and the onus is on the individual to play a constructive part in maintaining his or her health by practising healthy living habits (Sobel, 1979; Le Shan, 1984; Patel, 1987). While there are great differences of opinion within the movement as to what these health-giving practices might be, ranging from meditation and yoga through chiropractic and naturopathy to jogging and aerobics, there is general consensus that nutrition plays a central role in the maintenance of health, and that the optimum intake of vitamins is of particular importance. In the United States, a whole range of popular journals caters to this holistic focus on nutrition, led by the long-lasting and biggest-selling *Prevention*, which has a paid circulation of three million and allegedly derives an income of $10 million a year from food supplement advertising (Marshall, 1986). Some natural health food books by popular nutritionists such as Adelle Davis have sold by the million to a receptive public.

Orthomolecular medicine, and megavitamin therapy in particular, have thus been assured of a large and enthusiastic popular following, the extent of which may be judged by the great expansion of the vitamin market in the western world. A recent study reported that about forty per cent of the whole US population regularly consumes vitamin supplements of some kind (Koplan *et al.*, 1986). This trend has survived the long-term and continuing campaign by conventional nutritionists to the effect that the average American diet contains all the necessary vitamins and minerals (a claim based on the officially-determined RDAs and the assumption that individual requirements do not vary widely), and that vitamin supplements are not only unnecessary and expensive, but might be dangerous (Fried, 1984; Marshall, 1986).

Cancer has become the particular focus of dissident nutritional and holistic attention, and dietary manipulation and vitamin and mineral supplementation have become the norm in alternative cancer therapies. They are promoted by an ever-growing popular literature and by a network of organizations including the International Association of Cancer Victims and Friends (founded 1963), the Committee for Freedom of Choice in Cancer Therapy (founded 1972), the Foundation for Alternative Cancer Therapies (founded 1970), Project CURE (founded 1979), and the Cancer Control Society (founded 1973). These organizations disseminate information about self-help nutritional regimes and alternative 'suppressed' cancer therapies, and tell people where and how to obtain them through their journals, directories and telephone 'Hotlines'. They also organize conferences which provide a platform for dissident cancer therapists, and arrange bus tours of Mexican alternative cancer clinics.

Such organizations draw their members and support from the diffuse and broadly-based cancer counterculture in American society which traditionally has been suspicious of orthodox scientific claims about the 'dread disease' (Patterson, 1987). Generally, these organizations and their members attribute the opposition and hostility with which alternative therapies are treated by orthodox oncologists and institutions to a self-interested conspiracy by the 'cancer establishment'. This 'conspiracy' purportedly involves a cover up of its own failures (e.g., the fudging and misrepresentation of cancer statistics by the establishment) and its suppression and legal harassment of the too-competitive and successful alternative treatments and their practitioners (Petersen and Markle, 1979a; Moss, 1980; Long, 1983; Culbert, 1983; Markle and Petersen, 1987). Well-funded and politically active, the dissident cancer organizations are devoted to the defence of alternative practitioners against legal action or harassment, and to the promotion of the concept of freedom of choice in cancer treatments. Their more radical activists are the self-styled 'freedom fighters', who picture themselves as waging a guerrilla countercampaign for a pluralistic medicine against the 'quackbusters' of the monopolistic and monolithic medical establishment who have condemned all alternative treatments without fair trial (Moll, 1987).

It was such organized elements of the holistic health movement which, during the seventies, resisted the combined opposition of the National Cancer Institute, the American Medical Association, the American Cancer Society and virtually all of the American medical community to the testing of the purported anti-cancer drug, laetrile, and forced a number of evaluations of this 'vitamin' from the reluctant medical community (Petersen and Markle, 1979; Moss, 1980; Markle and Petersen, 1987). With the withering away of the laetrile movement in the early 1980s, promoters of the freedom of choice argument turned their attention to highlighting the failures of the orthodox biomedical model and conventional cancer treatments in particular. Among other initiatives they sponsored a number of television documentaries and films which dealt sympathetically with alternative treatments in the context of hard-hitting critiques of conventional medicine and its institutions (Chowka, 1988). Such publicity efforts have kept the issue of freedom of choice to the forefront of the public consciousness. In 1985 a national public opinion poll found that half of the 1,402 Americans surveyed believed that clinics using unorthodox cancer therapies should be permitted to operate in the U.S., even if the treatments they utilized were opposed by the medical community, while 52 per cent stated that they would themselves seek out such alternative treatments if they were seriously ill (Associated Press, 1985). These attitudes were given concrete political expression when, in the same year, the Bahamian clinic of Dr Lawrence

Burton, an American scientist and developer of the contentious immunological cancer treatment, immuno-augmentative therapy (IAT), was
closed, allegedly through pressure on the Bahamian government from
U.S. agencies, including the National Cancer Institute. The closure of the
clinic led to public protests and appeals from patients deprived of their
treatment for Congressional intervention. The freedom-fighting groups
joined forces around the issue to mobilize Congressional support for a
searching probe of national cancer policy with respect to alternative
cancer treatments. In 1986 some thirty-eight members of Congress peti-
tioned for a special investigation of Burton's therapy by the Office of
Technology Assessment (OTA), a nonpartisan analytical support agency
whose task is to analyse complex issues involving science and technology
for both Senate and House Committees. Their request was approved
and broadened into a comprehensive OTA review of unorthodox cancer
treatments with a view to developing 'objective guidelines for planning
evaluation' of such therapies, most of which have never been formally
evaluated. Freedom of choice advocates optimistically heralded the OTA
review (which was scheduled for completion in mid-1988, but as of
December 1989 is still unconcluded) as having the potential to make
the subject of alternative cancer therapies 'a legitimate field for scientific
and humanistic inquiry', and to pave the way for a 'sweeping review and
reform of the entire national cancer policy' (Chowka, 1988; Moll, 1987).

Holism is thus a potent force in American society, and it has achieved
a degree of political and governmental recognition. Senator George
McGovern is a prominent political patron of holistic health (McGovern,
1980). McGovern chaired the Senate Select Committee on Nutrition and
Human Needs which produced the controversial but influential report,
Dietary Goals for the United States, on the links between nutrition and
disease (Broad, 1979; see also section 3.3). Political supporters of holism
are not confined to liberal Democrats, but range across the whole
political spectrum, with the right wing strongly represented (Deutsch,
1977; Petersen and Markle, 1979a, b; Patterson, 1987). Ideological issues
aside, various analysts of holism have stressed the appeal of the holistic
emphasis on self help to those wanting government cuts in health
care expenditure (Guttmacher, 1979). Perhaps the most significant of
all the reasons for the social and political strength of the holists lies in
their concentration on individual rather than social solutions for health
problems. The advocates of holism have thereby provided new avenues
for corporate and entrepreneurial marketing efforts, of which the vitamin
business is indubitably one of the biggest and most profitable (Berliner
and Salmon, 1979a; Crawford, 1980).

Although its enthusiasts and advocates often refer to the holistic model
as the 'new health revolution' and depict it as a threat, even a 'haunting
spectre', to the dominance of the biomedical model, closer analysis

shows that the holistic model actually constitutes less of a challenge to than an extension of the biomedical model. Its critics have pointed out that both models deflect attention from the social, environmental, and economic determinants of health. By locating the individual at the centre of health problems, the holistic model fosters the rationale that the sick and disadvantaged suffer as a result either of biological inadequacy or their own indigence, and such rationalization fits the prevailing social and medical ideology of 'victim blaming' (Crawford, 1980, 1984; Berliner and Salmon, 1980; Coward, 1989). Further, the holistic model, through its entrepreneurial exploitation and its would-be professionalism, has shown its potential to replicate the social and structural aspects of orthodox medicine, and is actually, to some extent, becoming merged with it. I shall return to this discussion in section 3.7.

2.7 THE HEALTH FOOD INDUSTRY

In the United States, retail sales of vitamins have been estimated at from $1.2 to $3 billion annually, with a growth rate of 10 per cent (Senecker, 1979; Anon., 1984; Fried, 1984). Vitamin C is by far the biggest single seller, and the vitamin C market has grown phenomenally since the early seventies. When Pauling's book *Vitamin C and the Common Cold* first appeared in 1970, the demand for the vitamin outstripped supply, and for a time, until the pharmaceutical industry stepped up production and cashed in on what is known in the trade as the 'Linus Pauling effect', there was a flourishing black market in the vitamin (Anon., 1975). It has been estimated that in the United States (with a population of around 250 million), at least 50 million on any given day in the late 1970s were ingesting vitamin C tablets or supplements (Carpenter, 1986).

The Swiss-based company, Hoffmann-La Roche, one of the largest and most powerful of the pharmaceutical giants, is the world's biggest producer of vitamin C, supplying more than half of all vitamin C sold on the world market. Under the impetus of the 'Pauling effect', during the 70s Roche doubled its production of the vitamin through the construction of a number of multi-million dollar plants around the world, while the bulk price of vitamin C rose by more than 300 per cent (Senecker, 1977). In spite of this, the bulk price of the vitamin in real terms remains low (around $6 a kilogram in 1985), and the profits depend primarily on the size of the market, which is considerable. In the U.S. in 1985 the total market was 16,000 tons, and the consumption of the synthetic vitamin (which includes vitamin C 'fortification' of drinks and foods) corresponded to around 200mg per day per head of the entire U.S. population (Carpenter, 1986). Just how profitable Roche perceives the world vitamin market to be may be gauged by its tactics in maintaining control of it. In 1976 Roche was fined DM1.1 million by the EEC Commission for monopoly pricing of vitamins within the EEC member countries, amidst more serious allegations of establishing an illegal cartel with other major vitamin manufacturers (Anon., 1979; Adams, 1984). Not surprisingly, whereas Pauling has experienced great difficulty in getting funding for his vitamin research from government sources, Hoffmann-La Roche has contributed about $100,000 annually to the Linus Pauling Institute.

The greater proportion of the vitamin market is still in the hands of orthodox manufacturers and retailers (including drug stores and super-markets), but since the late sixties the health food industry has made increasing inroads on the retail market and now draws a considerable portion of its very large revenue from vitamin sales (some estimates place it as high as 60 per cent). There is thus an important economic dimension to the ideological alliance among the vitamin C 'believers', and this is most pronounced in the nexus between the holistic health movement and the health food industry via the National Health Federation (NHF). Together they can exert a fair amount of economic and political leverage in the U.S.A.

The NHF was founded in 1955, and had its origins in right-wing politics and non-orthodox health activities. It was originally a very small organization which promoted individual freedom of choice in matters relating to health and served a 'watch-dog' function on the attempts by the Food and Drug Administration to regulate and prosecute 'unproven' health practices, appliances and substances (Roth, 1976). Its leaders were allegedly closely involved in the manufacture and marketing of health foods and a number of them had themselves been prosecuted by the FDA. From the late sixties, as alternative health practices grew in popularity, the membership of the NHF grew to over 30,000 and took on a more liberal political orientation. During the seventies, the NHF became the focus of dissident nutrition ideas, and it spearheaded the major political agitation and activism against the persistent attempts by the FDA to reclassify high potency vitamins as drugs and so restrict their over-the-counter sales. The NHF worked in tandem with the consortium of health food manufacturers and retailers, the National Nutritional Foods Association (NNFA), to organize letter campaigns and lobby Congress against the proposed vitamin legislation. Their intensive lobbying and well-organized campaign led to a number of congressional hearings, and in 1976 resulted in a resounding political victory when President Gerald Ford signed a bill to restrict the FDA's proposed limitations on vitamin sales. The 'Proxmire Amendment' made it unlawful for the FDA to regulate vitamins as drugs on the basis of their potency alone, and FDA officials are still trying to sort out its full implications (Harper, 1977; Deutsch, 1977; Shapo, 1979; Fried, 1984).

Pauling was a prominent figure in this campaign, and was the star of the 1973 Congressional Hearings when he testified against the proposed regulations (Committee on Interstate and Foreign Commerce, House of Representatives, 1974). Along with the NHF and the NNFA, Pauling personally brought a suit against the FDA, successfully challenging the validity of the regulations and the authority of the FDA to promulgate them (Harper, 1977). More recently, he made a much-publicized appearance in court on behalf of a mail-order vitamin dealer who was being prosecuted by the FDA for making 'false and misleading claims' about his products, and offered a spirited testimony in defense of the dealer's therapeutic claims (Budiansky, 1983). Although he is sometimes critical of the health food industry, the nexus between Pauling and the industry is thus well-established, and he has received a number of industry awards.

3 The Vitamin C 'Non-Believers'

Our studies of high-dose vitamin C in patients with far-advanced cancer were motivated by the remarkable testimony of Dr Linus Pauling that such treatment would prolong the overall life span of cancer patients by more than tenfold and would produce tumour regression in some, and would essentially cure others. For such a message to be conveyed to desperate dying people, with the endorsement of a Nobel laureate, the presumption must be that it is based on impeccable scientific methodology. As a minimum, this methodology should include randomized assignment of treatment and, particularly when symptomatic improvement is claimed, double-blinding.

The only attempt at control made by Cameron and Pauling in their two reports was the selection and then the reselection of case histories from hospital files. . . . With such a method one can only presume that any favourable result of treatment could simply result from case selection bias. The medical therapeutic experience over the past century is littered with the derelicts of treatment claims based on history review studies that could not be confirmed by more rigorous scientific method.

Dr Charles Moertel, *Nutrition Reviews* (Moertel, 1986a)

It was reported in that eminent medical journal, *The National Enquirer*, that Linus Pauling and Cameron, working at a great international medical research centre in Scotland (which turns out to be, I believe, a nursing home in the Scottish Highlands), found that megadoses of vitamin C increase survival of terminal cancer patients four-fold. This was published in the *Proceedings of the National Academy of Sciences*, a prestigious journal. You have to realize, however, that the basic criterion for getting something published in this journal is to be a member of the Academy. In fact, what was being described, in my view and in the view of a number of cancer experts is the placebo effect. The fact that these patients lived an average of eight months instead of an average of two months, is simply due to the fact that the patients were in the hands of enthusiastic doctors who felt that they could help. This is true at every cancer center in the United States. Put a patient in Sloan–Kettering or in Roswell Park . . . and that patient is going to live longer.

Professor Victor Herbert,
Resident and Staff Physician (Herbert, 1978)

By contrast with the marginal medical positions of Pauling and Cameron, the eminent oncologist they identify as their leading opponent – Dr Charles Moertel (who directed both Mayo Clinic trials of vitamin C) – is very well-placed to represent conventional opinion on cancer therapy. Moertel's affiliations offer a guide to the complexities of the shifting coalition of interested parties who may be collectively identified as the vitamin C 'non-believers'.

3.1   DR CHARLES MOERTEL

Moertel is Professor of Oncology at the Mayo Medical School, and, until recently, Chairman, Department of Oncology, Mayo Clinic, and Director, Mayo Comprehensive Cancer Centre. He is a member of the editorial boards of the leading American cancer journals, including *Cancer*, *Cancer Research* (the journals of the American Cancer Society), *Cancer Medicine*, and *Current Problems in Cancer*. He also plays a strong professional role, being a member of the Council on Cancer of the American Medical Association, and is past-president and board member of the American Society for Clinical Oncology. In addition, Moertel has close affiliations with the FDA, where he has served on the Oncologic Drug Advisory Committee, and he has also served on the Board of Scientific Counsellors and various committees on cancer research for the National Cancer Institute (NCI).

Unlike the struggling and marginal Linus Pauling Institute, the long-established, privately-endowed, enormous, and highly prestigious Mayo Clinic is perceived, both publicly and professionally, as synonymous with scientific medicine at its very best. Founded by the highly-successful Mayo brother surgeons in the 1880s and incorporated into a non-profit organization in 1923, the Mayo Clinic served as the prototype for the development of high-technology, hospital-based scientific medicine in the United States (Starr, 1982). Moertel and his co-researchers at the Mayo Clinic and its associated teaching and research centres thus are assured of professional and media attention and respect by virtue of their institutional location alone.

Moertel achieved his high professional and public profile through his commitment to the furtherance and defence of the teaching and practice

Vitamin C Shown Ineffective Against Cancer; Pauling Disputes Results, Moertel Defends

By Serena Stockwell

ROCHESTER, MINNESOTA—Vitamin C is ineffective against cancer, even for patients who have not had prior chemotherapy, a second study by the Mayo Clinic here has found. "It is very clear that this study fails to show a benefit for high-dose vitamin C therapy of cancer," the senior author of the report, Charles G. Moertel, MD, chairman of the department of oncology and director of the Mayo Comprehensive Cancer Center, reported.

In the randomized, double-blind study, 100 patients with advanced colorectal cancer were given either high-dose ascorbic acid (10 grams daily) or placebo. Overall, the patients were in very good general condition, and none had received chemotherapy. "Vitamin C therapy showed no advantage over placebo therapy with regard to either the interval between the beginning of treatment and disease progression or patient survival," Dr. Moertel said. "Among patients with measurable disease, none had objective improvement."

Linus Pauling, PhD, sharply critical of the study, told ONCOLOGY TIMES that Dr. Moertel was "not at all justified in saying vitamin C has no value." The Mayo report "blatantly misrepresents" his own earlier studies with Dr. Ewan Cameron. Dr. Pauling said. The most serious difference was that the patients in the Mayo study were given vitamin C for a relatively short time (2.5 months

median), while the patients in the Cameron/Pauling studies were given the vitamin until they died.

Rebound Effect

"None of the Mayo patients died while on vitamin C. They all died after being taken off," he said. The reason they died, he claimed, is probably due to the "rebound effect," a dangerous reaction that occurs when large doses of vitamin C are suddenly withdrawn.

As Dr. Pauling explained in his book. *Cancer and Vitamin C*, this phenomenon is well known in bacteria and called induced enzyme formation. "In the case of vitamin C in human beings, we assume that there are enzymes that help to convert ascorbate to certain oxidation products. It is known that these oxidation products serve a useful purpose—they have been shown to have anticancer activity in mice, and presumably are

(Continued on Page 14;

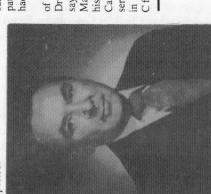

Dr. Charles G. Moertel

Lead article of *Oncology Times*, March 1985.

(Courtesy of *Oncology Times*, New York)

of a rigorously scientific medicine in the professional specialty of cancer research and treatment, or oncology. His area of expertise lies in the sub-specialty of cancer chemotherapy – primarily in the clinical evaluation of the efficacy of the cytotoxic drugs. He has an expressed antipathy to 'the mire of uncontrolled quackery', and is a leading professional advocate and practitioner of the definitive 'tightly controlled clinical trial performed in competent and experienced hands' (Moertel, 1978a). It was Moertel who led the NCI-funded multi-institutional team which officially 'closed the books on laetrile' (Relman, 1982a). With his two officially-endorsed negative trials of vitamin C, Moertel has emerged as the foremost professional demolition expert and vocal critic of alternative cancer treatments. In a recent interview he sweepingly condemned the evaluation of alternative cancer treatments as a 'waste of time and money . . . a waste of patient hope' (Moertel, 1989).

It is essential to note that Moertel has also brought his professional criticism to bear on certain conventional cytotoxic drugs, specifically 5-fluorouracil, although he has been a notably less effective critic of this established treatment (see section 8.1). He has been quoted as having compared cytotoxic chemotherapy with 'swatting at flies with a sledge-hammer' (Gupp and Neumann, 1981). Moertel has also been a critic of the cancer drug interferon, and, more recently, he made headlines when he called for a halt to the trials of interleukin-2 (interferon's succes-sor 'wonder drug'), citing disappointing response rates, 'unacceptably' severe toxic effects, and 'astronomical' costs (Moertel, 1986b).

Moertel has pursued his own campaign for reform, but it is reform very much within the dominant chemotherapeutic model, and it is to be achieved via the rigorous application of the professionally endorsed methodology. Even at his most critical, he has continued to defend conventional cytotoxic lines of research, and to insist on the necessity of keeping cancer patients out of the hands of 'quacks and charlatans' (Moertel, 1978b).

3.2 THE CANCER ESTABLISHMENT

In the USA, the management and direction of cancer research and treat-ment are shaped by a complex of interlocking government and private organizations, of which the giant government-funded National Cancer Institute is the most readily identifiable. Others are the extremely influen-tial American Cancer Society (ACS), the Food and Drug Administration (FDA), which oversees the regulation of all cancer treatments, and a variety of cancer research institutes, of which the privately-endowed Memorial Sloan–Kettering Cancer Center is the largest and most pres-tigious. A network of connections exists among these more visible bodies and other interested parties, such as the medical profession and its officially endorsed organizations and relevant specialties, various large and powerful business corporations, and, last but not least, the pharmaceutical industry (Strickland, 1972; Goodfield, 1975; Rettig, 1977; Moss, 1980; Studer and Chubin, 1980). Taken in all, this complex comprises what some critics have designated 'the cancer establishment'. While the term is misleading in so far as it suggests an organized and unified coalition, it serves the useful function of indicating a commonality of interests which sponsors and sustains officially endorsed or orthodox cancer research and treatment. There is, moreover, a significant economic dimension to this orthodoxy. Americans annually spend an officially estimated 6 per cent ($13.1 billion in 1980) of the total health care bill on cancer diagnosis and treatment (unofficial estimates are considerably higher), while current annual cancer research and prevention costs account for another 1 per cent (Page and Asire, 1985; NCI, 1985a). At the individual level, a study of the medical costs for children with cancer who died during the years 1975–79 found that total medical charges throughout the illness (median time 1.7 years), ranged from $8,000 to $53,000, with an average charge of $34,558 (Lansky *et al.*, 1983). The heavy economic and social costs, the bureaucratic ramifications, the high visibility, and the continuing political manipulation of the cancer problem have given it an overtly recognizable political aspect which is peculiar to this segment of medical treatment and research. The NCI, which in terms of size and dollars is the most powerful force in the cancer establishment, is also, because it is a government bureaucracy which is directly answerable to the President and Congress, most vulnerable to outside political pressure and manipulation.

3.3   THE NATIONAL CANCER INSTITUTE

The NCI was founded in 1938. Total budget appropriations to 1986 came to $15,436,730,283, with more than 85 per cent of that amount having been appropriated since the end of 1971 when the National Cancer Act was signed into law by President Nixon (NCI, 1985). In 1988, the NCI was spared the deep budget cuts suffered by other federal health agencies and allocated a budget of $1,468.4 million, a figure which is alleged to have barely kept ahead of inflation, but which still reflects the NCI's privileged and well-funded position in spearheading the government's war on cancer (Leary, 1989). From the start of this multibillion dollar war, the NCI came under intense political pressure to find a cure for cancer and concentrated its efforts in that direction. Its focus on cure and the linking of cancer research variously to the theory of viral aetiology, oncogene research, and the Biological Response

Modifiers Program (for which interferon was the prototype), conform with the orthodox biomedical model. Within this framework, the NCI has established a goal of reducing cancer mortality by 50 per cent by the year 2000, and promotes this in its official Fact Book as 'quite achievable both because of the promise of today's scientific opportunities and the record of accomplishments of the past decade' (NCI, 1985a). NCI officials have continued to defend this claim against the criticism of sceptical epidemiologists and biostatisticians.

Dr Vincent DeVita, Director of the NCI from 1980 until his resignation in August 1988 to become physician-in-chief at Memorial Sloan–Kettering Cancer Center, dealt directly with Pauling on behalf of the NCI during the two Mayo Clinic trials of vitamin C. DeVita's own background lies in the area of cancer chemotherapy, and he has received a number of high-ranking awards for his important contributions to this area, particularly the development of multiple-drug therapy for Hodgkin's disease and lymphoma (NCI, 1985a). He is a member of the Institute of Medicine of the National Academy of Sciences, and, like Moertel, is past-president and board member of the American Society of Clinical Oncology. He also serves on the editorial boards of numerous scientific and cancer journals.

By the time DeVita became Director of the NCI, the war on cancer had become, in the words of the then head of the FDA, 'a medical Vietnam' (Moss, 1980). From the mid-seventies on, the NCI has been subjected to a heavy barrage of public and political criticism of the poor returns on its pursuit of the elusive cancer cure, and its research and funding strategies became the target of a number of presidential and congressional investigations and interventions (Greenberg, 1974, 1975, 1981a, b; Moss, 1980; Patterson, 1987). In recent years, in response to such criticism and interventions, the NCI has modified its funding procedures and made some attempt to shift its focus from cure to prevention. But as late as 1988, only 5 per cent of the total NCI budget was earmarked for preventive efforts. In 1984 the NCI introduced a 'Cancer Prevention Awareness Program' which focuses on individualistic solutions to the cancer problem, primarily on the limitation of tobacco use and on diet (NCI, 1985a).

This NCI-sponsored investigation of the link between diet and cancer resulted directly from the public pressure (much of it orchestrated by Pauling and other dissident nutritionists, the health food lobby and the holistic health movement) which led to the setting up of the McGovern-chaired Senate Select Committee on Nutrition and Human Needs (see section 2.6). In 1980, following on the McGovern Report on the links between nutrition and disease, the NCI commissioned the National Research Council of the National Academy of Sciences to evaluate the role of diet in causing cancer, to identify dietary recommendations for the public, and to develop a series of recommendations for research and public education in the area. This study, when it appeared in 1982, generated a great deal of conventional medical and nutritional criticism (Committee on Diet, Nutrition, and Cancer, 1982; Marshall, 1986). Nevertheless, under continuing congressional pressure, the NCI endorsed the study, stepped up its research programmes in this area and proceeded to publicize its own dietary guidelines. These, as the director of the NCI Division of Cancer Prevention and Control stressed, are consistent with the RDAs set by the Food and Nutrition Board of the National Research Council. Accordingly, while these NCI guidelines acknowledge some preventive role for vitamin C (on the basis that there is epidemiological evidence that cancers of the stomach may be associated with diets low in vitamin C), they recommend that individuals should increase their intake of the vitamin through increasing their consumption of fresh fruit and vegetables. Their recommendation, they are careful to emphasize, is for *foods* rich in vitamin C, *not* tablets or vitamin supplements (Greenwald, 1986).

The politics of terminology are also evident in the title, 'chemoprevention', that the NCI has conferred on the associated studies of 'whether natural or synthetic agents – in pill or capsule form – can reduce the incidence of cancer'. The NCI currently has about two dozen such chemoprevention studies of human populations underway, including studies of vitamins C, A, E, and certain of the B vitamins (Greenwald, 1986). For the NCI, contrary to Pauling and the nutritional dissidents, vitamins taken in pill form are not to be classified as foods, and their role in cancer research and treatment is to be seen primarily as a preventive one. The NCI has thereby explicitly aligned itself with conventional nutritionists, and with the FDA and the ACS.

For all its much-publicized concern with dietary theories of cancer, the NCI allocated only 3 per cent of its total research budget in 1985 to nutrition. It still remains heavily oriented towards biological and chemotherapeutic research. It recently developed a centralized computerized data base on clinical trials, Physician's Data Query or PDQ. In 1986 PDQ listed over 1,000 active clinical trials accepting patients for new and highly experimental forms of treatment (NCI, 1986). PDQ also monitors and disseminates predominantly negative information on alternative cancer treatments to physicians and the public.

3.4 THE FOOD AND DRUG ADMINISTRATION

The role of the FDA in this area is to prevent harmful or useless methods of treating cancer from entering the marketplace. The FDA's mandate on drug regulation was legislatively set by the Kefauver-Harris

Amendments of 1962, which were stimulated by the thalidomide trag-
edy. These amendments require documented scientific evidence of a new
drug's efficacy and safety before it may be marketed in the U.S. It is
not the FDA's responsibility to generate this data. Its role is generally
limited to evaluating data supplied by developers and manufacturers
on the safety and effectiveness of new drugs. The 1962 amendments
also imposed regulatory controls on the advertising and promotion of
prescription drugs. In particular, drug firms are required to restrict
advertising and promotional claims to those approved by the FDA as
regards labelling and package inserts. The FDA is empowered to prosecute when 'false and misleading' claims are made on product labels,
and to block interstate commerce and the importation into the country
of unproven drug products.

While various critics have argued that such government regulation
is not sufficient to control the promotional and marketing activities of
the powerful drug companies (Silverman and Lee, 1974; Melville and
Johnson, 1983; Braithwaite, 1984), some economists and industry representatives have condemned the effects of the Kefauver-Harris legislation
on the development and marketing of new drugs (Grabowski, 1976;
Steward and Wibberley, 1980). Other critics have argued that the huge
costs associated with the development of a new drug, together with the
massive paperwork and the bureaucratic maze that new drug applications have to negotiate, favour the biggest and most powerful companies,
so that the effect has been to stifle the smaller and more innovative
applicants. Anti-cancer drugs, which are claimed to be among the more
expensive drugs to develop and therefore the highest priced, are dominated by a small number of the leading pharmaceutical firms (Moss,
1980; Temin, 1980).

In 1980, Americans spent an officially estimated $430 million for drugs
in cancer treatment (Rice and Hodgson, 1981). Supposedly serving only
a small market, the anti-cancer drugs are now claimed to be the fastest
growing segment of the pharmaceutical market. Their development has
been heavily subsidized by government monies allocated by Congress
and disbursed by the NCI. In certain instances, cytotoxic drugs have
been developed and marketed in conjunction with particular sections of
the cancer establishment, and this, it is suggested, has facilitated their
approval by the FDA (Moss, 1980).

Recently, as a response to the perceived severity of the AIDS crisis
(but also because of industry and consumer pressure), the FDA relaxed
its drug approval process. A new FDA ruling permits patients with
life-threatening or serious diseases to obtain 'promising new drugs'
that have not yet been approved by the FDA for marketing. Certain
investigational drugs, i.e., unapproved drugs being tested in clinical
trials under an Investigational New Drug (IND) application, may thus

be given Treatment Investigational New Drug Status (TIND), provided some evidence of the new drug's safety and activity is established. The FDA anticipates that most TIND applications will be submitted during Phase III trials, and the manufacturer must continue with these trials and actively seek final marketing approval for the drug to retain TIND status. Since the mid-1970s, some experimental drugs, including certain cancer drugs (termed 'class C' drugs), have, for experimental or compassionate reasons, been distributed to patients before final marketing approval. A major distinction between these drug classes and the new TINDs is that manufacturers may charge patients for the TIND. This has aroused the concern of some physicians and researchers. They fear that patients will not enter a randomized clinical trial, where they have only a fifty per cent chance of receiving the new drug, if they can purchase the same drug through a TIND. They have also argued that TINDs will promote poor medical treatment: patients will be treated with drugs whose efficacy and safety have not been fully evaluated (Mannisto, 1988; Young *et al.*, 1988).

One of the most potentially contentious effects of the new TINDs rule will be to legitimize the entrepreneurial promotion and marketing of experimental drugs which fall into this category (Monaco, 1987). The groundbreaking and most prominent example of such commercialization of experimental therapeutic research is Biotherapeutics, Inc., a private firm based in Tennessee and headed by an ex-NCI clinical oncologist, Dr Robert K. Oldham. Biotherapeutics, Inc. offers the experimental bio-logical response modifiers – such as the highly controversial interleukin-2 and lymphokine activated killer cells (LAK cells) – on a commercial basis to cancer patients who are not eligible or who choose not to par-ticipate in clinical trials involving these substances. LAK cell treatment is this company's best-seller, reportedly costing up to $19,400 per patient in laboratory expenses alone. During the five years of its controversial existence, the company has engaged in a running battle with the NCI, whose past director Vincent DeVita has charged Biotherapeutics, Inc. and its ex-NCI personnel with skimming the government's best ideas and selling them at a profit, rather than doing real research. In addition, the NCI finds it 'reprehensible' that these treatments are offered only to those with the cash to pay for them. In reply, Biotherapeutics, Inc. has rejected these ethical objections, claiming that they are merely a cover for the NCI's real concern: that the company threatens NCI's monopoly over the evaluation and distribution of experimental anti-cancer drugs (Boly, 1989).

The blurring of the distinctions between experimental and established treatments also blurs the lines conventionally drawn between the regu-lation of established and so-called 'unproven' or alternative cancer treat-ments, as their advocates have been quick to point out (Chowka, 1988).

Advocates of such 'unproven' treatments might be able to claim TINDs status for the treatment of their choice, arguing that their treatment is as 'proven' as some of the experimental drugs, and thus should be made available to cancer patients on the same basis. The TINDs rule offers new ammunition to those promoting the freedom of choice argument and seeking to challenge the regulatory powers of the FDA over unorthodox cancer treatments. To date, such challenges to the FDA have generally been mounted through campaigns for state laws exempting certain unorthodox cancer treatments from safety and efficacy requirements. In this way, the freedom of choice proponents have achieved some success in curtailing FDA jurisdiction over 'unproven' drugs. When the FDA, under the terms of its mandate, banned the use and sale of laetrile on the grounds of its inefficacy and toxicity, some seventeen states acted in opposition to legalize its sale, and supporters of the controversial cancer treatment were able to obtain an injunction from a federal district court judge in Oklahoma preventing the FDA from banning interstate commerce in laetrile (this decision was subsequently reversed by the Supreme Court on appeal by the FDA). A few states, in keeping with its claimed 'vitamin' status, declared laetrile not to be a drug, and therefore not to be subject to the regulatory requirements for drugs (Petersen and Markle, 1979a, b).

This is a significant distinction which has worked in favour of megavitamin therapy generally. Vitamins are not regulated as drugs, but as 'food supplements'. Since the passage of the Kefauver-Harris amendments, the FDA has attempted, without success, to label and regulate high-dose vitamin supplements as drugs. It has been supported in this struggle by the American Medical Association and orthodox nutritionists, who from the early sixties have issued regular warnings against 'nutritional quackery', and urged that the therapeutic use of vitamins be controlled by physicians and regulated by the FDA (Tatkon, 1968; Deutsch, 1977; Fried, 1984; Marshall, 1986). Their basic argument has consistently been that the distinction between vitamin preparations appropriate for food supplementation and those appropriate for therapy resides in potency. Those vitamin preparations in excess of one and a half times the officially determined RDAs should be reserved for use in therapy and regulated as over-the-counter drugs. Certain high-dose vitamins (A, D and folic acid) should be used only under close medical supervision because of their toxicity, and these should not be sold over-the-counter, but instead require a doctor's prescription. It was this definition of vitamins as drugs that the FDA subsequently attempted to employ in vitamin regulation, and that led to the congressional and court battles over the proposed legislation and to the political defeat of the FDA in 1976 (see section 2.7). As a result, the regulatory powers of the FDA were curtailed, but it is still empowered to prosecute when therapeutic claims are made on vitamin labels, or in the marketing of vitamins. However, the FDA cannot prevent the proliferation of such claims on talk shows, or in the burgeoning literature in the area, when it is not connected with the sale of specific products. By these means, it is alleged, the vitamin advocates have been able to evade regulation of their therapeutic claims (Marshall, 1986). It has been largely left to the American Cancer Society to lead the fight to protect the American public against the claims and inroads of the vitamin- and/or dietary-based 'unproven' methods of cancer management. Over the years it has played a very effective role in marginalizing and excluding unconventional cancer treatments. (Moss, 1980; Patterson, 1987)

3.5 THE AMERICAN CANCER SOCIETY

The ACS has played a key role in promoting 'cancer-consciousness' among the American public. Its politically and financially well-connected leaders, notably Mary Lasker (the philanthropist and patron of cancer research, dubbed 'the most powerful person in modern medicine'), were central to the campaign which led to the National Cancer Act and the war on cancer. Since its foundation by a group of wealthy philanthropists in 1913, the ACS has weathered a number of reorganizations and restructurings to become the nation's largest and most successful private fund-raising organization and, arguably, the single most influential member of the cancer establishment. It has, in the process, also weathered a good deal of criticism (some of it from within the medical profession) of its fund-raising publicity and 'scare tactics', of its mass screening campaigns, and of its research and funding procedures and priorities (Strickland, 1972; Chowka, 1978; Epstein, 1979; Moss, 1980; Patterson, 1987). In 1985, the ACS enlisted more than two million volunteers and raised over $200 million for the fight against cancer (ACS, 1985a).

The ACS maintains close ties with the NCI and the FDA. Its organizational structure incorporates leading cancer specialists along with businessmen (including prominent representatives of the pharmaceutical industry), bankers, and advertising men. This ensures the ACS's close affiliations with and support for orthodox cancer treatment and its research and marketing. The ACS has emerged as the most powerful opponent of cancer 'quackery', and it organizes and provides the resources for public and professional education in this area. Since 1954, the ACS has maintained a Committee on Unproven Methods of Cancer Management to monitor and investigate the claims of the efficacy of 'unproven' methods. The Committee formally liaises and shares information with the FDA, the American Society for Clinical Oncology, and the American Medical Association. Its educational programme aims at providing professionals and the public with information and criteria for recognizing and rejecting unorthodox cancer therapies which, according to the Society, are 'as much a part of the cancer problem as the disease's capacity to kill'. The possible harmful effects of unproven methods, as identified in the Society's publications in the area, are several: 'interference with prescribed treatment, both palliative and curative; financial cost to the patient and family; and diversion of important and expensive community resources' (Holland, 1982). The ideology of expertise and professionalism is constantly invoked in discrediting these 'unproven methods':

> Proponents of unproven methods of cancer management range from ignorant, uneducated, misguided persons to highly educated scientists with advanced degrees who are out of their area of competency. . . . (ACS, 1976)

The ACS further reinforces orthodoxy in cancer treatments through its promotion of state anti-quackery legislation for the prosecution of practitioners of illegal cancer therapies, and through the maintenance of files on 'unproven' methods and their promoters for use by the fifty-seven divisions of the Society and other interested professional groups. It also runs a telephone 'hot line' service for professionals and the public. ACS Statements on Unproven Methods are widely regarded as authoritative and are used as reference documents in litigation and insurance coverage decision-making (Mannisto, 1988). Once a researcher is 'quacklisted' by being placed on the ACS Unproven Methods List, it is alleged to be extremely difficult for that researcher to obtain grants, FDA approval for testing or research of the disputed treatment, or publication in orthodox medical journals (Moss, 1980; Houston, 1987).

The consistent ACS criticism of 'unproven' cancer treatments is that they are based on the unsupported testimony of their proponents or on anecdotal reports which carry no medical or scientific weight, and that such reports have not withstood the careful investigation and scrutiny of the Committee. These claims have been challenged by the medical journalist and cancer critic Ralph Moss. In his analysis of the 'unproven' methods listed in 1976 by the ACS, Moss found that no investigation at all had been undertaken of twenty-four of the fifty-eight methods listed, that seven of those evaluated had given positive results, and that in *no* case had the canonical clinical double-blind test been carried out on any of these procedures. Moss concluded that the methods had been condemned largely on *a priori* grounds (Moss, 1980).

Nevertheless, the ACS continues to urge physicians attending cancer patients to help their patients distinguish between such alternative 'unproven' methods and the 'experimental' therapies of orthodox cancer treatment. The difference, according to the ACS *Professional Education Publications*, is that the experimental therapies are the province of 'legitimate researchers', who carry out their work in a 'guarded, responsible fashion'. By contrast with the advocates of 'unproven' methods, legitimate researchers do not promote their methods publicly or profit commercially from their investigations; their work is peer reviewed and published in accepted medical forums; and above all, they use appropriate methods of testing: 'testable hypotheses, randomization of subjects, control groups, double-blind testing, statistical tests, peer review, full disclosure, replicability, and so forth' (Jarvis, 1986). Physicians treating patients whose disease is not controllable by conventional methods (and who are therefore vulnerable to exploitation by advocates of unproven cancer methods), are urged to recommend their participation in a 'properly conducted' clinical trial of a 'new and promising' treatment, as the preferred alternative to unproven treatments outside the medical system (Holland, 1982). Patients are exhorted to 'face reality and make altruistic decisions about submitting to an experimental program' (Jarvis, 1986).

The majority of unproven methods monitored by the National Unproven Methods of Cancer Management Committee of the ACS, and designated as 'active', i.e., currently in use in the U.S., are dietary and/or vitamin-based. Like the NCI, the ACS has also resolved the problem of the recent orthodox shift to recognition of a diet-cancer link by drawing the same professionally endorsed distinction – that vitamins within a balanced diet may confer protection against some forms of cancer but that vitamins in megadoses do not cure cancer, that indeed 'no diet cures cancer' (ACS, 1985b 1987; Jarvis, 1986). This claim has the full support of the orthodox nutrition scientists.

3.6 ORTHODOX NUTRITIONISTS, 'QUACKBUSTERS', AND THE FIGHT AGAINST 'NUTRITIONAL QUACKERY'

The most vigorous and outspoken opposition to the megavitamin therapists has come from those orthodox nutritionists who have felt their expertise directly confronted and threatened by the growth of orthomolecular medicine, which they satirize as 'paramolecular' or 'pseudomolecular' medicine (Jukes, 1986). Historically, nutrition has been a generally neglected area of medicine and medical education in the U.S., and dietitians and nutritionists have had to struggle for professional recognition and status. Their professionalization strategies have centred around their claims to a rigorously scientific disciplinary basis, and to the forging of close links with the established professional and regulatory bodies. With the strong backing of the American Medical Association, the FDA, and the professional association of clinical nutritionists, they have spearheaded the campaign against 'nutritional quackery' and 'food faddism' which they construe as the deception and financial exploitation of a gullible and misinformed public.

Nutritionists fought hard for the tighter regulation and control of vitamins, and they reacted with great bitterness to their 1976 defeat by the health food consortium and the nutritional dissidents (Harper, 1977; Shapo, 1979; Deutsch, 1977; Marshall, 1983; Fried, 1984). This political 'defeat of reason' ('Shades of the church fathers and Galileo!') and the ever-growing and 'scientifically irrational' consumption of vitamin supplements (Harper, 1977), have provoked the orthodox nutritionists to a more intensive educational campaign against nutritional quackery. The activists among them have founded a number of consumer protection organizations, such as the National Council Against Health Fraud, the Nutrition Information Center, and the Lehigh Valley Committee Against Health Fraud. These organizations produce publications, such as *Nutrition Forum*, devoted to the dissemination of 'factual' nutritional information and to the monitoring and exposure of 'health fraud'. Prominent 'quackbusters' such as Dr Stephen Barrett, Professor Victor Herbert, and Professor Thomas Jukes, all promote the Recommended Dietary Allowances as the working standard of optimal nutrition, and structure their campaigns around the assertion that healthy people eating a well-balanced diet do not need vitamin supplements. Against the benefits asserted by the megavitamin enthusiasts, they stress the risks and the need for controlled clinical trials, and they detail countervailing anecdotal reports of the deleterious effects of megavitamin consumption (Jukes, 1975; Barrett and Knight, 1976; Herbert, 1978, 1980a, 1980b; Herbert and Barrett, 1981; Yetiv, 1986).

Pauling, the most prominent 'defector from the ranks of reason', is their particular target and arouses their greatest hostility, primarily because he and his claims have proved much more recalcitrant to orthodox criticism and dismissal than the easier (though no less enduring) targets of the 'faddists', 'zealots' and 'food cultists'. The publication of Pauling's *Vitamin C and the Common Cold* sparked off an immediate furore. Since the early seventies, Pauling and a number of leading nutrition scientists have been locked in conflict over Pauling's common cold claims and their contradictory interpretations of the many controlled clinical trials (at least twenty published experiments) that have now been carried out on some thousands of volunteers.

The interpretations, counterinterpretations, and reinterpretations of these trials are a fascinating study in their own right, and in many ways they mirror the conflict over the interpretation of the vitamin C and cancer clinical trials. In a number of instances, successive randomized controlled trials carried out by the same group of experimenters have given bafflingly contradictory results. In some cases, where Pauling claimed benefits in shorter duration and lesser severity of colds, his critics alleged placebo effect and suggested that many of the volunteers became 'unblinded' by correctly guessing which pill they were getting. In other cases, Pauling's critics (and some of the experimenters themselves) have explained away apparently positive results as being more a function of the way in which the data were analyzed than of the vitamin itself. Certain trials with negative or marginal outcomes have been criticized by Pauling on the grounds that the experimenters misinterpreted or minimalized their own data. In other cases he has argued that the doses of vitamin C were too low for measurable benefits to be obtained. Pauling also alleges selective reporting and suppression of those trial results supporting vitamin C supplementation by journals such as the *Journal of the American Medical Association* (Pauling, 1970a, 1976, 1986; Doyle, 1983; Fried, 1984; Marshall, 1986; Carpenter, 1986; Levine, 1986; Truswell, 1986).

As Pauling has persisted with his claims and confronted and resisted the counterclaims of the professional nutritionists, and as vitamin C sales have continued to soar, his opponents have reacted with greater acrimony and frustration. Pauling's common cold claims have been reviewed and described by various prominent nutritional scientists and physicians as 'ridiculous', 'missionary', an 'embarrassment for an older scientist', a 'bummer', 'a nutritional fairy tale', and 'the most tragic example of [scientific] self-deception'. It has been suggested that he and his publishers benefit financially from the manufacture and sale of vitamin C, and that Pauling is a tool of the multibillion dollar vitamin and health food industry (Fried, 1984; Herbert and Barrett, 1981; Pauling, 1986). Even Eric Fried, the medical journalist who writes in support of the orthodox nutritional party line and against nutritional quackery, has criticized what he sees as the over-reaction of the profession. He interprets this over-reaction as the outrage of leading nutritionists over Pauling's 'excursions into the realm they consider their exclusive satrapy'. Fried argues that in the last few years, as the results of the more recent 'well-run' clinical trials have become available, 'the tide has shifted somewhat – not greatly, but perceptibly – in Pauling's favor' (Fried, 1984). However, it is notable, even from Fried's account, that where the orthodox have conceded some marginal benefits from extra vitamin C intake in the form of a slight reduction in the severity of colds, they have argued that these benefits are not outweighed by the potential risks. Although these latter (such as a postulated increased risk of kidney stones) have not so far been experimentally demonstrated and are as contentious as the alleged benefits of vitamin C, the majority of nutritionists are agreed, and have continued to warn the public, that a continued intake of vitamin C at megadose levels is neither desirable nor safe (Fried, 1984; Marshall, 1986; Carpenter, 1986; Yetiv, 1986).

Meanwhile, the anti-quackery crusaders amongst them have extended the battle lines into the vitamin C and cancer debate where they have strongly defended the orthodox oncologists and the results of the Mayo Clinic trials, and alleged the possible tumour-enhancing effects of vitamin C megadose (Herbert, 1978, 1980a, 1980b, 1986; Jukes, 1986; Marshall, 1986; Yetiv, 1986). The most extreme (and most colourful) of these attacks have come from the above mentioned Victor Herbert, who is board-certified in both internal medicine and nutrition, and is Chief of the Hematology and Nutrition Laboratory, Bronx VA Medical Centre, and Professor of Medicine at State University of New York Downstate Medical Centre. Herbert is also Past President of the American Society for Clinical Nutrition and is a member of the Food and Nutrition Board of the National Academy of Sciences and of its Recommended Dietary Allowances Committee. He is a well-known public defender and promoter of the RDAs that he helps to determine. In a fairly typical example of his punchy style of writing published in the *Resident and Staff Physician*, Herbert reduced the Vale of Leven Hospital to a 'nursing home in the Scottish Highlands' and airily dismissed Cameron's trial results as 'placebo effect' (Herbert, 1978). He subsequently claimed in a letter in the *American Journal of Clinical Nutrition* to have visited the Vale of Leven Hospital (while Cameron was on vacation) and to have been informed by the senior nurse on Cameron's ward that Cameron's patients usually discontinued their vitamin C because it made them nauseated or gave them diarrhoea. On this occasion, Herbert denigrated Cameron's trial results as 'typical anecdotal and testimonial citation, useful in advertising but scientifically worthless' (Herbert, 1980b). In yet another attack on 'The Vitamin Craze' in the *Archives of Internal Medicine*, Herbert invoked Arthur Robinson's allegations over the mouse experiments at the Linus Pauling Institute in discrediting Pauling's and Cameron's claims (Herbert, 1980a).

3.7   *THE NEW ENGLAND JOURNAL OF MEDICINE* AND THE PROFESSION OF MEDICINE

The debate between the 'believers' and the 'non-believers' in the pages of the *New England Journal of Medicine* has been a little more restrained in tone, but no less acrimonious. The *Journal* published both negative Mayo Clinic trials of vitamin C, but has consistently rejected papers by Pauling and Cameron. The *Journal*'s editor, Arnold S. Relman, was publicly identified by Pauling as among his leading opponents when, in the aftermath of the second Mayo Clinic trial of vitamin C, Pauling threatened to bring suit against Relman and the *Journal* on the grounds that he had published and therefore condoned this 'fraudulent' paper (see Chapter 6).

Relman's professional affiliations are fairly clear cut. The *New England Journal of Medicine* is the journal of the Massachusetts Medical Society, and Relman's own background is in medical practice and education in Massachusetts. He has edited the *Journal* since 1978, and holds the concurrent positions of senior physician at Brigham and Women's Hospital and professor of medicine at Harvard Medical School. The *New England Journal of Medicine* is the oldest and most prestigious and powerful of the medical journals in the United States. Its editorial policy is to provide an 'open forum' for the discussion of issues that are important to medicine and health. The media and the stock market look to it as the barometer of medical information and opinion in the United States. Its economic and social significance is immense. Its publication of studies on promising new therapies has sparked runs on the stock market and influenced funding, research, and treatment decisions (Chase, 1986; Powledge, 1988). In an effort to curtail the prepublication leakage of influential and potentially profitable information to the media and business sources, the *Journal* has imposed the so-called 'Inglefinger rule' promulgated by Relman's predecessor, which bars contributors from publicizing their articles before publication in the *Journal*. This has led to charges of monopoly of information and power-mongering and to conflict between the *Journal* and the media (Powledge, 1988).

As the moderator of the 'open forum' he espouses, Relman's own editorial powers are considerable. He makes the choices about which voices will be heard. It is a power he claims to exercise scrupulously and responsibly, keeping the *Journal* 'always open to all points of view'. But, as Relman also represents the situation, the *Journal's* primary responsibility is to the profession of medicine, and he explicitly identifies the profession's interests with the public interest: 'We are serving the medical profession, and through them we serve the public' (Powledge, 1988).

In his capacity as editor, Relman has sought to preserve the traditional professional values and, above all, professional autonomy. He has been outspoken in his criticism of the intrusion of industry, government, and the courts into the practice of medicine, and in his condemnation of the 'new medical-industrial complex' and the commercialization of health care. As Relman sees it, the medical profession is its own best regulator: 'The best kind of regulation of the health-care marketplace should therefore come from the informed judgments of physicians working in the interests of their patients' (Relman, 1980).

Relman's advocacy of professional self-regulation extends to a detailed defence of professional, as opposed to increased state bureaucratic, control of the evaluation and implementation of medical technologies and therapies. As a solution to the proliferation of untested or inadequately tested diagnostic and therapeutic procedures, he has proposed a national programme of health care evaluation to be funded by the private health insurance companies, which would put the responsibility for controlling costs and maintaining quality care in the hands of the medical profession. In the face of the scepticism of critics of current medical practices, Relman has affirmed his belief in professional integrity as the best moderator of 'the other perverse economic incentives that now influence the use of medical technology'. Doctors, he argues, will respond to clear, new information about technology by modifying their behaviour in 'whatever ways that are appropriately responsive to the facts. They always have done so in the past and I see no reason to doubt that they will continue to do so – provided that the new information is convincing and commands the support of the experts' (Relman, 1983, 1982b, 1988).

Relman, and the *Journal* he edits, therefore endorse what I have termed the standard view, whereby medicine represents itself as a group of responsible professionals trained in scientific, rational, neutral processes, and self-regulated by an ethical code. The definition of what is medically rational conforms with the accepted knowledge of the profession, and with its professionally-controlled evaluative procedures. The assumption, endorsed by Relman, is that all medical procedures, if they are to be employed in a way that is both efficacious and cost-effective (i.e., rationally), must be exposed to the 'merciless judgment of the objective data derived from controlled studies'. However, as Relman himself concedes, 'at least 10 or 20 per cent' of the diagnostic and therapeutic procedures carried out in the practice of medicine are either 'worthless or unnecessary or are being inappropriately and excessively used. There are probably an equal percentage, another 10 or 20 per cent, that are of questionable or borderline value' (Relman, 1983).

These comments suggest that Relman and the profession he serves have some difficulty in balancing their claim to a professionally-based rational and responsible medicine against such seeming irrationalities in the professional practice of medicine. But they have had no difficulty in dismissing most alternative therapies on the grounds of their 'irrationality', i.e., their failure to mesh with conventional medical theories and practices (ineffective or questionable as many of these are conceded to be), or to have been evaluated by the canonical controlled clinical trial (to which, it is also conceded, much of conventional medical practice has never been subjected).

As holistic medicine and health care have grown in popularity, many orthodox western physicians have begun to incorporate certain holistic approaches and procedures into their conventional practices, and this partial *rapprochement* has received a degree of professional acknowledgement (Relman, 1979a; Glymour and Stalker, 1983; Reilly, 1983; Smith, 1983; Cassileth *et al.*, 1984; Cassileth and Brown, 1988; Fink, 1988; Fulder, 1989). But, in the United States at least, this professional recognition is confined to reclaiming those aspects of holism which are affirmed to be legitimate to traditional health care, and does not generally extend to alternative therapies judged by orthodoxy to be 'irrational' and 'unscientific'. This professional strategy has been faithfully reflected in the editorial policy of the *New England Journal of Medicine*.

In keeping with its 'open forum' policy, the *Journal* has given a limited space to holistic medicine and monitored developments in the area with a cautious and sceptical interest. It broke new ground towards the close of 1976 when it published the highly controversial account by Norman Cousins, the editor of the *Saturday Review*, of how (after conventional medicine had failed to alleviate his ankylosing spondylitis) Cousins had discharged himself from hospital and cured himself with his own self-help regime of laughter, faith, and very high doses of vitamin C. Although Cousins' article was greeted with a good deal of scepticism about the claimed diagnosis, treatment, and cure, his arguments about the limitations and depersonalization of modern medical care and the need for a more self-reliant and broader holistic approach to health were generally well-received by his professional audience (Cousins, 1977). Three years later, the *Journal* ran an article by a young psychologist who underwent surgery and chemotherapy for cancer of the testis, and who supplemented this conventional treatment with a holistic regimen. The author argued that 'effective cancer therapy must treat the healthy portion of the patient's body and psyche as well as . . . the diseased cells', and urged programmes that 'offer patients an opportunity to participate actively in their own recovery, to take responsibility for their own health care, to regain a sense of control over their bodies' (Relman, 1979a).

'Who can quarrel with these insights?' asked Relman rhetorically in a supporting editorial, where he also noted the recent formation of the American Holistic Medical Association, and the sponsorship by the American Medical Association of a symposium on 'Holistic Medicine and Health Care' at its annual meeting. Every experienced physician, Relman asserted, knew that he must deal with patients and not just their diseases, that 'physical, psychologic and social factors are inextricably mixed'. And skilled physicians always tried, as far as possible, to involve their patients in their own treatment. 'If these are the lessons of holistic medicine, they should be welcomed as old friends.' What was less welcome, Relman made clear, was the 'irrational side of the holistic movement, with its mystical cults and all the paraphernalia of

sectarianism'. Relman gave his editorial approval to some 'notable exceptions' such as osteopathy, biofeedback and certain 'recognized kinds of
psychotherapy', but concluded that the 'valuable message' of holism was
'distorted' by the 'palpable quackery and silliness of much that calls itself
holistic' (Relman, 1979a).

Relman was challenged by holist supporters on the grounds that
he had engaged in 'rhetorical vilification' and 'condemnation without
credible scientific evidence' (Goldenring, 1979; Siegelbaum, 1979). Critics pointed out that 'curiously' what Relman designated rational was
'that which is most consistent with the paradigm of scientific medicine' (Berliner and Salmon, 1979b). From the other side, he was rapped
over the knuckles by an FDA spokesman for not emphasizing that the
remedies of holism, such as laetrile, were not only ineffective but also
dangerous (Nightingale, 1979). In response, Relman redeployed the same
professional stratagem of reclaiming holistic 'humanism' for orthodox
scientific medicine, while invoking the need for 'rigorous' orthodox
scientific evaluation of holistic therapeutic claims:

> The most important question is not whether orthodox medicine can
> be open-minded enough to consider 'alternative' approaches, but
> whether it will continue to live by the rules of scientific evidence
> that have brought us out of the age of medical superstition into the
> modern era. . . . In our zeal to put humanism back into the practice
> ˙of medicine we must not abandon science or forget the public's need
> for protection against quackery. (Relman, 1979b)

This is, in essence, the orthodox case for the subjection of alternative
therapeutic claims to orthodox methodology and to orthodox evaluators
who are the only assessors acceptable to the orthodox. It is espoused
by all participants in the controversy among those I have called the
vitamin C 'non-believers'.

Since 1979, the *New England Journal of Medicine* has been the chosen
professional forum for 'closing the books' on both laetrile and vitamin C,
the two most popular (and, inevitably, the most contentious) alternative
treatments for cancer (Moertel *et al.*, 1982; Relman, 1982a; Creagan *et al.*,
1979; Moertel *et al.*, 1985; Wittes, 1985).

Part II
Reconstructing the Vitamin C and Cancer Controversy

Which brings us right back to the shelves of the corner drugstore and the local health food shop and the predictable reactions of disbelief and scorn which will certainly come from my incredulous medical profession.

Cameron's first letter to Pauling, 30 November, 1971

There will no doubt be much scepticism about your conclusions, no matter how the observations are presented. If, however, you are able to make a comparison of your ascorbic-acid subjects and a matched set of control subjects . . . the evidence might be given greater consideration by the readers.

Pauling to Cameron, 5 February, 1973

Overshadowing such minor quibbling is the major obligation that both we and Dr Pauling must assume to cancer patients and the general public. On the basis of claims derived from speculation and non-randomized studies endorsed by the Pauling name, megadoses of vitamin C are being used by thousands of patients with cancer, and such treatment has been embraced by the metabolic therapy cults.

Moertel and Creagan, *New England Journal of Medicine* (Moertel and Creagan, 1980)

The Mayo Clinic doctors have refused to discuss this matter with me. I conclude that they are not scientists, devoted to the search for the truth. I surmise that they are so ashamed of themselves that they would prefer that the matter be forgotten. The Mayo Clinic used to have a great reputation. This episode indicates to me that it is no longer deserved.

Pauling, *How to Live Longer and Feel Better* (Pauling, 1986)

The Mayo Study is solid and we have no apologies whatsoever.

The Mayo Clinic Responds (The Mayo Clinic, 1985)

4 The Cameron–Pauling Hypothesis and the Vale of Leven Trials

It is my opinion that the attack you are making on the cancer problem is the most important and promising of all those I have heard about. It is essential that a thorough test be made of the value of ascorbic acid.

Linus Pauling's second letter to Ewan Cameron,
11 January 1972.

I am convinced that ascorbate produces a favourable shift in the host/tumour relationship. I think that we are achieving tumour retardation and prolongation of life in many patients even although I fully appreciate that these factors are notoriously difficult to measure. What is perhaps more important than mere prolongation of life, is that by symptomatic relief, we are improving the quality of life.

Ewan Cameron to Linus Pauling, 25 June 1972.

'Is Vitamin C an Effective Cancer Treatment?'
New Scientist, 1 July 1976 (Hanlon, 1976)

In his 1970 book, *Vitamin C and the Common Cold*, Pauling had suggested that ascorbate might be of value in the prevention and treatment of cancer. At this stage the all-out war upon cancer was being mobilized. To the accompaniment of a great deal of publicity, the National Cancer Act was passed at the end of the following year. In his well-timed address of November 5, 1971, at the opening of the Ben May Laboratory for Cancer Research at the University of Chicago, Pauling pushed for research into the link between nutrition and cancer. He outlined the ways in which he thought vitamin C might act as preventative and treatment for cancer. Apart from its anti-viral properties which should have linked it into mainstream cancer research, Pauling pointed out that vitamin C was essential for the synthesis of collagen fibrils in the ground substance (the jelly-like material in which all body cells are embedded), and that it might function in other ways to strengthen the ground substance and to prevent the infiltration of tissues by cancerous growths. He went on to argue that if, as he expected, proper nutrition were to decrease the incidence of cancer by ten per cent then this would be a most significant contribution to the attack on cancer. He urged scientists and medical men to turn their attention to this neglected area. The *New York Times* picked up Pauling's speech, and it was this indication that they might be thinking along 'broadly similar lines' which prompted Ewan Cameron to initiate the correspondence with Pauling which was to lead to and sustain their long-term collaboration.

On 30 November 1971, Cameron wrote a seven-page letter to Pauling in which he set out his theoretical views on the cancer process (which he had detailed in his 1966 book, *Hyaluronidase and Cancer*), explained his more recent views on the possible role of ascorbate in relation to these earlier ideas, and indicated the 'very encouraging' results of his administration of ascorbate to some of the untreatable cancer patients in his care at the Vale of Leven Hospital.

4.1 THE CAMERON–PAULING HYPOTHESIS: VITAMIN C AND PHI

In his book (a copy of which he dispatched to Pauling), Cameron had argued that the attempt to control cancer should be directed at control-ling its invasiveness rather than destroying the cancer cells. He sum-marized earlier work which supported the hypothesis that cancer cells appeared to modify the properties of the ground substance through the release of spreading factors or enzymes, specifically hyaluronidase, and that this allowed the malignant cells to proliferate and penetrate the ground substance and to invade surrounding tissues. In a state of health, the ground substance is relatively impermeable and suppresses such proliferation and penetration. Cameron put forward the hypothesis that in normal tissues the process of cell invasion was kept in check by the viscous environment, excess hyaluronidase activity being controlled by the existence in the tissues and blood of the 'physiological hyaluronidase inhibitor' (PHI). Cells, he argued, in becoming malignant, somehow acquire and are able to pass on to their descendants the ability to continu-ously produce hyaluronidase. This 'excess' hyaluronidase overwhelms the counterbalancing PHI, and so cancer cells are able to multiply and spread into the surrounding tissue.

Cameron had tried to show how this concept could explain all the puzzling features of cancer, from its inception right through the behav-iour patterns of growing tumours, to their response to various forms of treatment. But, above all, he had argued that the approach most likely to succeed in the treatment of cancer was by the employment of PHI, the naturally occurring substance which kept hyaluronidase production in check and which would directly neutralize the malignant capacity of the cancer cell. As he put it to Pauling, Cameron's hope in writing the book was that some cancer research institute or large drug company would take up his idea and isolate and define the PHI substance and prepare it in a form suitable for clinical use:

> I have waited five years for this to happen. And now I believe that part of the answer has been lying around the shelves of every drugstore in the country for years.

In the wake of the publication of *Hyaluronidase and Cancer* Cameron had begun to receive a long series of letters from a Douglas Rotman of Connecticut. Rotman, as far as Cameron could make out, was an amateur medical researcher, an enthusiast who began to bombard Cameron with long lists of substances which had been reported as interfering with the hyaluronidase system and to have some retarding effect on the growth of malignant tumours. It was Rotman who drew Cameron's attention to ascorbic acid in this context, and who directed him to the papers by McCormick, a Canadian physician who in the fifties and early sixties had postulated a relationship between vitamin C deficiency and cancer (McCormick, 1959). McCormick had also, rather confusingly it seemed to Cameron on first reading, argued the value of high dose vitamin C therapy in the treatment of many infectious diseases. However it did seem logical to Cameron (on the basis of his own hyaluronidase hypothesis) that there was a possible parallel between the tissue disintegration characteristic of scurvy and the erosion of ground substance in cancer, as McCormick argued, and that cancer patients might be helped by the administration of megadoses of vitamin C.

While he awaited more research on PHI, Cameron had been treating those patients beyond the hope of any conventional therapy with a 'hormone cocktail' which he hoped, on various grounds, would have the effect of rendering the host ground substance more resistant to malignant proliferation and thus indirectly retarding tumour growth. There had been, so far as he could detect, no measurable response to this experimental therapy. He now added high doses of vitamin C to his 'cocktail'. This time, he wrote to Pauling,

> the early results have been very encouraging indeed. . . . These first impressions are so striking that I have omitted the hormonal regime altogether and am trying to devise a suitable therapeutic programme using ascorbic acid alone. . . . The early clinical response is so impres-

sive that I cannot imagine the effect is being produced indirectly by modification of the ground substance. (Cameron to Pauling, 30 November 1971)

On the basis of the chemical similarity between ascorbic acid and glucuronic acid (a component of PHI), he and Rotman had arrived at the tentative conclusion that PHI might actually include ascorbic acid molecules in its structure:

We wonder whether PHI is a relatively simple long-chain polymer composed of alternating units of N-acetyl glucosamine (or N-acetyl galactosamine) and ascorbic acid with a configuration as follows:-

$$\sim \text{Ascorbate} \left[\text{N-Acetyl Hexosamine} \sim \text{Ascorbate} \text{N-acetyl Hexosamine} \right]^{n} \sim$$

My knowledge of organic chemistry is so rudimentary that I do not even know whether such a chemical configuration is possible, but if it is, and this is PHI, then the physiological and therapeutic implications are enormous. By its very structure (basic similarity but subtle difference from the natural substrate) we have produced a very powerful inhibitor of hyaluronidase. Suddenly all the missing pieces of the jig-saw fall into place.

This meant, as Cameron interpreted it, that given sufficient ascorbic acid, the body would synthesize its own PHI. This would not only explain why ascorbic acid was so effective in curing scurvy, stabilizing the intercellular environment and improving wound healing, but also suggested that it would act as an almost specific broad-spectrum antibiotic against all the pathogenic organisms which employ hyaluronidase to establish and spread themselves throughout the tissues. Above all, it would provide a 'rational and logical cure for cancer':

Which brings us right back to the shelves of the corner drugstore or the local health food shop and the predictable reactions of disbelief and scorn which will certainly come from my incredulous medical profession.

As Cameron saw it, it was this predictable professional reaction which represented the major obstacle to the presentation and acceptance of his views. He intended to submit his hypothesis to the *Lancet*, but because of its controversial nature, he doubted that it would be accepted. Even if it were, it would be many months before it appeared in print, and he felt the matter to be too urgent for such a delay. He asked Pauling's help in establishing the theory on a 'sound scientific basis' and in publicizing it as widely as possible:

> I have no doubt in my own mind that the basic facts are correct. I am presumptious enough to believe that between us, and not forgetting Mr. Rotman's contribution, we could soon cure cancer. (Cameron to Pauling, 30 November 1971)

Pauling (then Professor of Chemistry at Stanford University) responded quickly, expressing his interest and offering considerable encouragement for Cameron's theoretical views. He provided some support from his own views on enzyme activity and the action of inhibitors for the Cameron/Rotman hypothesis of the role of ascorbate in the synthesis of PHI. But the aspect of Cameron's work which clearly interested him the most (and he underlined these portions of Cameron's letter), was Cameron's therapeutic administration of vitamin C to his cancer patients and 'the striking clinical response' which he claimed to have observed. At that stage, as he explained to Cameron, Pauling and his principal associate Dr Arthur B. Robinson were working with a team of postdoctoral fellows and technical assistants on the development of improved techniques for analysis of body fluids. They were carrying out vitamin loading tests on patients with Hodgkin's disease and other forms of cancer, notably bladder cancer, and Pauling was attempting to persuade the clinicians at the Stanford School of Medicine to undertake a trial of ascorbic acid in the control of cancer. Cameron's observations, he wrote, would be of much value in helping to convince the clinicians, and he requested more detailed information on the clinical response of Cameron's patients.

As for Cameron's publication worries, Pauling referred to his own difficulties in getting his papers on vitamin C and the common cold published and how he had resolved them. After having had two papers rejected by the editor of *Science*, Pauling had rewritten them and published them in the *Proceedings of the National Academy of Sciences (PNAS)*. As an Academy member he had the right to publish a certain number of papers in the *Proceedings*, and to submit papers by other authors for publication. Publication, he assured Cameron, was reasonably rapid – about two months (Pauling to Cameron, 14 December 1971).

Cameron had been working hard on the hypothesis over the Christmas and New Year period, and he responded to this encouragement with a seventeen page letter plus three hefty attachments. His major and most pressing concern remained 'the publication problem', i.e., 'how to disseminate and publicise this idea as soon and as widely as possible but without attracting all the wrong kind of attention too early'. Attachments 1 and 2 comprised copies of a letter to the *Lancet* (co-authored by Cameron and Rotman) which contained a preliminary notice of the ascorbate/PHI hypothesis, and a detailed presentation of the hypothesis by Cameron which he had also submitted to the *Lancet* just prior to receiving Pauling's letter. Cameron now expressed some regret that he had not taken up Pauling's offer of supporting its publication in the *PNAS*. He was concerned that his manuscript might be retained in the *Lancet* offices for many months and then rejected, and he again stressed the urgency for speedy publication of such a promising theoretical contribution to the understanding of the control of cancer.

Cameron was now obviously intent on relating his work more closely to Pauling's. His hypothesis manuscript included Pauling's term 'orthomolecular' in its title and concluded with a tribute to Pauling's 'brilliant concept', visualizing the control of cancer by vitamin C as a 'supreme triumph' for orthomolecular medicine. In his letter, he explained to Pauling in some detail why he regarded his own approach to the cancer problem as having all along fallen within the orthomolecular framework, and why he now accepted the term 'orthomolecular' as being more expressive of this general concept of the employment of intrinsic physiological mechanisms in the control of abnormal disease patterns. The manuscript itself summarized Cameron's hyaluronidase hypothesis, drew together the evidence for the role of ascorbate in the synthesis of PHI, and argued the case for the therapeutic use of ascorbate in the treatment of a wide range of diseases, including bacterial and viral infections, inflammatory and auto-immune diseases, and, of course, cancer.

Attachment 3 contained the information that Pauling had been awaiting – Cameron's preliminary report on his early clinical experiences with the use of high dose ascorbic acid in terminal cancer. By this stage, Cameron had been treating patients with ascorbate for only seven weeks, ie., since about mid-November 1971. In the earlier patients treated, he had administered 5 grams of ascorbic acid per day by intravenous infusion for a period of from 5 to 7 days, followed by oral medication of around 2 grams per day. Seeing that this was well tolerated, for more recent patients he had increased the daily intravenous infusion to 10 grams for variable periods of a week or more, followed by a daily oral dose of 8 grams. In his manuscript to the *Lancet*, and here again in his introduction, Cameron had set out the expected clinical response to ascorbate treatment on the basis of his theoretical understanding of the cancer process and the role of ascorbate in the synthesis of PHI. As it was this issue of the expected clinical response to ascorbate which was to become so contentious in the course of the controversy, it is important to understand exactly what Cameron initially expected of ascorbate therapy.

As he repeatedly emphasized, he did not expect ascorbate treatment to cure cancer, but rather to control it. He thought that ascorbic acid in adequate doses might prove to be the ideal 'cytostatic' agent, i.e., that it would act to 'disarm' rather than kill cancer cells, by preventing their proliferation. It would be important, Cameron stressed, for any clinician who proposed to try this form of therapy to realize that he was employing a 'carcinostatic' (cancer-stabilizing) and not a 'carcinocidal' drug (i.e., cancer-killing, like the standard cytotoxic drugs employed in the treatment of cancer). Even if the treatment were successful, pre-treatment malignant masses would still remain palpable and visible on x-ray. But it would be hoped that all further malignant invasive growth would be arrested – that malignant ulcers would heal, that pre-existing tumours no matter how widely disseminated would become 'benign' and encapsulated, and that pain, haemorrhage, weight loss, and all the other secondary distressing effects of cancer would be brought under control. In a 'very very few' patients with very rapidly growing tumours proliferating at the very limits of available blood and nutrient supply, the administration of ascorbic acid might be sufficient to actually kill the cancer cells, to induce tumour necrosis and bring about dramatic regressions. 'Although it must be appreciated', reiterated Cameron, 'that such a dramatic therapeutic response could only be expected as a very fortuitous occurrence in a very few patients.'

In this first clinical report to Pauling, Cameron gave details on eleven cases and offered the following tentative conclusions: that the administration of high-dose ascorbic acid was well tolerated and harmless in seriously ill cancer patients, and that it had alleviated some of the more distressing symptoms in these terminal patients. In one patient he thought there was evidence of some tumour regression on palpation. Overall, there was just enough evidence of a possible therapeutic effect in many of the patients to regard the procedure as at least promising, although he emphasized that these results must be regarded as quite inconclusive at this stage. The major ground for a trial of ascorbate treatment remained the theoretical argument he had evolved and the evidence he had brought to its support.

In his letter, Cameron expressed the hope that clinical trials of ascorbate treatment in cancer would be undertaken at Stanford and that his work would help Pauling's advocacy. In return, Cameron hoped to be able to invoke Pauling's name in persuading his clinical colleagues at the Vale of Leven Hospital to try this form of treatment and to set aside a special unit within the hospital for its study. Nevertheless, for all the promise of ascorbate, Cameron's own hopes remained pinned on PHI as the ultimate cure for cancer. He urged on Pauling the need to define the pharmacology of PHI, discover its structure and establish its method of manufacture, routes of administration and dose schedule:

I think ascorbic acid is going to be a very valuable drug in controlling cancer. I still believe that PHI will be the cure.

With the greatest possible respect for all your past magnificent work, I sincerely believe that if you could give the clinicians of the world pure PHI, it would be your greatest contribution to the health and happiness of mankind. (Cameron to Pauling, 5 January 1972)

Pauling in response made it very clear that he was less interested in PHI than in the role of ascorbate in cancer treatment. Apart from Cameron's encouraging clinical observations, what particularly interested him was Cameron's intention of pursuing these on a larger and more systematic scale at the Vale of Leven Hospital, and he heavily scored the margin against this section of Cameron's letter. He wrote Cameron of his own lack of success in convincing the Stanford clinicians to experiment with ascorbate treatment, endorsed Cameron's efforts to set up a trial at the Vale of Leven Hospital, and indicated his intention of visiting Cameron within the next few months in order to make their collaboration more effective. 'It is my opinion', he wrote,

that the attack you are making on the cancer problem is the most important and promising of all those that I have heard about. It is essential that a thorough test be made of the value of ascorbic acid. (Pauling to Cameron, 11 January 1972)

He urged Cameron to employ even larger doses, citing published evidence that no severe side effects had resulted from the use of amounts as large as 50 grams per day. To underscore his emphasis on the need for a clinical trial, Pauling wrote Cameron again the following day to pass on his son Peter's suggestion that Cameron should apply to the British Medical Research Council for financial support for his work on vitamin C, and offered to write a statement supporting his application.

Meanwhile, Cameron had undergone a depressing period of 'unmitigated clinical disaster', as he hurriedly wrote Pauling. No fewer that three of the patients in his small series who had seemed to be doing so well, had died suddenly of advanced cancer. They included the case of ovarian cancer which Cameron had thought to be in regression, and the death of this patient was Cameron's major clinical disappointment. He sent clinical details and autopsy reports of all three patients for inclusion in his earlier report. For all his disappointment Cameron managed to salvage some hope from the autopsy findings. The patient with ovarian cancer had died from massive abdominal adhesions and consequent intestinal obstruction, but autopsy revealed no such abdominal masses as had been described at laparatomy some months previously and which had been palpable when she was admitted to Cameron's care. Another patient who had received only 20 grams of ascorbic acid in 48 hours had died of a very rapidly growing, widely disseminated testicular cancer, and his autopsy report suggested to Cameron that his short burst of ascorbate therapy had induced widespread tumour necrosis. Had his tumour been less advanced and more localized at the onset of treatment, this patient's response might have fallen within the predicted category of the very few who experienced a dramatic therapeutic response to ascorbate treatment. Still, Cameron sounded a note of caution to Pauling:

> It would seem that until we have all the basic guide-lines worked out as regards dosage and route of administration, I am perhaps being far too ambitious in trying to treat the most difficult cell-proliferative disease of all, cancer, and to be in a position only to try this form of treatment in the most difficult terminal stages of the disease. It would seem that even if this form of treatment is successful there will be many major clinical problems to be worked out with regard to possible complications of this form of therapy. (11 January 1972)

Yet, in spite of this clinical setback, Cameron still felt strongly that the theoretical argument in favour of ascorbate treatment justified his persistence with its therapeutic evaluation. When shortly afterwards the *Lancet* accepted the Cameron-Rotman letter but 'flatly rejected' Cameron's manuscript, he wrote to Pauling of his 'bitter disappointment' at their lack of courage and imagination. Any reservations he may have had about the safety of ascorbate therapy for cancer patients were overridden by his indignation at the stated reason for rejection – that he had not presented any evidence for or reasoning behind the idea of ascorbic acid belonging in the PHI molecule. 'I would have thought', commented Cameron,

> that the reasoning was fairly strong and if we had the evidence I would not have submitted the paper to their hypothesis section. . . . With all humility I think that it is the paper that clinicians all over the world have been waiting for; a theoretical basis for trying an extremely safe substance in the treatment of an incurable disease, and many other diseases besides. (24 January 1972)

He asked Pauling's help in obtaining publication in the United States, but doubted whether in its present form ('being written by a non-scientist in non-scientific terms') his paper was suitable for publication in the *PNAS*. Could Pauling suggest how it might be modified? Better still, would Pauling revise the manuscript and come in as co-author? Again Cameron stressed the closeness of their views. 'It would be a very great honour for me and I would not even need to see the modifications because I know that we are both thinking along exactly similar lines'.

Spurred on by Pauling's mention of a prospective visit to Vale of Leven, Cameron was able to assure Pauling that he and most of his colleagues were anxious to participate in a clinical trial at the Vale of Leven Hospital. It was at this crucial stage that Cameron argued against the necessity for a full-scale double-blind trial (which he conceded was the 'only real way to obtain scientific information' and which would be perfectly ethical in the situation where the value of ascorbate to cancer patients was still unknown). However, Cameron put it to Pauling that cancer is a very special situation where the 'blind' part of such a trial is all around us. Cancer is almost invariably a relentlessly progressive fatal disease, so the arrest of progressive tumour growth and invasion in even quite a small group of patients would, in Cameron's opinion, achieve the objective of demonstrating the therapeutic efficacy of ascorbate (21 January 1972).

Pauling, for his part, favoured the idea of a double-blind trial:

> In this unusual situation, where the investigator might well have difficulty in deciding whether it is better for the patient to receive the ascorbic acid or better for him not to receive the ascorbic acid, it is, I suggest, worth while to set up a double-blind test.

However Pauling agreed that a double-blind trial was not really essential. If Cameron felt it to be best for his patients to supplement their conventional treatment with ascorbate, then, 'in the course of time the statistical analysis of the results should show whether the treatment is helpful or not' (4 February 1972).

It was around this time that Cameron, mulling over the distinctions between conventional chemotherapy and vitamin C treatment, amused himself by dashing off a short paper for the popular presentation of the ascorbate/PHI hypothesis, which he mailed to Pauling. As Susan Sontag has stressed in her well-known analysis of the culture of cancer, the controlling metaphors in cancer descriptions are drawn from the language of warfare. Cancer cells do not simply multiply, they 'invade'; the body fights back with its 'defences'. Patients are 'bombarded' with toxic rays and drugs. Treatment aims to 'kill' cancer cells: 'It is a rousing call to fight by any means whatever, a lethal, insidious enemy'. As Sontag structures it, this militaristic imagery justifies the deployment, to their full heroic extent, of the conventional methods of cancer warfare: slashing, burning and poisoning (Sontag, 1983). In his manuscript, Cameron specifically counterposed his and Pauling's approach to cancer treatment to such militaristic ideology, and aligned it with peaceful coexistence and disarmament:

> Cancer is not a simple 'military' situation with a simple decisive

answer. It is a complex multifactorial behaviour problem requiring a political solution.

To treat cancer intelligently demands a rethink of our whole therapeutic philosophy. We should abandon our futile and illogical policy of trying to kill cancer cells. Instead we should endeavour to understand the cause of their discontent and seek a compromise solution. If we are prepared to accept that cancer cells too have a right to survive, we could be well on our way to a negotiated peace and an end to the cellular rebellion. (Cameron, March, 1972)

But the famous anti-war activist did not respond immediately to Cameron's request for comment on this political restructuring of the conventional cancer metaphor, having taken on board the more serious and pressing task of revising Cameron's manuscript for submission to the *PNAS*. As he reminded Cameron, he had the right to submit papers to the journal, providing another member of the Academy certified their suitability for publication. But this requirement did not apply where Pauling himself was an author. Over the next few weeks he redrafted the manuscript, and at Cameron's insistence attached his name to the paper. He made some minor changes which located the paper more clearly within the orthomolecular framework, but the major change introduced by Pauling was to downplay Cameron's emphasis on the incorporation of ascorbic acid into the PHI molecule. Pauling's own work on the inhibition of enzyme activity suggested that ascorbic acid might be involved in the synthesis of PHI in some other way than by inclusion of an ascorbic acid residue in the inhibitor, and, as he put it to Cameron, the elimination of this unnecessary assumption strengthened the argument. Cameron quickly agreed that his original version was 'dangerously over-precise and potentially vulnerable', and that Pauling's version was a 'tremendous improvement' (29 March 1972). In any case the *Lancet* had finally published his and Rotman's letter and the original hypothesis was already in print (Cameron and Rotman, 1972).

Now that publication seemed imminent, Cameron confessed to some symptoms of cold feet. He re-emphasized to Pauling their lack of anything approaching irrefutable clinical proof of the validity of the hypothesis:

I could summarize the present clinical position in two completely contrasting ways. I could report in all honesty that more than half of the original patients who commenced treatment in November-December 1971, are now dead. I could offer many plausible explanations for each individual death (co-existent cardio-vascular disease, death from 'mechanical' causes such as intestinal, vascular and airway obstruction, and even failure to take their medication after leaving hospital), but the harsh statistical fact remains true.

In contrast I could report with equal sincerity that we have an increasing number of patients in the terminal stages of a fatal illness who are still alive, and who remain, if not exactly 'well', at least by clinical standards 'very much improved'. I am very conscious that this is only a clinical impression to balance against a hard statistical fact. (29 March 1972)

He urged Pauling to disregard these preliminary clinical observations altogether and to consider carefully whether or not the paper should be published in its own right, on the basis of its logic and its relation to Pauling's own experimental findings and publications.

To counterbalance his 'canny Scot' caution, in the very same letter Cameron enthusiastically detailed his plans for the projected trial. His work-load as senior consulting surgeon made it impossible for him to give the project his undivided attention, but he had managed to persuade the Board of Management to allocate one thousand pounds from Endowment Funds to employ a Clinical Research Assistant to supervise and document the terminal cancer patients receiving ascorbate therapy, and Dr Gillian Baird had begun work on March 21. Cameron had also approached the Medical Research Council for funding, but discovered that the MRC would only support ongoing research projects which showed strong evidence of promising results, which he could not at this point provide. His discussion with Professor Kay of the Chair of Surgery at the University of Glasgow (and a member of the MRC committee) had reinforced his earlier opinion that a double-blind clinical trial was not appropriate in 'this special situation'. According to Cameron, Kay had thought the proposal worth investigating, and had agreed that Cameron and his colleagues should continue to treat 'hopeless' cases with ascorbate therapy and, for the meantime, ignore all the failures. The immediate objective must be to find a relatively small number of ascorbic-acid induced regressions, but the evidence of diagnosis and regression in these patients must be indisputable. To this end, Kay had offered free access to the more sophisticated diagnostic facilities in his Department.

Cameron thought that if he could find ten or so undoubted regressions among the terminal patients in Vale of Leven, this would convince his regional colleagues of the need to set up a large-scale randomized trial on earlier and more favourable patients. Only through such large-scale trials would the hypothesis be proved, but they would require a great deal of organisation and resources, as well as a great deal of persuasive advocacy. 'The present intention,' Cameron wrote Pauling,

is that we continue to treat every cancer patient that comes our way by perfectly conventional methods. There will be no intention of conducting a trial in the usual sense, or of any experimentation with these patients. However with these conventional methods we record some 340 cancer deaths a year in this area, and most of these patients have at least been documented at some stage of their clinical career in this hospital. Some patients are beyond the scope of any conventional form of therapy when first diagnosed, many more suffer widespread recurrence and relapse into this 'untreatable' category. We intend to offer ascorbic acid therapy to this 'terminal' group. We appreciate that we are dealing with the unfavourable end of the therapeutic spectrum, but ethical considerations leave us no other choice. . . . We know that we are going to encounter many failures (in a situation, however, where they would all have been 'failures' without our intervention) but we believe that if we can only find and record 20 or even 10 undoubted regressions in this 'terminal' group, the preliminary phase of the investigation will have been triumphantly accomplished. (29 March 1972)

Careful records would be kept and every form of patient monitoring that could be utilized would be employed. These would include all the standard forms of histological, biochemical, haemotological, and radiological assessment, plus procedures such as clinical photography, mammograms, cystograms, etc. (all available at Vale of Leven), and even isotope liver and bone scans and ultrasonograms (available through Kay's offices at the University of Glasgow). As well, Cameron intended to set up some laboratory investigations, such as ascorbic acid urine and serum assays, and perhaps serum PHI assays. He also discussed the possibility of setting up a suitable animal experiment, using the guinea pig with its well-known inability to synthesize ascorbic acid. All of this evidence, together with what might be collated from library searches, would go towards establishing the ascorbate-PHI hypothesis.

On 5 April 1972, Pauling wrote back to say that he had submitted the paper to the *PNAS*, and that he expected it to be published in two or three months. 'From your letter', he wrote drily, 'with its rather restrained statements, I have the impression that you are satisfied that some of the terminal cancer patients who have received the ascorbic-acid therapy have made surprising progress.' To Cameron's elation, he added a hand-written postscript, 'I am very happy to be associated with you in publishing this paper'.

4.2   THE PILOT VALE OF LEVEN TRIALS

With the problem of publication now apparently resolved, Cameron focussed on the organization of the essential clinical trials at the Vale of

Leven Hospital. But his optimistic scenario proved much more difficult to translate into practice than he had anticipated. From the beginning, the clinical problems he encountered and Cameron's limited resources at Vale of Leven were a source of frustration, much of which he poured out in lengthy letters to Pauling. The major problem was that he was only able to employ ascorbic acid in the treatment of terminal cancer patients. These patients were gravely ill and suffering from disseminated cancer, and often with associated cardiac and renal problems. They manifested so many individual, pathological and emotional variables, as to almost defy quantification. His 'failures' died with a sharp, definable end point. His possible 'successes' were far more nebulous and ill-defined. Vale of Leven was a relatively small hospital with only a relatively small number of cancer patients, and in a clinical situation full of so many variables as terminal cancer, it was very difficult for Cameron and his colleagues to measure and compare degrees of therapeutic response, particularly the lower levels of response that Cameron generally expected from ascorbate therapy. As he explained to Pauling, the predicted grades of response ranged over the following therapeutic spectrum (5 May 1972):

(1) NO RESPONSE, or at least a response so slight as to be undetectable

    (2) RETARDATION OF TUMOUR GROWTH

        (3) CARCINOSTASIS

           (4) TUMOUR REGRESSION

              (5) TUMOUR NECROSIS

Because of the near impossibility of extrapolating growth rates backwards, Grade 2 and Grade 3 responses were very difficult to measure and evaluate, and the reliance on shifting clinical impressions and the lack of any measurable progress in the short term were discouraging. Cameron ran into further difficulties when he tried infusing a few terminal patients with very high levels of sodium ascorbate (about 45 grams per day) in an attempt to achieve a more positive response. The gross fluid retention and generalized oedema which resulted convinced him that such megadoses could be harmful to terminal cancer patients with limited renal and cardiac resources.

He had difficulty in securing sufficient supplies of ascorbic acid in a form suitable for infusion, and wrote to Pauling that he had virtually cornered the entire British stocks of sterile aqueous solutions of ascorbic acid. He spent a good deal of wasted effort attempting to persuade Hoffmann-La Roche to provide a sterile, stable, preservative and sodium-free solution of ascorbic acid for his trial, before he finally managed to secure a supply from Antigen International of Ireland. The serum PHI assays proved more recalcitrant than expected and Vale of Leven lacked the technological resources and biochemical expertise to carry them out. Funding was a continual problem. The guinea pig experiment was delayed for lack of funds, and the continued employment of Dr Baird on the project required all Cameron's ingenuity in finding grant money. At the beginning of 1973, Cameron, with Pauling as referee, managed to obtain a Scottish Home and Health Department grant of £4,000 for research into the 'Orthomolecular Treatment of Cancer'. This sum, together with the initial grant of £1,000 from Vale of Leven Hospital, financed the pilot Vale of Leven trials.

Throughout, Pauling encouraged the continuance of the trials, even, to Cameron's embarrassment, sending his personal cheque for $300 towards the expenses of the guinea pig experiment. Pauling had been having his own problems at Stanford where he could not find laboratory space or funding for his and Robinson's orthomolecular research. Nor was he making much headway with the Stanford oncologists. As the possibility of a Stanford-based clinical trial of ascorbate receded, Cameron's Vale of Leven trials took on even greater significance. Pauling urged Cameron not to be discouraged at his failure to achieve measurable response to ascorbate therapy. He cited a long extract from his Ben May speech of the previous November, where he had argued that even a ten per cent decrease in the incidence of cancer would be a most significant contribution to its control. 'You might have difficulty', he exhorted,

> in recognizing what could be called a 'ten per cent response'. The problem is such an important one that it would be wrong to give up with a reasonable new attack until it has been shown quite clearly that even a small degree of control of the disease cannot be achieved. (11 May 1972)

When Cameron, at the height of his discouragement and frustration, began to query the ascorbate/PHI hypothesis and to cast around for alternative hypotheses, Pauling kept him on course. 'I myself was sceptical', he wrote,

> about ascorbic acid, as having value for so many different disease states, until I formulated the general argument that is presented in my paper 'Evolution and the Need for Ascorbic Acid'. Having convinced myself by this argument that the optimum intake of ascorbic acid for good health is far larger than the usually recommended intake,

I can now believe that this optimum intake might be of some value for almost every disease state.

I do not think of its being a wonder drug, in the sense of its having very powerful activity (except, of course, in the prevention of scurvy). It seems to me that its greatest value might be in prophylaxis. . . .

But there is also, I think, the possibility that certain disease states would react in a very striking way to very large amounts of ascorbic acid, and that it might for these disease states act as a powerful drug. (12 June 1972)

4.3 THE *PNAS* AFFAIR

But even Pauling confessed himself temporarily at a loss, when, in an unprecedented move, the Editorial Board of the *PNAS* rejected their manuscript. He was informed by the Chairman, John Edsall, that the Board had concluded that papers advocating therapeutic procedures, particularly in such an emotive area as cancer, were out of place in the *Proceedings* and belonged in medical journals where they would be properly refereed (Edsall to Pauling, 26 April 1972). In effect, the Board had changed its publication rules in mid-play. Pauling (who had himself served as Chairman of the Editorial Board for a number of years), was confounded. He thought this to be the first time that a paper with a member of the Academy as author had been rejected, and he expressed some concern that its rejection might reflect the opinion that he was becoming somewhat 'senile' in his promotion of vitamin C therapy (Pauling to Cameron, 6 May 1972). Cameron in his turn now reassured:

It is rather good to know that hidden away in private correspondence we have all the facts to make such scurrilous attacks ridiculous. (30 May 1972)

After some toing and froing, it was agreed that Cameron should submit the hypothesis paper in their joint names to the *British Medical Journal*, which he did in late June.

Pauling, in the meantime, kept his ear to the ground. His opportunity for action came when he learnt that the rejection of the hypothesis paper by the *PNAS* was about to be publicised in the journal *Science*. On 24 July he returned the paper to the *PNAS*, along with a trenchant letter to the new Chairman (Robert Sinsheimer) requesting its publication 'without further delay' on the grounds that the Editorial Board had no right to refuse publication of a paper authored by a member of the Academy. As some concession to the Board, he made a few revisions in the paper.

These amounted, as he explained to Cameron (31 July 1972), to changing a couple of the subheadings to eliminate the expression 'therapeutic use', and he also changed the title to remove the emphasis on treatment. He did not expect that they would run into complications through having submitted the same paper to two journals concurrently, because he thought that the *PNAS* would again reject the paper. It was a question of 'principle', and Pauling felt strongly that medicine would benefit from the publication and discussion of theoretical papers, even in the absence of any experimental support.

The *PNAS* did not, as Pauling had predicted, share his view. The Council of the Academy affirmed the Editorial Board's rejection of the paper (Sinsheimer to Pauling, 22 August 1972). In a contradictory way, however, the *PNAS* affair did achieve the objective of publication of the hypothesis.

The rejection of a Pauling paper and the revision of the Academy's publication rules was given widespread publicity by *Science* (Cullitan, 1972), followed by *Newsweek* and *Time*, and almost immediately Pauling received an offer of publication by telegram from *Oncology*, an international periodical devoted to clinical and experimental cancer research. Alexander Wolsky, who edited the theoretical section of the journal, wrote a follow-up letter, deploring the action of the Academy and explaining that he would be most happy to accept the paper sight unseen on the basis of the Pauling reputation and his own enthusiastic advocacy of vitamin C as a cure of collagen weaknesses (Wolsky to Pauling, 8 August 1972). Two weeks later, having learnt that the paper had been rejected yet again by the Academy and turned down by the *British Medical Journal*, Pauling accepted Wolsky's offer (Pauling to Wolsky, 24 August 1972; Cameron and Pauling, 1973).

At the same time Pauling pursued his case with the National Academy of Sciences. *Science* had published some statements purportedly by Edsall (who had initially turned down the Pauling–Cameron paper) to the effect that Pauling's previous papers on vitamin C had been published in the *PNAS* only with 'extreme mental reservations', and that most members of the Academy took issue with their scientific validity. Pauling made it clear that he considered these remarks 'derogatory and damaging to his reputation'. He disputed them with Edsall and Sinsheimer and in the pages of *Science* (Pauling, 1972). Over the next few months he obtained expressions of 'regret' from Sinsheimer and the President of the Academy that the rejection of his paper had become public knowledge, and Edsall wrote to *Science*, dissociating himself from the deprecatory comments attributed to him (Edsall, 1972).

More important, by appealing against the decision of the Academy and persistently restating his case, Pauling forced the Academy to soften and define more clearly its revised editorial policy. His point – that members of the Academy whose papers conflicted with the new ruling should be given the opportunity for revision and not have their papers summarily rejected – was conceded. Belatedly, Pauling and Cameron were formally invited to revise and resubmit their manuscript (Handler and Sinsheimer to Pauling, 3 November 1972). By this time the paper was already in press for *Oncology* and it was too late for publication in the *PNAS*. But Pauling's confrontationist stand and the adverse publicity engendered by the whole affair meant that the *PNAS* in future would handle any Pauling manuscript, however controversial, with the utmost care. As Cameron, who was an appreciative onlooker, commented to Pauling, it was good to know that such a powerful ally was on *his* side in the struggle.

Struggle it now undoubtedly was. Getting the hypothesis into print was one thing; stimulating the interest of orthodox oncologists quite another. Even Pauling's persistence, ingenuity and sheer clout were severely tried by the almost united lack of interest of the cancer establishment in the vitamin C and cancer hypothesis and their resistance to Cameron's clinical findings.

4.4   CAMERON'S PILOT TRIALS FINDINGS AND HIS PRESENTATION STRATEGY

From around late June 1972, in spite of his continuing problems with assessment, Cameron had been indicating to Pauling that he had acquired enough clinical experience to be in 'no doubt whatsoever . . . that ASCORBIC ACID IS A VALUABLE REMEDY IN THE GREAT MAJORITY OF PATIENTS WITH TERMINAL CANCER'. After some trial and error, he had settled on a dose regimen of 10g/day intravenous ascorbic acid for up to 10 days, followed by oral doses of 10g/day 'indefinitely'. While this form of medication was clearly not a cure for terminal disseminated cancer, 'I am convinced', Cameron wrote Pauling,

> that [it] produces a favourable shift in the host/tumour relationship. I think that we are achieving tumour retardation and prolongation of life in many patients even although I fully appreciate that these factors are notoriously difficult to measure. What is perhaps more important than mere prolongation of life, is that by symptomatic relief, we are improving the quality of life. (25 June 1972)

He described for Pauling what he had come to recognize as the 'standard response' to large-dose ascorbic acid in patients with advanced cancer. Patients entered his series dying from the relentless progression of their tumour, usually heavily sedated and steadily losing weight. They did not show any immediate improvement, in fact they sometimes got worse (which in Cameron's opinion ruled out placebo effect), but about a week after commencement of therapy the majority of patients began to experience subjective improvement – they had a feeling of well-being and improved appetite and began to gain weight. Around the same time, Cameron and his colleagues began to get some objective evidence of improvement. Some patients had experienced striking relief from the bone pain of skeletal metastases and had been able to dispense with their heavy sedation regimes. 'To be able to do this alone,' wrote Cameron, 'with nothing more striking than ascorbic acid seems to me to be tremendously important'. Other complications of advanced cancer, such as the accumulation of malignant effusions, jaundice and respiratory distress were alleviated or arrested. The standard biochemical indices of malignant activity such as the Erythrocyte Sedimentation Rate (ESR) and serum mucopolysaccharide levels, instead of rising relentlessly, remained stationary, and in many patients gradually fell – in a few patients to normal levels. This 'standstill' phase was of variable duration: in some patients only transient, in others this symptom-free 'well-being' phase continued for weeks or months before the patient suddenly succumbed to death from fulminating cancer. The manner of death was unusual in Cameron's experience. Instead of the characteristic long-drawn-out decline, patients went through a 'whirlwind' reactivation of their cancer and usually died within a few days.

By the end of October, Cameron was better able to substantiate these clinical impressions, and he began work on a clinical paper. He presented Pauling with a set of serial x-rays which demonstrated tumour regression with bone regrowth in a 55 year old man who had presented with cancer of the right kidney which had subsequently metastasized to his bones. Apart from surgery to remove the affected kidney, this man had received no other treatment than ascorbic acid for the previous six months and was now free of bone pain and 'fit and well' (31 October 1972).

However, Pauling's attempt to interest the Chairman of the Stanford Department of Oncology in Cameron's x-rays failed. Nor was the Chairman impressed by Pauling's arguments, and Pauling, having by this stage decided to move off the Stanford campus, finally abandoned all hope of help from the Stanford oncologists. He wrote Cameron of his intention of going to the Scientific Advisory Panel of the National Cancer Institute (NCI) in an effort to 'get some work started on ascorbic acid in relation to cancer in this country. It seems to me that it would be justified to start a good sized programme of investigation in this field' (6 December 1972).

He immediately contacted the Director of the National Cancer Institute and the Chairman of the Board of Advisors, and was invited to Washington to talk with some of the officials on 6 March 1973. Cameron had sent him the first draft of his clinical paper on the first fifty patients to receive vitamin C (who now included several 'apparently genuine' regressions) and Pauling summarized these results for the NCI officials. He also presented various supporting arguments such as the anti-viral action of vitamin C and, of course, the ascorbate/PHI hypothesis, in an effort to convince the NCI officials of the desirability of setting up a double-blind control trial, but in vain: 'I think that I failed nearly completely', he wrote Cameron. The response of the officials was that there had to be thoroughly convincing animal evidence before any trials were made with humans (Pauling to Cameron, 28 March 1973). In return, Cameron reported on his own lack of success in trying to stimulate interest in full-scale clinical trials through his correspondence with Canadian researchers and his local contacts with Scottish oncologists: '[I]t seems for the moment we shall have to go it alone with perhaps "a little help from our friends" ' (15 April 1973).

Although both Cameron and Pauling disputed the NCI insistence on prior animal experimentation – on the grounds that there was no need for tests to establish the safety of ascorbic acid and that animal experiments might give quite misleading results on its anti-cancer potential (since most animals synthesise their own ascorbic acid) – they conceded its necessity if they were to establish the need for large-scale clinical trials in earlier and more favourable cancer patients. The guinea pig trial that Cameron had initiated had 'petered out', but Pauling had already applied to the NCI for funding for a controlled experiment involving the study of the effect of vitamin C on the incidence of cancer in guinea pigs. Following Pauling's visit to the NCI, the proposal was supported by NCI assessors but given such a low level of priority that it was not funded.

Early in 1973, Pauling and Robinson had established the Institute of Orthomolecular Medicine near Stanford, and for most of its first year of existence the Institute was plagued by financial problems. It was a difficult period for Pauling. Apart from his fund-raising efforts, he was embroiled in controversy over his common-cold claims and had taken on a heavy schedule of American-wide lectures and talks on vitamin C and peace. He had had, as he wrote Cameron, a 'hard time keeping my head above water'.

Nevertheless he doggedly persisted with his pursuit of NCI funds for an animal experiment involving vitamin C and cancer, and he did not give up on his attempt to arouse establishment interest in Cameron's clinical trials of vitamin C.

Cameron, for his part, became even more circumspect with respect to the ethics of his pilot study of terminal cancer patients. All along he had stressed to Pauling (and Pauling had concurred) that the study should not be vulnerable to ethical criticism – that it should be concerned with 'good doctoring' rather than 'experimentation'. Accordingly, vitamin C had been offered only to those patients deemed 'untreatable' by at least one other attending physician not involved in the study, and wherever Cameron thought that even for such patients any other form of medication 'could possibly do any good' it had also been offered. Hence, in the interests of good doctoring but in a muddying of the therapeutic waters, a number of patients had been treated by ascorbic acid in conjunction with irradiation or hormone therapy, and in a small number of cases with cytotoxic drugs. These patients had to be excluded from the study. However his experiences with such combination therapy did lead Cameron early in the piece to the significant conclusion that the combination of ascorbate and cytotoxic drugs was not very effective, perhaps because of the leucopenia (low level of circulating white blood cells which maintain the immune mechanisms in the body) induced by the cytotoxic drugs (Cameron to Pauling, 9 September 1972).

Overall, his clinical experience with ascorbate inclined him more and more to the ethical position that it was 'just good doctoring' and that it should not be withheld in otherwise hopeless cases. In June 1973, while on a visit to the United States where he and Pauling met for the first time, Cameron visited the National Cancer Institute and in the company of one of the senior residents spent some time visiting various wards and looking at patients. He found the experience, he wrote to Pauling, 'very distressing'. He thought that the aggressive surgery, irradiation and chemotherapy were being pushed to the very limits of human tolerance: 'I do not know what kind of "results" they are achieving but they are certainly causing much mutilation and human suffering along the way' (12 July 1973). This visit, and his later experiences with some of the desperate patients who had run the gamut of conventional therapies and sought his help, reinforced Cameron's commitment to the vitamin C programme and hardened his ethical position that it represented 'good doctoring'.

There can be no doubt, as he himself conceded, that Cameron's own first flush of enthusiasm for vitamin C had been tempered by his clinical experiences (12 April 1974). He experienced increasing difficulty in retaining the interest of his Vale of Leven colleagues who did not share his commitment to making the necessary adjustment of their clinical expectations to this different form of cancer treatment which did not 'cure' but 'controlled'. They were not interested in drawing the finer discriminations in patient response that its evaluation entailed and that had become Cameron's stock-in-trade. He and Pauling had never expected 'miracle cures', but the fact that they did not predict them and Cameron could not produce them told against them:

When I first suggested that we use ascorbic acid in advanced cancer, [my colleagues'] natural first reaction was one of incredulity. However they gave it a cautious trial, and became very enthusiastic and some were even making far greater claims for its efficacy than I was. In fact I found myself in the rather odd position of having to restrain their enthusiasm and high expectations, and having to warn them that most of their patients would probably die. And as their patients have died, I am sorry to report that most of them have tended to lose interest. (12 April 1974)

The problem was, as Cameron put it to Pauling, they were dealing in different shades of grey rather than the dramatic contrasts of black and white that his medical colleagues had been taught to look for. Fortunately, the occasional 'dramatic miracle' of regression did occur to buoy up flagging spirits. The most outstanding of this handful of cases was that of a forty-five year old truck driver who had been progressively ill for some months with increasing listlessness and weight loss and enlarged glands of his neck, armpits and groin. His liver and spleen were also enlarged and x-ray revealed massive chest gland enlargement. His seromucoid and ESR were grossly elevated and he was anaemic. He was diagnosed after biopsy of a neck gland as having 'lymphosarcoma of reticulum-cell type' – a cancer of the lymphatic system. This is usually treated by chemotherapy or radiotherapy or a combination of both, but there was some administrative delay in admitting this patient to a treatment unit, and he was started on intravenous ascorbate ('more or less as a stop-gap'). Within two weeks this man was clinically completely well. All the palpable glands had disappeared, his enlarged liver and spleen became impalpable and his chest x-ray reverted to normal. His elevated ESR and seromucoid fell dramatically, and a second neck gland biopsy was reported to show 'normal architecture'. He pronounced himself fit and returned to work, having received no other treatment than ascorbic acid.

This patient had been treated in a neighbouring hospital where Cameron had managed to interest some of the clinicians in ascorbate therapy, and in view of the unexpected outcome, the original pathologist had some understandable second thoughts about his diagnosis. However, the original slides were examined by a number of pathologists, including a leading authority on reticulosis, and pronounced to be 'undoubtedly malignant'. The physicians who treated this patient had no doubt whatever that ascorbic acid had 'cured' him. Cameron was more cautious on the basis of his own more moderate expectations, pointing out to Pauling that it was far too early to predict how long this remission would last (26 December 1973). He thought these particular colleagues to be going through the same 'over-enthusiastic phase' as he had himself experienced when he first began treating his patients with ascorbate, and predicted that 'time and increasing experience' would modify their views as they had his (12 April 1974).

Nevertheless there was no doubt in Cameron's own mind that many of his patients had survived far longer than any reasonable clinical expectation and had gained considerable symptomatic relief. And these were valuable gains in cancer treatment. The difficulty was how to present this in the most convincing way to sceptical editors and oncologists (15 April 1973). Of course, their greatest handicap was the 'sheer simplicity' of their proposal:

It is just too simple for the average conditioned medical mind to comprehend and accept. . . . The sheer familiarity of vitamin C and a thought process that thinks only in terms of vitamin deficiency is probably the greatest barrier we have to overcome. (20 May 1973)

He and Pauling discussed the problem at length in their letters and at their June meeting, where Pauling had persuaded Cameron to publish a brief report on the potential of vitamin C for giving relief from bone metastasis pain and reducing dependency on opiates in terminal cancer patients (Cameron and Baird, 1973). However, the larger problem remained, and Cameron was doubtful about Pauling's suggestion of finding comparable untreated controls from the Hospital records. 'There will no doubt be much scepticism about your conclusions,' Pauling had written,

no matter how the observations are presented. If, however, you are able to make a comparison of your ascorbic-acid subjects and a matched set of control subjects (possibly more than one per ascorbic-acid subject), the evidence might be given greater consideration by the readers. (5 February 1973; 28 March 1973)

Cameron, though, thought it would be almost impossible to find exactly matched controls for comparison, and that in any case their selection might involve a degree of bias (11 February 1973; 15 April 1973). He finally settled on presenting a rewrite of the draft of the paper he had earlier sent Pauling. It would be based on a table of fifty patients as before, but, as he explained to Pauling, a few of the original patients whose diagnosis might be queried would be replaced by patients whose diagnosis could be histologically verified. Great care would be taken to ensure that the overall effect remained the same: 'I mean that we would not just pick fifty of our "best" patients and exclude the failures.' They had to tread a very careful path and make no exaggerated claims: 'Somehow we have to get the message across that ascorbic acid is no miracle cure drug in advanced disseminated cancer, but that it does, in our opinion at least, check the relentless progression of the disease in an appreciable proportion of such patients' (24 October 1973).

To this end, Cameron decided on a 'low-profile presentation'. He thought it advisable to shift their ground a little at this stage. The strategy he eventually adopted was that they should not advocate ascorbic acid as a treatment in its own right, but rather promote it as an 'adjuvant supportive therapy' and talk in terms of 'enhancement of host resistance' and 'containment'.

> If we can get that message across and this form of treatment widely established, then it would be my hope that as general experience grows, some of the definitive 'eradicative' drastic forms of therapy will be found to be unnecessary in earlier and more favourable patients. Perhaps someday we shall be able to write a book 'NO MORE SUR-GERY!' but that is a long time in the future.   (18 August 1973)

In keeping with this strategy, the PHI/ascorbate hypothesis was moved off centre stage. Cameron marshalled all the evidence and arguments that he and Pauling had sifted and sharpened in the course of their two-year correspondence and that could serve to rationalize the use of ascorbate in the supportive treatment of cancer. In this way, the role of ascorbate in stimulating the immune system and generally enhancing resistance to cancer was given greater theoretical prominence. This also had the advantage of allying ascorbate treatment with the currently fashionable interest in immunotherapy. As well, the clinical results of Cameron's pilot trial were modulated around the low-key claim that ascorbate therapy could 'lighten varying shades of grey' (Cameron to Pauling, 20 February 1974) or 'palliate' terminal cancer, and this in turn suggested its use as a standard supportive measure to reinforce established methods of treatment in the general management of earlier and more favourable cases.

Overall, it was a fairly neat balancing act, because, for all his strategy of not poaching on the preserves of conventional oncologists, Cameron had still to get the message across that the conventional methods of cancer treatment had their limitations and that he and Pauling had something new and different to offer that did not fit the prevailing therapeutic policy of trying to eradicate every cancer cell in the body. Vitamin C was therefore offered as 'supportive care' which would strengthen the intrinsic defence mechanisms of the patient and so bring about 'striking improvement' in the response to standard forms of treatment (Cameron and Pauling, 1974). Its therapeutic promise was that it would not replace or threaten conventional treatments but actually *improve* their efficacy.

In the end Cameron decided that two papers were necessary, one summarizing the reasons behind employing ascorbate in cancer and the other follow-up paper dealing with the clinical evaluation of ascorbate. Dr Baird had by this stage left Vale of Leven and Cameron asked Allan

Campbell, a consultant physician who had attended some of the patients to join him as co-author of the clinical paper. He invited Pauling to co-author the other, pointing out that the ideas contained in it had evolved through their joint correspondence and that Pauling's authorship would increase its chances of publication. Pauling this time demurred on the grounds that it was primarily Cameron's work.

For some time Cameron had been intending to submit the papers to *Cancer*, the leading journal in the field and published under the auspices of the American Cancer Society, but now he hesitated over taking this definitive step. Then, unexpectedly, the two papers were given a professional vetting at one of the most prestigious cancer centres in the world, Memorial Sloan–Kettering Cancer Center in New York. This came about as a result of Pauling's lobbying of the Director and his subsequent telephone conversation with Dr Lloyd J. Old, Vice President and Associate Director. At this stage, as a result of the public campaign on its behalf, Sloan–Kettering was involved in the testing of laetrile, the controversial cancer 'cure', and subject to a good deal of public pressure to broaden their approach to the cancer problem (Petersen and Markle, 1979a, b; Moss, 1980). Unlike the Chairman of the Stanford Oncology Department (who became 'quite rude' on the telephone when Pauling, undaunted by his previous reception, again approached him), Old gave Pauling a hearing, and both he and Cameron were invited to Sloan–Kettering on 12 March 1974, to discuss their views on ascorbate and Cameron's clinical findings.

Their meeting went well, with Old and some of the clinicians apparently impressed enough by Cameron's findings to carry out some observations of their own at Sloan–Kettering. Cameron was sufficiently encouraged by Old's response to finally post the two papers off to *Cancer* in April, with himself (at Pauling's insistence) as sole author of the paper dealing with the justification of ascorbate therapy. Not, as he disclaimed to Pauling, that he expected much from such an 'establishment-orientated' journal: 'Indeed, if they are accepted, it will be a case of "The Marines have Landed"' (15 April 1974).

The marines did not land; at least, not quite how Cameron had envisaged they might. A month later, *Cancer*, with what Cameron felt to be 'almost inordinate haste' and only a 'very cursory reading' of the manuscripts, rejected them, because in the opinion of their editorial advisers the material was 'not of sufficiently high priority to warrant publication space' (18 May 1974). At that point, Pauling and his wife, Ava Helen, made their long-promised and long-delayed visit to Vale of Leven to stay with the Camerons, and Pauling again came to the rescue. He and Cameron spent some time revising the manuscripts; Pauling came in as co-author of the first paper and almost immediately found a home for both papers in a non-medical but respected scientific journal,

Chemico-biological Interactions. By 20 July 1974, they had been accepted 'as they stand' and the printing queue rearranged so as to guarantee their publication in that same year.

At Pauling's suggestion, a third paper detailing the case of the truckdriver with the reticulum cell sarcoma was commissioned by the same journal. This case had now become, as Cameron put it to Pauling, one which 'might almost have been designed to prove our contention' (18 May 1974). This man's initial response to ascorbate therapy had been dramatic enough, with the complete regression of his cancer. But the case unfolded in an even more spectacular fashion when some months later the patient, having seemingly recovered, discontinued his daily ascorbate medication and relapsed. After four weeks with no ascorbic acid, he complained of a recurrence of lassitude and a slight cough. His ESR and Seromucoid levels were found to have risen again and x-ray showed unmistakable signs of recurrence of his malignancy. His oral medication with ascorbic acid was recommenced, and when after two weeks he showed no signs of improvement, he was hospitalized and treated by the continuous infusion of 20g/day of ascorbic acid for 14 days, followed by oral ascorbic acid (12.5g/day) thereafter. This time he did not respond so dramatically to ascorbate therapy, but slowly improved until his chest x-ray showed normal again and there was no evidence of active disease. He resumed his heavy employment on a continuous daily dose of 12.5g/day of ascorbic acid, a living and well 'cast iron case' for the efficacy of vitamin C, as Cameron jubilantly reported to Pauling. His initial diagnosis had been confirmed by a leading cancer pathologist and accepted by Sloan–Kettering, and the case had been fully documented by serial x-rays. The first occasion might have been merely a 'spontaneous' regression which happened to coincide with the administration of ascorbate, but Cameron knew of no case in the whole literature who had the good fortune to go through two spontaneous regressions in the course of a cancer illness, and both these remissions had coincided in time with ascorbate treatment, with relapse when the medication was withdrawn. The patient had virtually acted as his own control, and it was almost indisputable that his double remission was a direct therapeutic response to ascorbate treatment (Cameron to Pauling, 20 July 1974).

When this third paper was submitted, Cameron had some difficulty in convincing a referee of this 'somewhat remarkable claim' in that to the referee's knowledge no case of reticulum cell sarcoma had been known to undergo 'spontaneous' regression. The referee also quibbled over the particular kind of malignancy diagnosed and cast doubt on the ethics of withholding conventional treatment from such a patient. A somewhat exasperated Cameron explained that the 'remarkable claim' was the point of the whole paper and that the reason why the patient had not received conventional treatment was because there was no 'slot' available for him and he was given ascorbic acid as a holding operation. The referee was eventually 'silenced' and the paper accepted. To Pauling, Cameron gave vent to his real feelings:

> If there were the least doubt about the diagnosis (which there is not) would it not have been criminally unethical to submit this man to irradiation and cytotoxics? . . . How does he suggest we treat [the patient] now? – stop his ascorbic acid, irradiate him! The point seems to have been lost somewhere along the line that this dying man is now extremely fit and well. (13 April 1975)

4.5   REFINING THE VALE OF LEVEN TRIALS

With the Pauling-engineered publication of this trio of papers, the biomedical community, if not the cancer specialists, began to take note of the Vale of Leven trials (Cameron and Pauling, 1974; Cameron and Campbell, 1974; Cameron et al., 1975). Cameron was now inundated with requests for reprints and the overflow of correspondence was redirected to the Orthomolecular Institute, now renamed The Linus Pauling Institute of Science and Medicine. The alliance between Cameron and Pauling had been consolidated – they were no longer Professor and Doctor, but Linus and Ewan to one another. Cameron's trial findings were an acknowledged boon and drawcard for the Linus Pauling Institute, still hard-pressed for funds. Cameron had been made a Non-Resident Fellow of the Institute at the beginning of 1974, and the last three publications had stated this affiliation. In mid-1975, as some measure of the significance of the Vale of Leven research to the Institute, Cameron was awarded $10,000 of their slender resources for the continuance of his research. When Cameron indicated that he had some idea of using this Institute grant for the employment of a postgraduate student to look into the role of ascorbic acid in the hyaluronidase/hyaluronic system (5 July 1975), he was advised by Pauling to 'leave the biochemistry to the biochemists' and redirected to the task in hand:

> I suggest that you use it in whatever ways seem to you most effective in your clinical studies of ascorbic acid in relation to cancer. (15 July 1975)

For some time Pauling had been urging Cameron to refine his analysis of his clinical findings, and he revived his earlier suggestion that Cameron might use the hospital records to make a comparison of the clinical histories of his ascorbate treated patients with those of similar patients treated by conventional methods (12 August 1974).

The need for some sort of comparative analysis had become more pressing when he and Cameron received the first report on a preliminary trial of ascorbic acid at Sloan–Kettering. In January 1975, Dr Charles Young of Sloan–Kettering had written, enclosing the case histories of sixteen patients he had treated with ascorbic acid without any evidence of benefit. Young himself had conceded that his group of patients was small and that all had had 'extremely far advanced disease' that had been treated with extensive prior therapy. This represented an obvious difference between his patients and Cameron's, the majority of whom had received ascorbate as initial therapy. He could not therefore rule out the potential useful activity of ascorbate, and he proposed to continue the trial (Young to Cameron, 22 January 1975). Cameron, in discussing Young's results with Pauling, described his patients as a 'highly selected group of failures' and thought they need not be too discouraged by his results (12 February 1975). Nevertheless, Young's failure to replicate Cameron's findings pointed up the need for a controlled study of some kind, and Pauling continued to press for one.

During a flying visit to Scotland at the end of 1975, Pauling pushed hard for a comparative clinical study using the Vale of Leven records. Early in the new year Cameron complied with a rough draft of the format of the proposed paper (17 January 1976). With Pauling's ready endorsement, and using part of the Pauling Institute grant money, he hired a young New Zealand doctor, Dr Fran Meuli, whose task it was to go through the hospital records and find ten matching controls for each of one hundred ascorbate treated patients.

As Cameron explained to Pauling, the test cases, i.e., the ascorbate-treated patients, comprised the first consecutive 100 patients listed in the hospital's pharmacy ledger. He eliminated a few patients from this list who had discontinued their medication on the advice of some other doctor, but argued that this did not represent 'selection' of test cases, as the 100 test patients retained included some who were strongly suspected of non-compliance. For each patient, Cameron stencilled out a pro-forma sheet recording sex, age, tumour type and a synopsis of the extent of tumour spread at the time that ascorbate was commenced. Survival times were deliberately excluded from these data. Then for each test case, the hospital record clerks found at least ten case records belonging to patients of the same sex, within ten years of the same age, and with the same type of tumour. These constituted the controls who had not received ascorbate treatment. Next Dr Mueli, quite independently of Cameron, went through all the case records of the controls. She matched them to the clinical synopsis of the test cases on the Proforma Sheets, and using her own judgement to ascertain the date of 'untreatability', recorded their survival times. Dr Mueli, of course, did not know the survival times of the test cases. Finally, after all the other information had been collated, these survival times were filled in and a comparison of the relative survival times of test cases and controls was made. '[B]y going about things in this way', Cameron wrote optimistically, 'I think we can forestall any criticism of "control case selection"' (15 May 1976).

Cameron had 'confidently expected' that the study would demonstrate a significant advantage in life expectancy for the ascorbate treated test cases, and this expectation was fulfilled when the final results were analysed. 'The results', he wrote Pauling in June, 'have worked out rather better than I would have expected with a near four-fold gain in survival times in the Treated Group.' The patients receiving ascorbate had survived for a mean of 210 days (and some of them were still alive), while the mean survival time for the controls was 50 days (5 June 1976).

The final selection of test cases was not random, as Cameron had 'rightly or wrongly' felt it necessary to include the 50 patients whose case histories had already been published in *Chemico-biological Interactions*. He had done this on the grounds that some people might ask 'whatever happened to so-and-so?' The other fifty test cases were randomly selected, and Cameron reassured Pauling that the selection of the controls was entirely random and that his tactic of having Dr Mueli compute the control survival times without foreknowledge of the test case survivals had removed 'any element of personal bias or selectivity of controls from the final figures'. Moreover, even if they were criticized for the random selection of a significant number of 'early deaths' among the controls, it was possible to remove those patients who had survived less than ten days from the date of 'untreatability' from the control group and still demonstrate a three-fold gain in survival times in the treated group. 'Either way, we are certainly showing a substantial degree of benefit, and I am convinced that this would be greater and greater if we deal with earlier and earlier patients.'

After rewriting Cameron's draft paper to include the details on patient and control selection procedures and demonstrating the statistical significance of his data, Pauling submitted the manuscript in their joint names to the *Proceedings of the National Academy of Sciences*. At the same time, he sent a copy to Dr John C. Bailar, Editor in Chief of the *Journal of the National Cancer Institute*. This was a deliberate testing of the establishment waters. 'It will be interesting to see what happens', he wrote Cameron, referring to their earlier problems with the *PNAS* (14 July 1976). Pauling was also keen to provoke some feedback from the National Cancer Institute and, if possible, obtain some exposure for his and Cameron's findings in a specialist cancer journal. 'It is astounding to me', he had written Cameron some six months earlier on learning that the NCI had yet again rejected his annual application for funding for his animal experiment, 'that the people in the National Cancer Institute should be so lacking in enthusiasm about the possible value of vitamin C in controlling cancer' (19 November 1975).

Bailar, for his part, responded courteously and at some length to Pauling. As he carefully explained, he had read the paper as a scientist interested in statistical aspects of treatment evaluation rather than as an editor. The major problem he identified in the paper was whether the ascorbate-treated patients were sufficiently similar to the controls. In particular, he queried the designation of 'terminal' in both cases, and whether such a designation was made at similar points in the progress of the disease. He thought that if Pauling and Cameron could provide satisfactory evidence that the patients and controls were classified as 'terminal' by nearly identical criteria, their paper should be published. But he warned that this would not be easy. Even independent review of the ordinary medical records would not be enough, if the records themselves could reflect the hopes of the attending physicians that ascorbate would be beneficial (Bailar to Pauling, 13 July 1976).

As Bailar had intimated, the *PNAS* referees (both 'eminent physician-scientists with long experience in the care of cancer patients' and each associated with a 'leading research hospital') took what Sinsheimer understatingly described in his covering letter to Pauling as 'severe exception' to the basic design of the Cameron/Pauling experiment. Their major criticism was that randomized concurrent controls had not been used, and that this methodological inadequacy invalidated the study. Hopefully, wrote Sinsheimer, Pauling could rebut these comments. Of course, he might simply choose to stand his ground, which would place a difficult decision before Sinsheimer and the Board of Editors (Sinsheimer to Pauling, 6 July 1976).

Within the week, Pauling, having followed Bailar's advice and obtained further details from Cameron on the assignment of patients to ascorbate treatment and the determination of the date of 'untreatability', sent Sinsheimer a revised version of the paper, following this up with a letter which dealt summarily with the objections of the referees. He explained Cameron's reluctance to carry out a double-blind control trial as ethically based, and detailed the factors influencing the assignment of patients to ascorbate treatment at Vale of Leven. Although Cameron was the chief surgeon, he alone did not make the decisions about treatment. The physician who brought the patient to the hospital, the other clinicians in the hospital, outside consultants (in all, some 19 professionals), and the patient's family, were all involved. Pauling and Cameron felt that these various factors operated in such a way as to cause the assignment of 'untreatable' patients to ascorbate treatment in 'essentially a random way'. This should also rebut the criticism that patients assigned to ascorbate therapy were categorized as 'untreatable' at a significantly earlier stage of the disease than the controls. There was no such case selection bias and this could not explain the four-fold increase in the survival times of the ascorbate cases. No matter how the results were analysed (and Pauling gave several examples including the method suggested by the referees), the difference in survival times between the controls and the test cases was statistically significant.

'[A] double-blind study,' pointed out Pauling, quoting Louis Lasagna, an eminent American expert on clinical trials, 'is one that is described by the investigators as double-blind.' In other words, the credibility of the results of even the most rigorously conducted investigation hinges on the trustworthiness of the investigators:

> Both of these two referees talk about the failure to use a process of randomization. Here we have to rely on the judgement by Dr Cameron that in fact the ascorbate-treated patients represented essentially a random selection from the entire group of 'untreatable' cancer patients. Some readers of the paper, like the two referees, are sure to complain. It would be too bad if they did nothing but complain. For over four years I have tried to get oncologists in the United States to carry out some sort of trial of ascorbic acid in relation to cancer, without success. . . . I trust that publication of this study will stimulate some of them to make a trial of the sort that they like.
>
> Every month some 30,000 people die of cancer in the United States. If 10 per cent of them could be put back in good health by treatment with ascorbic acid, 3,000 lives would be saved per month. This thought makes me determined that this paper will be published with the minimum delay. If the National Academy of Sciences rejects it, it will be published somewhere else, just as our earlier paper, rejected by the National Academy, was published in *Oncology*. . .
>
> I am beginning to think that the attitude of oncologists toward new ideas is largely responsible for the fact that, despite the expenditure of billions of dollars during the last 20 years, there has been essentially no change in survival times of cancer patients. Your referees behave as though they do not want any change to be made. Instead of being interested in the possibility that a discovery has been made that might lead to significant improvement in the treatment of cancer, they strive to suppress the publication of our paper. You may never have looked at the leading cancer journals. A more depressing display of mediocrity and pedestrianism is hard to find. I feel that we have written a scientific paper, an interesting and important one, which should be published in a scientific journal. (Pauling to Sinsheimer, 13 August 1976)

If there was an acerbic edge to Pauling's criticism of conventional treatments and oncologists, it may be attributable to the fact that he now had even more of a personal stake in the credibility of the Vale of Leven trials. Four weeks earlier, Pauling's wife, Ava Helen Pauling, had been diagnosed as having stomach cancer and had undergone surgery. She had decided to refuse back-up radiotherapy or chemotherapy and was now on the high dose vitamin C regime of ten grams per day. This may well have sharpened Pauling's determination that Cameron's clinical findings should be brought more forcefully to the attention of the cancer establishment, and he stepped up his public and political campaign to this end.

4.6   PUBLICITY

While Sinsheimer deliberated over whether or not to publish the revised version of the manuscript and Pauling lobbied from behind the scenes, the contents of the paper had already received an airing in *New Scientist*, and the publicity ball was rolling. *Prevention*, the wide-circulation magazine of the alternative circuit in the United States, had 'pirated' the earlier papers from *Chemico-biological Interactions*, and made the Vale of Leven trials known to the American holistic health movement. But the *New Scientist* publicity was the first from a more conventionally-oriented popular science journal, and the greatly-increased survival times claimed for vitamin C-treated cancer patients attracted considerable attention. Pauling's public references to these favourable trial findings had been picked-up by a *New Scientist* journalist in connection with a proposed BBC programme on the vitamin C debate, and he had approached Cameron for more detailed information. In order to support their claims, Cameron had released the figures and some details of the new trial on the understanding that they would not be cited in the article. He was rather disconcerted when they were not only published, but also publicly dissected and criticised by two British cancer specialists, Richard Peto and Kurt Hellman (Hanlon, 1976). This was followed a few days later by the BBC broadcast which also discussed the Vale of Leven trials. Several British dailies including the *Guardian* followed suit, and Cameron was concerned that this burst of publicity might prejudice the publication of their paper. Pauling, having had a hand in it himself, was less perturbed: 'It [the publicity] would have had to come sooner or later' (14 July 1976).

In the event, Sinsheimer, after prolonged negotiations with Pauling and the two referees, finally decided to publish the contentious paper. It appeared, as Pauling had requested, 'with minimum delay' in the *PNAS* of October 1976, and sparked off a round of generally favourable publicity in the American press, notably in the *New York Times* and the *Washington Post* (Cameron and Pauling, 1976). *Prevention* also alerted the alternative network to the latest results from Vale of Leven, and the Institute's direct mailing programme for contributions towards continuing this promising line of research snowballed.

Things were now looking decidedly better for the Cameron-Pauling hypothesis, the Vale of Leven trials, and the Linus Pauling Institute. But Pauling was convinced they could be made even better. Even before the *PNAS* paper appeared, he pressed for a more thorough statistical analysis of the trial results which would resolve the criticism concerning the comparability of the ascorbate-treated patients and the control patients (27 August 1976). At the same time, in the light of the favourable publicity the trials had received, he and Robinson geared up for a major fund-raising effort ('perhaps running to a couple of million dollars over the next three years') for research on vitamin C and cancer. They were optimistic that a good part of this sum might come from the National Cancer Institute; and they lobbied politicians in Washington and NCI officials to this end. Pauling also undertook a heavy public lecturing schedule and made a number of appearances on radio and television in which he 'spread the gospel' (9 September 1976; 14 December 1976). Things were helped along considerably by the public statement from Dr Theodore Cooper, Assistant Secretary of the Department of Health, Education and Welfare (HEW), that he thought that megadoses of vitamin C were valuable in controlling both the common cold and malignant disease and that he himself took large doses (Pauling to Cameron, 14 December 1976).

4.7   A TIME OF OPTIMISM

Cameron was at first rather alarmed at the publicity generated by these activities and overwhelmed by the magnitude of the grant sought. But he was soon convinced that he too might become involved in the application for NCI grant money. After a visit from the Paulings in October, he enthusiastically joined in the preparation of a detailed submission to the NCI. This included a proposal for animal experiments at the Linus Pauling Institute, carefully designed prospective clinical trials as an extension of the Vale of Leven trials, and biochemical research on the role of ascorbate in altering the cell/matrix inter-relationships. He was also readily enough persuaded that more might be made of the existing Vale of Leven trial data and he began work on its revision for another paper.

As well, although Pauling failed in two attempts to breach the barriers of the prestigious *New England Journal of Medicine* with a short paper on 'Vitamin C and Cancer' (Ingelfinger to Pauling, 3 March,

1977, 8 June, 1977), he had finally managed to gain entry to one of the leading cancer journals. Dr Sidney Weinhouse, the editor of *Cancer Research* (also published on behalf of the American Cancer Society) had invited Pauling to submit a review article on vitamin C and cancer. Pauling and a graduate student, Brian Leibovitz, set to work on a paper summarizing the evidence for the rationale and efficacy of vitamin C in cancer treatment. Cameron, who by this stage was 'drowning in mail from cancer patients and their close relatives', was drawn in as senior author of this major analysis of over three hundred and fifty reports in the literature (Cameron *et al.*, 1979). By this stage, some further significant evidence had accumulated in favour of ascorbate's anti-cancer and immune-enhancing properties.

This included recent research to the effect that cancer patients generally exhibited diminished immunocompetence and that their lymphocytes (the circulating blood cells which maintain the immune mechanisms in the body) almost invariably had low ascorbate content (Yonemoto *et al.*, 1976). The implication of this finding for the Cameron-Pauling hypothesis was the 'common sense view' that lymphocytes rich in ascorbate should be able to conduct their protective business more efficiently than those that were not; therefore this constituted a sound theoretical argument for increasing the ascorbate intake of cancer patients (Cameron *et al.*, 1979). As well, it had been shown that ascorbate inhibited the carcinogenic effects of nitrosamines (the carcinogens formed from the processing of certain foods such as bacon and ham). Recent epidemiological studies of large population groups also supported the cancer-preventive role of foods rich in vitamin C (Bjelke, 1974). On the clinical side, there was further evidence of the role of ascorbate in retarding human bladder cancer (Schlegel, 1975). It had been reported also that ascorbate had induced some regression in familial colorectal polyposis (an inherited and well-recognized premalignant condition); ascorbate was now being recommended as a prophylactic measure for this condition (DeCosse *et al.*, 1975). Even more encouraging support for the Vale of Leven trial results had come from a recently concluded Japanese study, which compared the survival times of apparently terminal cancer patients who had been given varying doses of ascorbate, and which found that the death rate of the low-ascorbate-treated patients was about three times that of the high-ascorbate patients, a result that meshed with the Vale of Leven findings (Morishige and Murata, 1979; Cameron and Pauling, 1979a). These recent reports, together with the forthcoming *PNAS* paper, now comprised a substantial body of evidence in favour of vitamin C.

This favourable collective clinical and experimental evidence was further enhanced by vitamin C's 'unique advantage' relative to other remedies for cancer: its safety. It was, according to Pauling and Cameron 'almost completely safe and harmless even when given in sustained high doses for prolonged periods of time'. Its risks, as they had discussed them in their correspondence and previous publications, were 'acceptable'. These were: (a) a 'clinical suspicion' that, in the very rare patient with a very rapidly growing tumour existing at the very limits of nutritional support, the sudden exposure to high-dose vitamin C might precipitate widespread tumour haemorrhage and necrosis with real danger to the patient (for this reason they recommended that patients should *gradually* increase their intake of ascorbate to the appropriate level), (b) a 'much stronger suspicion' that the sudden discontinuation of an established regimen of ascorbate could produce a 'rebound effect' of a precipitous drop in tissue ascorbate and so reactivate the hitherto controlled neoplastic process (as, for instance, they thought had happened in the case of the truck driver who stopped his vitamin C), and (c) the 'theoretical but extremely remote' risk that a few susceptible patients might develop urinary oxalate stones (Cameron and Pauling, 1973; Cameron and Campbell, 1974; Cameron and Pauling, 1974; Cameron *et al.*, 1979). All of this added up to the need for extensive studies of ascorbic acid in cancer, of the kind for which Pauling and Cameron had applied for NCI support.

They now received some much-needed peer support from the Canadian researcher, Dr T. W. Anderson, who had himself recently directed two large-scale controlled clinical trials of vitamin C's effect on the common cold. In an article on 'New Horizons for Vitamin C' in *Nutrition Today*, Anderson wrote:

> The risk/benefit ratio relative to the severity of the disease as well as to other available treatments in cancer is so heavily weighted in favour of vitamin C in this situation that validation or refutation by other groups will presumably occur quite quickly. (Anderson, 1977)

This passage was now pressed into the service of the Pauling-Cameron rationale for large-scale ascorbate studies (Cameron *et al.*, 1979).

4.8   THE CONCLUSION OF THE SLOAN–KETTERING TRIAL

All of this optimistic and heady activity overshadowed Dr Charles Young's report from Sloan–Kettering that he had now given 23 patients an 'adequate trial' with high dose ascorbic acid with no obvious response (except for one patient where minimal therapeutic response had occurred) (Young to Pauling, 8 April 1976). In reply, Pauling referred Young to the forthcoming *PNAS* study. In addition, he pointed out that Young's patients had discontinued their ascorbate treatment after periods ranging from 5 to 64 days, whereas Cameron's patients took their vitamin C 'indefinitely'. He suggested that Young's patients might have experienced the above-described 'rebound effect', and that this might have permitted their cancers to develop more rapidly than otherwise (Pauling to Young, 24 August, 1976). Young responded courteously, but he did not pursue Pauling's suggestion and dropped his clinical investigations of vitamin C. Sloan–Kettering was now at the centre of the bitter controversy over laetrile, and in full retreat from its earlier liberal position on unorthodox cancer treatments (Moss, 1980).

The Sloan–Kettering study, limited as it was, foreshadowed the interpretative difficulties of the Mayo Clinic trials. In a number of significant ways, it served as a testing ground for the subsequent exchanges between Pauling and Cameron and the Mayo Clinic team.

5 The First Mayo Clinic Trial: Pauling's Head-On Collision with the Scientific Method?

No vitamin-C benefit found in Cancer trial.
Dr Linus Pauling's much publicized claim that vitamin C can prolong and improve the lives of terminal cancer patients has collided head-on with the scientific method.
Medical World News, 25 June 1979 (Anon. 1979b)

Mayo Study: Pauling Wrong on Vitamin C for Cancer
Post-Bulletin, Rochester, 12 September 1979 (McCracken, 1979)

Early in 1977, Pauling heard that the NCI grant application would not be approved, and he stepped up the pressure on Dr Vincent DeVita, then Director of the Division of Cancer Treatment, and subsequently Director of the NCI. He disputed the NCI evaluation of the Vale of Leven data as not being of sufficient scientific quality to warrant further investigation and funding. In particular, Pauling confronted a written assessment of the Cameron-Pauling *PNAS* study of 1976, made by Dr Brian J. Lewis, Special Assistant to DeVita. Lewis had criticized the study on a number of grounds, arguing that had the article been submitted to a 'more severely edited journal, it never would have been accepted for publication'. The study was not acceptably randomized, the determination of a patient's status as terminal was 'ill defined and unreproducible', and the authors' 'vague description of the initial antitumor therapy of the cancer patients before they were entered into the study . . . would make it impossible for any other workers in the field to do a comparable study.' Lewis concluded his report with the recommendation that:

[T]he authors have violated two of the most essential tenets of sound scientific research: they have made it impossible for the reader to

111

determine which variables were responsible for the longer survival of the treated group, and likewise their lack of specificity and consistency in the study design would frustrate any attempt to do a comparable experiment.　(Lewis, 1976)

Pauling did not agree. Lewis's statement, he wrote, had 'no basis in fact':

Inasmuch as in the paper by Cameron and Pauling evidence is presented that ascorbic acid in amount 10 grams per day has some effectiveness in controlling essentially all kinds of cancer, control experiments could be carried out by use of this amount of ascorbate with a randomly selected subgroup from a group of patients with one or another of the various kinds of cancer, with the remaining subgroup of patients serving as controls.

He urged DeVita to consider changing the funding strategies of the NCI so that a portion of grant money might be reserved for promising ideas that fell outside mainstream research.

It is my opinion, which has grown stronger and stronger during the past four years, that the use of ascorbic acid in controlling cancer may well turn out to be the most important discovery about cancer that has been made in the last quarter century. Ewan Cameron deserves the credit for having made this discovery. The National Cancer Institute has not contributed to it. (Pauling to DeVita, 5 January 1977)

The Pauling–Cameron grant application was not funded. But in the face of Pauling's continued representations and public criticism, DeVita approached 'one of our premier investigators', who agreed to undertake the proper double-blind controlled clinical trial. DeVita wrote that the NCI wanted to be sure that the trial met the criteria Pauling thought to be necessary for the effective use of vitamin C (DeVita to Pauling, 10 March 1977). In April Pauling visited the NCI and, in discussing the proposed trial with DeVita, he learned that the principal investigator was Dr Charles Moertel of the Mayo Clinic.

5.1　THE FIRST MAYO CLINIC TRIAL

On 28 April 1977, Pauling wrote to Moertel, giving details on dosage and tolerance and stressing that the trial should not be carried out with cancer patients whose immune systems had been damaged by radiation and chemotherapy:

There is evidence that ascorbic acid is effective against cancer largely through the potentiation of the immune mechanisms of the body. It is accordingly important and essential that a double-blind study not be carried out with patients whose immune systems have already been destroyed or seriously damaged by earlier courses of therapy. I emphasize that it is essential that the trial be made with patients with intact immune systems, and not with patients who have received large doses of high-energy radiation or cytotoxic drugs.

In addition, Pauling pointed out that the case of the truck driver, whose cancer had recurred when his vitamin C was temporarily discontinued, indicated that 'patients should continue with the oral dosage for an indefinite time. The cancer may return if the ascorbate is stopped' (Pauling to Moertel, 28 April 1977).

In reply, Moertel agreed that every effort should be made to duplicate the conditions which existed in Cameron's clinical trial, but that a randomized prospective study design would be employed rather that the historical controls in Cameron's trial. While in the main he thought that he and Pauling were in agreement on the methodology to be employed, he indicated some difference of opinion with Pauling over the patient group selection. He pointed out that it was possible that the salutary effect on survival claimed by Cameron in preterminal patients could have occurred through the restoration of immune processes previously depressed by the various modalities of cancer therapy to which they had been previously exposed. He quoted from the *PNAS* paper to the effect that patients selected for the Cameron study had been established as showing untreatability by such conventional standards as the establishment of inoperability at laparotomy or the abandonment of any definitive form of anti-cancer treatment. Moertel proposed to use these same criteria for selection of patients in the Mayo Clinic study (Moertel to Pauling, 6 May 1977). The inference to be drawn from this was that Cameron's patients had undergone conventional radiation treatment or chemotherapy, so that Pauling's insistence on choosing patients who had not been exposed to such treatments was misplaced.

In response, Pauling wrote of his 'impression' that there were significant differences between the treatment of patients in the United States and Scotland, where cytotoxic drugs were not employed to the same extent as in the United States (Pauling to Moertel, 10 May 1977).

Pauling's sudden insistence on the incompatability of cytotoxic chemotherapy and vitamin C treatment requires some explanation. Prior to this point, as we have seen, he and Cameron had promoted vitamin C as a standard supportive measure to reinforce established methods of treatment. Their published papers were consistent with this strategy, and contained no reference to any incompatability of vitamin C and standard cancer chemotherapy. In their personal correspondence, Cameron had as early as 1972 concluded that the combination of ascorbate and cytotoxic drugs was not very effective, and speculated that this might be because of the leucopenia (the low level of circulating white blood cells, especially the lymphocytes, which maintain the immunocompetence of the patient) induced by the cytotoxic drugs. But neither he nor Pauling had discussed the implications of this finding for Cameron's trials or the treatment of cancer patients generally.

It would appear that Pauling's recent discussions and exchanges with NCI officials had alerted him to the differences in conventional cancer practices between Scotland and the United States and their implications for any U.S. replication of Cameron's Vale of Leven work. As well, he and Cameron had recently given greater prominence to the role of ascorbate in stimulating the immune system and generally enhancing the patient's resistance to cancer. The review paper on vitamin C and cancer that they were currently writing for *Cancer Research* emphasized this aspect of ascorbate's role in cancer therapy, and was consistent with recent research on the low lymphocyte ascorbate content of cancer patients (Cameron *et al.*, 1979). To these reasons should be added Pauling's increasing exasperation with and scepticism of the official claims for the benefits of conventional cytotoxic chemotherapy, which are evident in his correspondence with NCI officials and Sinsheimer of the *PNAS*. By the late 70s, the War on Cancer was running into some harsh public and political criticism, and the official figures on cure rates were being forcefully challenged by critics such as science journalist Dan Greenberg (Greenberg, 1975, 1977). All of these factors, therefore, combined to reinforce Pauling's reiterated message to Moertel that a proper trial of vitamin C could only be carried out on patients who had not received prior immunodepressive chemotherapy.

Cameron initially welcomed the trial. He wrote, 'This is something we have needed for years and I am quite sure that [Moertel's] results will vindicate our claims' (23 May 1977). But he was soon sharing Pauling's concern:

> The point you make about ascorbate potentiating the immune system while cytotoxics depress it, is a very important one, and should be considered by the investigators before embarking on their trial. It seems possible to me that they could be embarking on an X – Y Zero situation, with any benefit from one regime cancelling out the other. (Cameron to Pauling, 13 August 1977)

At Pauling's prompting, Cameron also wrote to Moertel, explaining that the practice at Vale of Leven was to refer patients for whom radiotherapy or cytotoxic therapy was indicated to the Glasgow Regional Centre of Radiotherapy and Medical Oncology:

As a result our local clinical experience in the use of cytotoxic chemotherapy is really quite limited.

Cameron offered some further details about patient selection in the Vale
of Leven trials, and concluded by assuring Moertel that he would be
'delighted' to let him have any further information that he required from
Vale of Leven Hospital (Cameron to Moertel, 30 May 1977).

Moertel failed to respond to this invitation, and there matters stood
until August 1978, when Pauling was 'provided' by a correspondent with
a copy of the protocol for the Mayo Clinic trial. He was concerned to note
that there was no mention in the protocol of earlier chemotherapeutic
treatment as a contra-indication for patient elegibility, and again wrote
to Moertel reiterating his emphasis on this point:

> ... if you hope, as you stated in your letter, to repeat the work of
> Cameron as closely as possible, you should be careful to use only
> patients who have not received chemotherapy.

Pauling suggested that if the study was already underway and contained
patients who had received chemotherapy, then it would be valuable to
compare the progress of those patients who had received chemotherapy
alone with those who had received vitamin C alone, and those who
received vitamin C plus chemotherapy. Such a comparison would give
'interesting information about the value of chemotherapy itself and about
the interaction of chemotherapy and vitamin C' (Pauling to Moertel, 9
August 1978).

Moertel, however, was clearly not interested in making such comparisons, and persisted in perceiving vitamin C's most valuable potential
as adjuvant treatment (as indeed Cameron and Pauling had initially
represented it), not as a substitute for conventional treatment. He pointed
out the difficulty of selecting patients who had not been exposed to prior
chemotherapy, since chemotherapy was routine practice in the United
States. Moreover, Moertel did not think the problem to be crucial. He
reiterated his argument that if vitamin C did operate by potentiating
immune mechanisms, then it might be of greatest potential benefit for
patients whose immune mechanisms *had* been suppressed by chemotherapy. In any case, in a passage which was subsequently quoted by
Pauling in the pages of the *New England Journal of Medicine*, he assured
Pauling that in the analysis of the data, he and his colleagues would
distinguish between those patients who had received prior chemotherapy
and those who had not:

> Certainly in any presentation of this data I can assure you we will call
> attention to the fact that the majority of our patients had had prior

chemotherapy, whereas in the study conducted by you and Dr Cameron it was clearly stated that none of the patients had had prior chemotherapy. (Moertel to Pauling, 15 August 1978; Pauling, 1980)

Moertel also assured Pauling that patients would not have their vitamin C treatment interrupted, and informed him that the study should be completed within the next six months.

Pauling expressed his satisfaction with this reassurance, but within a few weeks was disconcerted to receive a press clipping from the *San Diego Union* of an interview with Dr Edward Creagan, one of the Mayo Clinic investigators. According to the report, all of the original participants in the study were dead and Creagan was 'cautiously pessimistic' about the value of vitamin C as a cancer treatment. The report also stated that the Mayo Clinic study of patients who had been 'treated extensively with surgery, radiation and chemotherapy' was 'duplicating the Pauling therapy administered at the Linus Pauling Institute' (Scarr, 1978).

Pauling wrote immediately to Moertel, alleging that the statements were 'damaging to me and to this Institute'. If the Mayo Clinic patients had received prior chemotherapy, it was 'not proper' to say that the study was a duplication of Cameron's work (20 October 1978).

Moertel quickly wrote an apologetic reply, assuring Pauling that many of the statements attributed to Creagan were taken out of context or were erroneous, and again offered the reassurance that the Mayo Clinic team was fully aware that only a small minority of the Vale of Leven patients had received chemotherapy. He could not provide any details on patients until the code was broken at the completion of the trial in about six months time. Until then the study remained blinded and no conclusions could be drawn (Moertel to Pauling, 27 October 1978).

Enough had been said to alert Pauling to the likelihood of a negative result. Even before he had received the results of the trial from Moertel, he publicly predicted that the trial would not settle the issue, because it was not a replication of Cameron's study (Shurkin, 1979). In the meantime, he worked to strengthen the credibility of the Vale of Leven studies. Apart from their forthcoming review article in *Cancer Research*, he and Cameron had finally completed their revision of the comparison of ascorbate and non-ascorbate treated patients at Vale of Leven, and this was published (but 'only after the statutory hassle' with highly critical referees, Cameron to Pauling, 24 June 1978), in the *PNAS*, September, 1978.

The original group of 100 ascorbate-treated patients had been revised to exclude those patients with unusual cancers for whom it was difficult to find matching controls, and other patients randomly selected from the hospital records had been substituted in their stead. In addition, a new group of 1000 controls was randomly selected, as data on some of the initial control patients were discovered to be unreliable and incomplete. Most of the new controls, though, were drawn from the original control population (Cameron to Pauling, 11 March 1977; 27 November 1977). In order to overcome the earlier criticism, this revised and updated analysis measured survival times not only from the date of 'untreatability', but also from the date of first hospital attendance for the condition. It gave even more encouraging results than the previous *PNAS* study:

> The ascorbate-treated patients were found to have a mean survival time about 300 days greater than that of the controls. Survival times greater than 1 year after the date of untreatability were observed for 22 per cent of the ascorbate-treated patients and for 0.4 per cent of the controls.

Moreover, eight of the ascorbate-treated patients were still alive some 3.5 years after untreatability (Cameron and Pauling, 1978b).

The *PNAS*, having again lost the 'statutory' publication battle with Pauling, dampened the impact of the publication of such promising results by juxtaposing a critical statement by Dr Julius H. Comroe (a member of the Editorial Board), to the effect that the study was not based on 'well-established rules for clinical investigation'. Comroe urged the need for a 'well-designed' double-blind, randomised, prospective controlled study which would 'confirm or disprove' the observations reported by Cameron and Pauling (Comroe, 1978). Pauling immediately dispatched a response to Comroe, signing it with both his and Cameron's names. He referred to the forthcoming Mayo Clinic study, but, with a sideswipe at the National Cancer Institute, pointed to the difficulties he and Cameron had experienced in obtaining grant money or arousing official interest in the need for just such a study. They had been forced, wrote Pauling, with the limited resources available to them, to get as much information as possible out of the Vale of Leven case histories (Cameron and Pauling, 1978c).

If they had not yet managed to secure a scientific and medical audience for their views, it was clear from the daily volume of mail and telephone calls that came their way that Pauling and Cameron had succeeded in reaching a large and far-flung popular audience. At the close of 1977, Cameron had estimated that 'many thousands of cancer patients in very many countries are now ingesting supplemental ascorbate, and from the self-selected return correspondence arriving here, a significant proportion of them are deriving benefit' (Cameron to Pauling, 19 December 1977). Towards the end of 1978, Cameron took a year's leave of absence from Vale of Leven and took up the post of Visiting Research Professor at the Linus Pauling Institute, primarily to work full-time with Pauling on a popular book on vitamin C and cancer, which would make the Cameron–Pauling hypothesis and the Vale of Leven data more accessible to cancer patients and their relatives.

It was at this point that the schism between Pauling and Robinson became public. A year earlier, an article in *New Scientist* by Farooq Hussain had suggested that all was not well at the Linus Pauling Institute. Hussain had alleged a good deal of internal dissension and, among other things, implied that Robinson was an inept administrator and was mismanaging federal funds (Hussain, 1977). After Pauling and those involved had threatened litigation, *New Scientist* published Pauling's and Robinson's lengthy rebuttals. For a time, these quelled adverse publicity. But behind the scenes the tensions between Pauling and Robinson mounted, and on 15 August 1978, the Board of Trustees voted to install Pauling as President in Robinson's stead. In November, Robinson brought suit against Pauling and the Institute, and the breach became public knowledge. This was followed by Robinson's public allegations of fraud in Pauling's conduct of the mouse experiment (Grant, 1979; Robinson, 1979; Carroll, 1979).

At the height of his confrontation with Robinson, Pauling received word from Moertel that the Mayo trial had failed to demonstrate any evidence of therapeutic benefit from vitamin C. Of 123 patients enrolled in the study, 60 had received vitamin C (10 grams orally per day), and 63 placebo. There had been no significant difference in symptomatic improvement between the two treatment groups. As he and Pauling had previously agreed in correspondence, Moertel wrote that he and his co-workers intended to emphasize the fact that the overwhelming majority of these patients had been subjected to previous cytotoxic drug and/or irradiation therapy. Only five of the patients assigned to vitamin C had not been previously treated with these modalities. The study could therefore in no way be interpreted as representing results that might be obtained in patients not previously exposed to immunosuppressive treatments. Conclusions could only be drawn regarding the specific population of patients that had been tested (Moertel to Pauling, 26 April, 1979).

Pauling initially was not too perturbed at the news. After all, he had more or less predicted such an outcome. He wrote a memo to Cameron stating that the result was consistent with their theoretical views and clinical expectations:

> I think that the conclusion to be drawn from this result, together with your observations, is that cytotoxic chemotherapy destroys the immune system to such an extent as to prevent ascorbate from being effective by potentiating this system.   (Memo, Pauling to Cameron, 7 May 1979)

He suggested that Cameron should carry out a detailed analysis of the Vale of Leven data to determine whether they supported this conclusion.

The information would be important in connection with their forth-coming book, because it would be necessary to make a decision as to how strong their statements should be about cytotoxic chemotherapy in relation to ascorbate therapy. Cameron agreed, but confessed 'I am still puzzled that Dr Moertel could show no effect in his test patients'. Until they received the full details of the trial it would not be possible to draw conclusions. Chemotherapy could have been stopped in the trial patients either because of bone marrow exhaustion, or because of a positive clinical decision that it was failing to do any good. Those patients in the latter category might be expected to show some response to ascorbate (Memo, Cameron to Pauling, 16 May 1979).

Pauling did become seriously disturbed when, following on the public presentation of the Mayo trial results to a joint meeting of the American Society of Clinical Oncology and the American Association for Cancer Research, *Medical World News* ran a report headed 'No vitamin-C benefit found in Ca trial. Dr Linus Pauling's much-publicized claim that vita-min C can prolong and improve the lives of terminal cancer patients has collided head-on with the scientific method' (Anon., 1979b). Although the report cited Pauling's claim that the Mayo study was not a replication of Cameron's work, it dealt with it dismissively, quoting Moertel to the effect that although the majority of the patients in the Mayo study had received prior chemotherapy, 'they were all capable of an immune response'.

On 12 September, Pauling finally received the long-awaited pre-publication copy of the Mayo study, and was utterly disconcerted to discover that it was headed (in his opinion, misleadingly), 'Failure of High-Dose Vitamin C (Ascorbic Acid) Therapy to Benefit Patients with Advanced Cancer'. Worse, from Pauling's point of view, the all-important abstract made no mention of the fact that the patient population was not comparable to that of the Vale of Leven trials. And, in the body of the text, it was asserted that 50 per cent of the Vale of Leven ascorbate-treated patients had 'previously received irradiation and chemotherapy'. In their discussion of the trial results, the Mayo Clinic team used this to dispute Pauling's argument that prior chemo-therapy might have obscured any benefit provided by vitamin C:

It is ... impossible to draw any conclusions about the possible effectiveness of vitamin C in previously untreated patients. ... Since vitamin C may have an impact on host resistance to can-cer, we recognize that earlier immuno-suppressive treatment might have obscured any benefit provided by this agent. Nevertheless, the non-randomized study [Cameron and Pauling, 1976] that showed a fourfold enhancement of survival with vitamin C included patients who had received conventional cancer treatment (i.e., cytotoxic agents and radiation therapy). This improvement could not be substantiated by our study.

The implication was that the Mayo Clinic trial had indeed replicated and undermined the Vale of Leven studies. Creagan, Moertel, and their co-researchers went on to finish the job by undercutting the Cameron-inspired strategy of presenting vitamin C as a standard supportive measure to reinforce established modes of cancer treatment:

> One might expect . . . that vitamin C would exert some restorative influence in patients whose immune apparatus has been compromised by earlier treatment efforts. If such an effect did occur in our patients, it was not seen in their clinical improvement. We cannot recommend the use of high-dose vitamin C in patients with advanced cancer who have previously received irradiation or chemotherapy.   (Creagan *et al.*, 1979)

In effect, as such treatment was routine in the United States, this meant that vitamin C was useless for cancer patients.

After a hurried study of the paper, Pauling and Cameron immediately telephoned Moertel. According to Pauling's memorandum of this telephone conversation, Moertel agreed to contact the *New England Journal of Medicine* (where the paper was to be published), requesting that a 'correction' be made to the statement that 50 per cent of the Vale of Leven ascorbate patients had received prior chemotherapy. As Pauling now explicitly informed him, only 4 per cent of the patients had been so treated (Pauling, Memo, 12 August 1979). However, when Moertel contacted the *Journal*, he was informed that the paper was too far along in the printing process to allow such a correction to be made. He assured Pauling that every effort would be made to publish a correcting statement at the earliest possible time (Moertel to Pauling, 18 September 1979; telephone conversation, 21 September 1979).

With this assurance Pauling set about counteracting the mounting adverse international publicity with a news release from the Institute, and by writing personal rebuttals to the more important newspapers, including the *New York Times*, the *Washington Post*, and the *Wall Street Journal*. But the damage had already been done, and the Mayo Clinic negative results were now being linked with the Robinson allegations (Carroll, 1979). Matters were exacerbated by the refusal of the *New England Journal of Medicine* to publish the promised correction by the Mayo Clinic team (Moertel to Pauling, 16 October 1979). It was argued that the publication of such a letter from those who had conducted the experiment did not conform with *Journal* policy, and that the information should be conveyed by Pauling himself in the standard form of a letter to the editor. This Pauling categorically refused to do, asserting that the onus was on the Moertel team to correct their 'serious error' (Pauling to Relman, 7 November 1979). He and Arnold Relman (editor of the *Journal*) remained locked in conflict until the intervention of Pauling's long-term friend, Dr Arthur Sackler, editor of the *International Medical Tribune* (Sackler to Relman, 16 October 1979; Pauling to Sackler, 19 October 1979). Finally, Relman wrote Pauling to state that the letter from Moertel addressing Pauling's assertion of inaccuracy would appear in the next issue of the *Journal* (Relman to Pauling, 14 December 1979).

Up to this point, relations between Pauling and Moertel had been reasonably cordial. Although they could not reach agreement about the conduct of the trial, they had courteously negotiated their differences. Moertel had responded to Pauling's requests for information, and Pauling had scrupulously refrained from making public statements based on the trial preprint until it had been published. At Pauling's insistence, Moertel had made the attempt to correct the 'error' in their paper. But now their relations took a marked turn for the worse, and their exchanges were no longer politely negotiated in personal correspondence, but acrimoniously conducted in the pages of the *New England Journal of Medicine*.

One of the precipitating factors was a report in the *Post-Bulletin*, Rochester (home town of the Mayo Clinic), headed 'Mayo Study: Pauling Wrong on Vitamin C for Cancer' (McCracken, 1979). Pauling insisted on an article of correction and the publication of a clarifying letter from himself, threatening a libel suit if the newspaper did not comply. But neither Pauling nor Moertel was satisfied with these when they were published. Pauling considered that the paper had taken only enough action to protect itself against litigation, while Moertel was annoyed by Pauling's implication that Moertel had applied to Pauling for guidance in setting up the protocol for the trial, and that Moertel 'chose to ignore [Pauling's] advice' against including patients who had previously received chemotherapy in the Mayo study (Moertel to Pauling, 16 October 1979; Pauling to Moertel, 19 October 1979).

There can be little doubt that Moertel was becoming exasperated by Pauling's persistence with what Moertel was shortly to denigrate publicly as a 'valid' but 'scientifically trivial' point (Jacobs, 1980). Equally clearly, the point for Pauling was far from trivial, and was of crucial significance to the defence of his and Cameron's claims. Moreover, Pauling was by now seriously worried about media coverage of the Mayo trial and its possible impact on the fund-raising activities of the Institute. Cameron, who had recently returned to Vale of Leven Hospital where he was pursuing his vitamin C research alongside his routine surgical work, wrote to Pauling that media reports on Moertel's 'uncorrected paper' had 'done a great deal of harm' to cancer patients, who might discontinue their vitamin C. Cameron also was of the opinion that the adverse publicity had cost him a substantial research grant for his vitamin C work (Cameron to Pauling, 14 November 1979).

Relations deteriorated further when the promised letter by Moertel and Creagan finally appeared in the *New England Journal of Medicine*. This gave the information insisted upon by Pauling, but followed it up with a forcefully expressed rebuttal of the Pauling interpretation:

> We must of course stand by our conclusion that high-dose vitamin C is of no value in patients who have been treated in a conventional manner according to accepted standards of cancer management in the United States today. Any contention that previous chemotherapy prevented our patients from achieving the extraordinary survival increase claimed by Drs. Cameron and Pauling must be considered highly speculative at best. Our patients were entered into the study only when they were well past any acute immuno-suppressive effects of previous therapy.
>
> On the basis of available evidence, we do not consider it conscionable to withhold oncologic therapy of known value to give the cancer patient large amounts of vitamin C. Any claims of benefit from high-dose vitamin C at any stage of malignant disease remain to be established by properly designed prospective, randomized, and concurrently controlled studies. We hope that Drs. Pauling and Cameron will agree that such scientifically acceptable evidence should be obtained before this treatment is publicly advocated for clinical use. (Creagan and Moertel, 1979)

This managed to cast doubt on the methodological adequacy and credibility of the Vale of Leven trials (a sensitive issue in the context of the Robinson allegations), and on the ethics of Pauling and Cameron for promoting a scientifically unproven cancer treatment. Their book, *Cancer and Vitamin C* had just been published, and, in spite of the Mayo Clinic trial, was selling well (Cameron and Pauling, 1979b). But, more important, this published letter by Moertel and Creagan firmly categorized vitamin C as an unorthodox treatment. The Mayo Clinic trial had scientifically established that vitamin C was of no value in conjunction with conventional cancer treatments, and this relegated it to the province of those who rejected professionally accredited treatments of 'known value' and opted for scientifically questionable alternatives.

From this point on, relations degenerated to what the science journalist Paul Jacobs was shortly to describe as a 'running feud' (Jacobs, 1980). The next letter published in the *New England Journal of Medicine* was by Cameron, who pushed a line of his own by arguing that the results of the trial were consistent with surreptitious ingestion of the readily available vitamin C by the controls, who were participating in the study with their informed consent (Cameron, 1980). This was rebutted in the same issue by Moertel and Creagan, who stated that they had randomly checked ascorbate levels in urine samples, and that these indicated a high level of patient compliance with the trial protocol. At the same time they took the further step of defending their patients against Cameron's implied slur on their integrity:

> We do not think that it is naive to trust in the sincerity of their altruism or in the honesty of their replies to our regular inquiries regarding compliance. (Creagan and Moertel, 1980)

Pauling's letter, when it eventually appeared on 20 March 1980, contained excerpts from his correspondence with Moertel in demonstration of his claim that he had alerted Moertel to the problem of the incompatability of vitamin C treatment and chemotherapy even before the Mayo Clinic trial was organized. Pauling now alleged that the Mayo Clinic team had 'misrepresented' the Vale of Leven studies and had not refuted Cameron's findings. The implication was that Moertel's professional ethics were questionable. He had not stood by his assurance to Pauling that he would 'call attention' to the crucial distinction between his and Cameron's patients, and had published a 'misleading' report (Pauling, 1980). Once more, Moertel and Creagan were given the right of reply alongside Pauling's letter, and strongly defended the morality of their position. They asserted that by publishing their subsequent 'statement of clarification' of this scientifically 'trivial' point in the *Journal* they had adequately discharged their 'voluntarily assumed obligation' to Pauling. The one whose ethics were questionable was Pauling who persisted in promoting an unproven cancer treatment, and Moertel and Creagan publicly exhorted him to behave more responsibly:

> Overshadowing such minor quibbling is the major obligation that both we and Dr Pauling must assume to cancer patients and the general public. On the basis of claims derived from speculation and non-randomized studies endorsed by the Pauling name, megadoses of vitamin C are being used by thousands of patients with cancer, and such treatment has been embraced by the metabolic-therapy cults. Our randomized double-blind study indicates that for at least one segment of the population of cancer patients, such treatment is of no value.
> The name of Dr Pauling is one of the most revered in American science, and rightly so. We hope very much that Dr Pauling will join with us in discouraging patients with cancer from using high-dose vitamin C or any other cancer treatment unless it has been proved to be of value by properly designed scientific study. (Moertel and Creagan, 1980)

Behind the scenes, Pauling in vain protested Relman's 'unfair' policy in permitting Moertel the 'first and last word', alleging a lack of symmetry in the *Journal*'s treatment of the Mayo Clinic and the Linus Pauling Institute:

[I]n each case the Mayo Clinic publications will have been made without our having had the opportunity to see them first, and our publications will have been examined beforehand by the Mayo Clinic. (Pauling to Relman, 22 February 1980)

His reiterated complaints finally evoked an exasperated four page response from Relman who structured the situation as follows: Pauling had attacked Moertel who had published a paper in the *Journal*, and the *Journal* had simply allowed Moertel to defend himself. And that was the end of the matter, as far as Relman was concerned (Relman to Pauling, 14 March, 1980).

5.2   THE SECOND MAYO CLINIC TRIAL IS ANNOUNCED

But Pauling, on this occasion, *did* have the last word. A week after the final exchange between Pauling and Moertel in the *New England Journal of Medicine*, it was officially announced that another NCI-funded trial of vitamin C would be undertaken by Moertel at the Mayo Clinic, this time involving patients who had not had prior chemotherapy or radiotherapy (Jacobs, 1980).

Even before the Mayo study had been published, Pauling had begun the campaign for another NCI-sponsored trial which would replicate the conditions of Cameron's Vale of Leven studies. He pressured Vincent DeVita and other senior NCI officials, urging on them vitamin C's non-toxicity, cheapness and other potential benefits. To DeVita's objections that it was very difficult to ethically justify using ascorbic acid before more effective chemotherapy, he counterposed Moertel's own recently published assessment of the inefficacy of the conventional chemotherapy of gastro-intestinal cancers (Pauling to DeVita, 24 September 1979; 23 November 1979). Pauling also made the point that vitamin C had been shown to increase the synthesis of interferon under antigenic stimulation, and that it offered a 'very inexpensive' alternative to interferon, currently undergoing evaluation by the NCI at a reported cost of sixty to seventy thousand dollars per patient (Pauling to Macdonald, 7 January 1980).

But Pauling's most effective tactic was the recruitment of a number of members of Congress, including President Jimmy Carter himself, to these eventually successful negotiations. At this stage the NCI was under some pressure from the Senate Subcommittee on Nutrition, headed by

Senator George McGovern, to initiate research on the link between diet and cancer, and was therefore vulnerable to political criticism on this particularly sensitive issue (Broad, 1979).

Cameron, however, was less than enthusiastic about the announcement of the new Mayo Clinic trial. He wrote to Pauling that he could see 'endless pitfalls ahead in our joint struggle to establish the truth'. He thought it would be good if he and Pauling could 'establish some early control and cooperation' in this forthcoming Moertel trial. For one thing he was doubtful about Moertel's scientific integrity. He had not kept his earlier promises to Pauling in publishing his results of the first trial. His research methods were 'sloppy' – he had clearly not read the earlier published papers by Cameron and Pauling, or he could not have stated that fifty per cent of the Vale of Leven ascorbate-treated patients had previously received irradiation and chemotherapy. He had only reluctantly and incompletely corrected this mistake in the *New England Journal of Medicine*. Nor could Cameron believe Moertel's statement in the *Journal* that 24-hour urine specimens from advanced cancer patients in their trial group contained 'very high levels of ascorbate'. This contradicted all Cameron's own experience and published reports. With reluctance, Cameron had to conclude that Moertel was not a 'reliable independent investigator', but was the protector of an 'established cancer industry', determined to discredit what he regarded as a 'transient irritation of quackery'.

Another problem that Cameron foresaw was the compliance of the Mayo Clinic patients. In contradiction of Moertel, Cameron thought that the Mayo Clinic team had been naive to trust in the altruism of dying cancer patients who would comply with the trial protocol 'in the hope that they [by dying] could contribute knowledge of value to others'. There were few such 'saints' in the real world, in Rochester or anywhere else. Regular, accurate tests must be incorporated in the protocol of the new trial in order to ensure that the test patients were actually taking their ascorbate and that the controls were *not* taking self-prescribed ascorbate. Cameron's own experience indicated that blood estimations were more accurate than 24-hour urine samples, because of the high retention of ascorbate by cancer patients and the rapid deterioration of urinary ascorbate.

To sum up, it would be much better if he and Pauling 'could possibly become involved at the pre-trial planning stage, rather than be asked to give comments just a few days before the findings were due to be published.' Cameron would be pleased to make a journey to the Mayo Clinic, if Pauling thought it would be of any help (Cameron to Pauling, 20 April 1980).

Pauling, who had checked off Cameron's points as he read them, wrote forthwith to Moertel, informing him, that if Moertel agreed, Cameron would come to the Mayo Clinic to discuss the plans for the second clinical trial:

> He and I believe that it is important that your second clinical trial provide a significant check on the Vale of Leven studies, and there are many questions in connection with it that could profitably be discussed by him with you.

Pauling also pointedly asked for detailed information on how the ascorbate levels in urine specimens from the patients in the first trial had been tested, and for copies of the results that were obtained (Pauling to Moertel, 12 May 1980).

Moertel did not respond to this offer of collaboration, nor to Pauling's request for information. And there matters rested for the time being.

In spite of the unfavourable publicity following on Arthur Robinson's allegations against Pauling and the negative results of the first Mayo Clinic trial, *Cancer and Vitamin C* continued to sell well, and Cameron continued to be inundated with transatlantic calls from those seeking further information about vitamin C therapy. In an effort to generate more political support, one thousand complimentary copies of the book were distributed to all members of Congress and to senior government officials in health-related areas. As well, a $40,000 donation to the Institute from the wealthy Japanese industrialist, Ryoichi Sasakawa, permitted the distribution of about fifteen thousand copies to American physicians. In the Institute *Newsletter*, Pauling reassured donors that the Mayo Clinic trial had not invalidated the Vale of Leven trial results, but that, on the contrary, its negative results confirmed his and Cameron's hypothesis about the mechanism of action of vitamin C:

> The Mayo Clinic study seems to have answered an important question. Dr Cameron and Dr Pauling have pointed out that chemotherapy badly damages the body's natural protective mechanisms, especially the immune system, and that, inasmuch as vitamin C is effective against cancer largely by potentiating these mechanisms, patients who have been treated with chemotherapy probably would not respond well to treatment with vitamin C, but Dr Cameron and Dr Pauling did not have reliable information as to how great this effect would be. The Mayo Clinic study seems to show that patients who have received treatment with chemotherapy respond very poorly to subsequent vitamin C therapy. (Pauling, 1979)

The administration of the Institute was stabilized with the election of Dr Emile Zuckerkandl to the joint positions of President and Director. But the Institute was still faced with the heavy financial costs of defending itself and senior personnel against the suits brought by Robinson. As well, Pauling's differences with Robinson were delaying publication of the results of their earlier mouse experiments, the extension and funding of which Pauling was still pursuing with the National Cancer Institute.

5.3 PAULING, MOERTEL, AND THE LAETRILE CONTROVERSY

Since government funding for orthomolecular research was not forth-coming, Pauling was moving into closer alliance with the alternative health movement and its sponsors. He went on a number of fundraising trips, including one to Japan where he met with the above-mentioned Sasakawa and caused a run on vitamin C in Tokyo pharmacies. He was a featured speaker at an international alternative medical conference in New York, 'Cancer Dialogue '80'. This was sponsored by a coalition of holistic health interests: the Omega Institute (a holistic medical education centre in the Berkshires), the American College of Preventive Medicine, and the American Holistic Medical Association, and was an attempt to establish dialogue between orthodox and unorthodox cancer researchers. It was Pauling's intention to engage some of the leaders in the cancer field in an 'open discussion of the reluctance of the cancer establishment to become interested in the question of how valuable large doses of vitamin C, used either with or without conventional therapy, would be in the treatment of patients with cancer'. However, his intention was frustrated when Frank Rauscher (Senior Vice-President of the American Cancer Society and former Director of the NCI), and a number of other senior cancer researchers and administrators withdrew from the proposed 'Dialogue', allegedly under pressure from the American Cancer Society, on the grounds that the controversial drug laetrile would be prominently discussed at the four-day meeting (Treaster, 1980).

Laetrile, a compound extracted from apricot kernels, had been at the centre of a fierce conflict over its 'vitamin' status and anti-cancer properties since the early 1970s. Amidst charges and countercharges of 'quackery', 'prejudice' and 'suppression', laetrilists and the cancer establishment had battled it out in the courts, state legislatures, and the media. By the mid-70s, an estimated 70,000 people had used laetrile for cancer treatment, it had been legalized in some seventeen states, and public interest in the drug was still growing. The NCI, under heavy public and media pressure, finally undertook a 'retrospective review' of documented case histories of patients claiming objective responses to laetrile (Ellison *et al.*, 1978). Pauling had never been a proponent of laetrile as a cancer treatment, having heretofore resisted attempts by the laetrilists to enrol him publicly in its defence. In their book *Cancer and Vitamin C*, he and Cameron had dismissed it as having but 'little value', and had advised cancer patients against its use. But Pauling was necessarily involved in the laetrile controversy, partly because of his role of prestigious defender of holistic medicine, but more because of the fact that the so-called 'laetrile treatment' was usually combined with a vegetarian diet and vitamin and mineral therapy, including large doses of vitamin C. It was Pauling's opinion that the perceived benefits of the 'laetrile treatment' in improving the health and wellbeing of the patient were more attributable to vitamin C megadose than to the laetrile (Cameron and Pauling, 1979b).

Charles Moertel had also been heavily involved in the laetrile controversy since 1978 when, in his role of leading advocate of the double-blind, randomized clinical trial, he had called for a 'properly designed, tightly controlled clinical trial' of laetrile in the pages of the *New England Journal of Medicine*. Moertel had argued that the exposure of 'hundreds of thousands' of desperate cancer patients to this drug 'of unknown effectiveness, unknown safety and poor manufacturing quality', could not be effectively challenged by the 'case-history-review type of study' proposed by the National Cancer Institute:

> It is foolhardy to deny that Laetrile is a dominant unresolved problem for American medicine today. It is naive to take the attitude that this problem will somehow go away if we simply ignore it. The image of the physician in the eyes of the American public will scarcely be enhanced if we stand imperiously on our ivory towers while they wallow in the mire of uncontrolled quackery. The Laetrile problem can only be successfully combated if we fight on familiar grounds, using the tools that we have known to be most trustworthy: a tightly controlled clinical trial performed in competent and experienced hands (Moertel, 1978a).

As Moertel had predicted, the NCI-organized retrospective analysis of laetrile treatment was inconclusive. Only 93 cases were submitted for evaluation; 26 were rejected because of incomplete data; and the remaining 67 cases gave no clear-cut evidence of effectiveness when reviewed by an independent team of twelve clinical oncologists (Ellison *et al.*, 1978). So in September 1978, the NCI announced plans to test laetrile in cancer patients. It was decided to use the 'same systematic approach for laetrile as that used to evaluate and document the efficacy of all currently available anti-cancer drugs.' Under the direction of Moertel, a multi-institutional team of investigators designed a protocol patterned after laetrile usage in Mexico and the U.S. The protocol combined laetrile with the 'metabolic therapy' programme indicated above, which contained megadoses of vitamin C. The FDA granted NCI approval to conduct three clinical trials: (1) a limited pharmacology/toxology study of laetrile, (2) a study to test the efficacy of laetrile as an anti-cancer agent, and (3) a study to test laetrile's effects on cancer symptoms, such as relief of pain, increase of well-being, weight gain, and prolonged survival (NCI, 1981). This third and final study was never carried out.

After the initial pharmacology/toxicology test had indicated that it was safe to proceed to the second stage of testing, the multi-centre trial to test the efficacy of laetrile as an anti-cancer drug began in July 1980. On 30 April 1981, Moertel presented a well-publicised paper at a meeting of the American Society of Clinical Oncology, in which he announced: 'Laetrile has been tested. It is not effective'. Moertel's report was featured in leading US papers, including the *New York Times* and the *Washington Post*, and Pauling re-entered the fray. He immediately reopened his correspondence with Moertel, asking him for a copy of the paper on which his public statement had been based. 'I am, of course,' he concluded pointedly, 'especially interested in knowing about the controls' (Pauling to Moertel, 8 May 1981).

Two weeks later, Pauling was able to determine from a more detailed discussion of the trial in *Science* that the study had been uncontrolled (Sun, 1981b). Of the 156 patients analysed, only one patient showed a transient partial reduction in tumour size. Only twenty per cent of the patients were alive after eight months, and of these five were 'stable'. One fifth of the patients claimed some improvement in subjective symptoms, but Moertel was quoted as stating that 'placebo trials achieve similar results', a statement heavily underscored by Pauling in his copy of *Science*. Pauling also underscored that section of the article which dealt with the special group of fourteen patients who had received 'even larger amounts of Laetrile and huge doses of vitamins', and Moertel's comment that even at such doses, laetrile [and the vitamins] appeared to be 'inactive' against cancer.

On 26 May 1981, Pauling again wrote to Moertel, this time, somewhat heavy-handedly, throwing down the gauntlet. He requested a copy of the paper in which he assumed that Moertel, 'in accordance with accepted scientific practice', had presented the detailed results of the patients and their control group:

> I am interested in making a proper statistical analysis of your study. . . . I want also to check your statement that Laetrile at higher doses together with huge doses of vitamins appears to be inactive.

On the basis of the information given in the *Science* article, Pauling calculated for Moertel's benefit the 'high statistical significance' of the difference in survival rates for the two groups studied, i.e., those given smaller amounts of laetrile in addition to a special diet of fresh fruit and vegetables did not appear to have done so well as those given larger amounts of laetrile in combination with vitamin megadoses:

It is accordingly not justified to state that Laetrile plus huge doses of vitamins is ineffective. I, on the basis of other studies, would anticipate that the huge doses of vitamins would be effective.

This provocative letter elicited a response from Moertel, but no copy of the requested paper. Moertel wrote that according to accepted scientific practice, he and his co-researchers had presented a progress report of an ongoing study. They would prepare a definitive manuscript only when all their observations had been completed. The trial had been carried out in accordance with accepted scientific means of drug evaluation as a Phase II study. If any reasonable evidence of therapeutic activity was obtained, a randomized controlled double-blind study of laetrile would be undertaken (Moertel to Pauling, 29 May 1981).

On 10 July, Pauling, having just returned from an overseas trip, caught up on his correspondence by firing off three separate letters to Moertel, gathering force as he proceeded. He cited what he had gleaned from various newspaper reports and pressured Moertel for detailed information on the trial. He did not think it 'proper' for Moertel to write to him that he must wait 'for perhaps a year' until his paper was published. In another letter, Pauling made it clear that he was 'not interested in laetrile', but in the 'possible value of vitamins, fresh fruits, and vegetables':

I know that you have made statements to the effect that investigations that are not prospective randomized double-blind controlled studies are completely unreliable, and accordingly I am asking for details about the laetrile study on which you have commented publicly.

For good measure, Pauling had also complained to DeVita at the NCI of Moertel's 'irresponsible statements' about the laetrile trial, suggesting that the NCI should 'look into the matter':

[I]t is rarely possible from a study of this sort to make the flat statement that one treatment is not effective, in comparison with another. Instead, some statement about statistical significance of the observations needs to be presented. . . . Dr Moertel's own statements about the subgroup that received huge doses of vitamins (as well as increased amounts of Laetrile) . . . not benefit[ing] from the treatment seem to be incorrect.   (Pauling to DeVita, 26 May 1981)

DeVita delegated responsibility for responding to Pauling's complaint to Dr Jane E. Henney (Special Assistant for Clinical Affairs, Division of Cancer Treatment). Dr Henney confirmed to Pauling that the trial had been uncontrolled in accordance with the standard procedure of Phase II studies supported by the NCI. The study was therefore endorsed by the NCI, as failing to confirm the claims of the laetrile advocates about the efficacy of laetrile when it was tested in humans using the same methodology that had been employed to identify effective antitumour agents (Henney to Pauling, 9 June 1981).

In July Pauling wrote to Henney, pulling out all the stops. He stated that Moertel had refused to send him the detailed report of the study. Under the Freedom of Information Act, he demanded the 'complete information about the tests in humans using the same methodology that has been employed to identify effective antitumor agents' (Pauling to Henney, 17 July 1981). On the same day, Moertel wrote again to Pauling, reiterating his claim that there was no prepared manuscript on the laetrile study, but that once the data collection had been finalized, he would be happy to make it available to Pauling at the same time it was made available to the scientific community at large. In the meantime, he offered a few details on patient selection and the metabolic therapy programme used in the study, including the information that the patients in the high dose category had been given the standard Vale of Leven dose of 10 grams per day of vitamin C (Moertel to Pauling, 17 July 1981). This, however, did not satisfy Pauling, and he continued to press Moertel and the NCI for more detailed information, citing the contradictions in press reports. He impatiently rejected Moertel's judgment that their differences were philosophical and unresolvable, keeping doggedly to the point at issue:

In your letter you say that we have a philosophic disagreement on the level of evidence required to decide that a cancer treatment programme has sufficient evidence of effectiveness to justify further study. This is not what I am interested in now. I am interested, instead, on the extent to which the statements that you made were justified by the observations.   (Pauling to Moertel, 31 July 1981)

The pattern of their exchanges was set. Their correspondence had now lost all veneer of politeness. Pauling's demands and criticisms were couched ever more bluntly. More often than not, Moertel failed to answer, or he responded with a few lines scrawled across the bottom of Pauling's letter. Pauling's file on Moertel now had a note pinned to the cover, 'Keep after Moertel'. In August, Pauling, ever vigilant and potentially litigious, was annoyed to read an article in *Oncology Times* in which Moertel was quoted as having referred to the 'non-randomized study conducted in the little hospital, Vale of Leven, in Scotland'. As Pauling forthwith informed Moertel, there was a description of Vale of Leven Hospital in his and Cameron's book *Cancer and Vitamin C*, to the effect that it was a 'large hospital, with 440 beds' which registered about 500 new cancer patients each year. Stanford University Hospital, considered to be one of the leading hospitals in the United States, had only 420 beds. Pauling warned Moertel that he considered his description of Vale of Leven as a 'little' hospital to have been used 'for the purpose of derogation' (Pauling to Moertel, 31 August 1981).

Pauling's attempt to extract the data he wanted from the NCI under the Freedom of Information Act also failed. As the NCI finally informed him, the raw data generated in clinical trials utilizing Federal funds belonged to the grantee, not the Government. Moertel was not obliged to release the data of the study (Henney to Pauling, 7 December 1981). In the end, Pauling managed to obtain a copy of the complete trial press kit originally released by the NCI on the occasion of Moertel's address to the Oncology Society – not from Moertel or the NCI, but from the Science and Medicine correspondent for the *Washington Post*. And with this he had to be content until such time as the study was published.

On 5 December 1981, Ava Helen Pauling died of her cancer at the age of seventy-seven. Receiving no other treatment than initial surgery and a daily vitamin C megadose, she had survived for a little more than five years after diagnosis, for a condition for which the official NCI 5–year relative survival rate was only 13 per cent. She had continued in reasonably good health for most of that time, accompanying Pauling as usual on his heavy lecturing and travelling schedule, and delivering her own lectures on sexual equality and disarmament. Pauling had regarded her response as further evidence of the beneficial effects of vitamin C for all cancer patients. Her death, although it devastated Pauling, seems to have hardened his determination to fight on, on behalf of vitamin C (Serafini, 1989).

Within a few days of the long-awaited publication of the laetrile study in the *New England Journal of Medicine* on 28 January 1982 (Moertel *et al.*, 1982), Pauling gave notice to Moertel that the battle was far from over. He challenged Moertel's statement that the survival times of the laetrile-treated patients appeared to be consistent with the anticipated survival in patients receiving placebo or no treatment: 'Would you send me the references to the papers in which survival times of these comparable patients are reported?' As well, he requested information on the fourteen patients treated with the high-dose schedule, and further details of the patients who had not received prior chemotherapy. Tongue-in-cheek, he concluded:

> I look forward to receiving this information from you, and I now express my thanks to you for your willingness to give me the information, now that your paper is published. (Pauling to Moertel, 2 February 1982)

More important, Pauling pursued the argument in the pages of the *New England Journal of Medicine*. The trial results had been accompanied by an endorsing editorial by Relman, 'Closing the Books on Laetrile', in which Relman had argued that the Moertel-led study had produced a 'decisive conclusion':

> Laetrile doesn't work. Even when combined with the 'metabolic' therapy (vitamins and a 'natural diet') so enthusiastically touted by the anti-establishment cancer therapists, Laetrile produced no discernible benefit in a group of 178 patients with a variety of types of advanced cancer.

Relman also defended the methodology of the trial, which he conceded, 'was not designed in the classic mold':

> The lack of concurrent controls was partially offset by the fact that all patients were in the advanced stages of a disease known to be almost uniformly and rapidly fatal. Any objective responses in tumour size or apparent prolongation of survival could be identified by comparison with historical controls.   (Relman, 1982)

This, of course, stood the persistent orthodox criticism of the historically-controlled Vale of Leven trials on its head. Pauling (who underscored and bracketed this statement with a large question mark in his personal copy of the editorial), immediately fired off a letter to the *Journal*, turning this to his own tactical advantage. In a covering letter to Relman, he expressed his 'astonishment' on seeing in the *Journal* a paper on an important clinical trial in which there was no control group of patients similar to those who received the treatment (Pauling to Relman, 3 February 1982). In his published letter he used the above quotation from Relman's editorial to dispute the negative interpretation of the laetrile trial by reference to the survival times recorded for the patients in the first Mayo Clinic trial of vitamin C. 'As one of the touters', Pauling wrote, 'I wish to point out that these conclusions are not justified by the evidence:

> It is my opinion that there probably was a beneficial effect, including prolongation of survival. Other studies have shown that the median survival time in patients with cancer 'for which no standard treatment was known to be curative or to extend life expectancy' was about 1.4 months; an example is the control group in the study by [Moertel], Creagan, *et al*. The observed median of 4.5 months accordingly constitutes a substantial increase. In any case it is improper to announce a negative result without performing a careful statistical analysis of the treated group and a suitable control group.   (Pauling, 1982)

This had the desired effect of forcing Moertel into print in defence of his methodology. Moertel readily agreed that a randomized, controlled clinical trial was essential before the superiority of any new treatment approach could be claimed. Such a study would avoid the 'obviously fallacious claim' made by Dr Pauling for a benefit of 'metabolic therapy', based on a 'comparison of 'two totally dissimilar patient populations'. However, in the case of laetrile:

> Any drug, orthodox or unorthodox, must be discarded from further clinical evaluation with such grossly inadequate performance in a Phase II trial. It would be unconscionable human experimentation to randomize people between exposure to such a drug and standard therapy which would hold a known potential for cure or extension of life span. No ethical physician would conduct such a study; no institutional review board would approve it: no rational, truly informed patient would submit to it.

Nevertheless, although he rejected Pauling's comparison of the laetrile with the vitamin C-treated patients of the first Mayo Clinic trial, Moertel was goaded (by what he referred to disparagingly as Pauling's 'venerable dramatic licence') into displaying for *Journal* readers the comparison of survival curves of laetrile-treated patients with colorectal cancer with that of a 'comparable' group of Mayo Clinic patients who were given treatment with new chemotherapeutic agents which were later discarded because of inactivity. As readers could see for themselves, this comparison did not provide any encouragement for further investigation of laetrile plus 'metabolic therapy' (Moertel, 1982).

Even though he had scored some points, it cannot be said that Pauling won this round. His attempt to reopen public debate with Moertel backfired when their published exchange prompted a spate of newspaper reports, headed 'Pauling Backs Laetrile'. Pauling and the Institute were kept busy dissociating him from such an interpretation:

> Dr Pauling does not 'back Laetrile', but does feel such an important clinical test should have included an adequate control group to allow valid conclusions to be drawn on the effectiveness of the treatment.   (Pauling, 1983)

Indomitable as ever, Pauling turned his attention to the animal experimentation which he optimistically foresaw as reinforcing his and Cameron's claims of the anti-cancer properties of vitamin C.

5.4   OF MICE AND MEN

In mid-1981, after repeated annual applications by Pauling, the NCI had announced a grant of $204,000 for his proposed two-year study of the effects of vitamin C on breast cancer in mice. This was allegedly decided only after a good deal of internal dissension at the NCI. According to a report by Marjory Sun in *Science*, Pauling had managed to antagonize a number of senior personnel by his resistance to criticism and impatience with standard NCI experimental protocol requirements (an interpretation which is disputed by the Linus Pauling Institute). According to Sun, in view of Pauling's stature, not to mention his persistence and political clout, the NCI had gone to 'extraordinary lengths' in helping him revise his grant submission (Sun, 1981c). A special ad hoc subcommittee (which comprised a number of prominent cancer researchers, including the British biostatistician Richard Peto) had made a site visit to the Linus Pauling Institute. They recommended various changes to Pauling's experimental design with which he complied, and the grant was finally approved.

Under pressure from Pauling, the NCI had already tested vitamin C in animal models without any positive outcome. But the interpretation of these results was complicated by the problem that the animals conventionally used to screen drugs for anti-cancer activity also produced vitamin C within their own bodies. As Pauling and Cameron (and Arthur Robinson also, before his falling out with Pauling) argued, the administration of vitamin C to such animals might suppress the internal production of the vitamin, so that considerably higher levels had to be administered before this negative effect was counterbalanced and vitamin C could exert its presumed anti-cancer effects.

Pauling had initiated his and Robinson's earlier controversial mouse experiments more for their propaganda value in demonstrating that he was complying with the NCI demand for controlled animal experimentation before clinical trials of vitamin C could be carried out in human subjects. But by the end of 1979, he was convinced that these experiments on the incidence of skin cancer in 'hairless' mice which had been irradiated with ultraviolet light demonstrated a statistically significant protective effect for vitamin C. The ramifications of the ongoing Robinson affair precluded publication of these results in Pauling's usual venue of the *Proceedings of the National Academy of Sciences*. In September 1980, Pauling presented a preliminary paper on the results of these studies at the Hoffmann-La Roche-sponsored 'Third International Symposium on Vitamin C' at Sao Paulo in Brazil. This paper was subsequently written up for publication in the Conference Proceedings. It listed various Institute research personnel who had been involved in the mouse experiments as co-authors, but not Arthur Robinson. Around this time, Robinson, still engaged in litigation against Pauling and the Institute, made a television appearance on the Walter Cronkite 'Universe' programme to reiterate his claim that vitamin C doses at the mouse equivalent of 10 grams per day, the level recommended by Pauling and

Cameron for their human patients, had actually caused an *increase* in the incidence of skin cancer in mice. Pauling now proceeded to publish these contentious data in the conference proceedings, arguing that they lay within the expected statistical variation and did not contravene the overall finding of the studies that vitamin C had a pronounced effect in decreasing the incidence of malignant skin lesions in the mice. As a result of the NCI visit to the Institute, he could call on some heavy ammunition in support of his claim. As this publication stated, the statistical analysis of the mouse data had received the benefit of advice from the cancer expert Richard Peto, and was in conformity with the method endorsed by the International Agency for Research on Cancer (Pauling *et al.*, 1982).

Encouraging as these results might be, their out-of-the-way place of publication could not be expected to counteract Robinson's allegations, which continued to attract publicity. This came to a head with the out-of-court settlement in mid-1983, which ended the bitter five-year legal battle between Robinson and the Institute (see 2.4). All of Robinson's allegations were revived again in the widespread coverage this received in the press and in *Nature*, the leading international scientific journal (Anon., 1983a).

To add to the adverse publicity, a few weeks later, under the heading 'Pauling Backs Wonder Cures' (complete with an apposite cartoon of Superman about to take the witness stand), *Nature* gave extended coverage to Pauling's testimony in court on behalf of the mail-order vitamin dealer, Oscar Falconi, who was being prosecuted under a statute prohibiting the use of the mail to obtain money by false representation. According to *Nature*, Falconi had claimed among other things that vitamin C 'probably offers 100 per cent protection against bladder cancer', and had promoted a 'Drug Rehabilitation Kit' which included three pounds of vitamin C powder with instructions for its use in overcoming drug addiction and counteracting drug overdose (Budiansky, 1983). Pauling, as leading defence witness, invoked Ewan Cameron's clinical trial results in support of Falconi's claims. This thoroughly disconcerted Cameron who, from the standpoint of his conventional medical background, was outspoken in his condemnation of those 'para-medical zealots, self-seeking entrepreneurs and opportunists' who were attempting to jump on the bandwaggon of his and Pauling's research.

As if this were not enough for the beleaguered Pauling Institute, in August 1983, *Medical World News* featured a report on a multi-institutional double-blind controlled study of vitamin C in 144 patients with advanced cancer. 'As a treatment for advanced cancer, vitamin C has flunked again', the article stated. Neither Pauling nor Cameron had known of the existence of the trial up to this point (nor, as they subsequently discovered, of the involvement of Mayo Clinic researchers in it). According to the article, a preliminary report of the trial's results to the American Society of Clinical Oncology had stated that the vitamin C treated patients (most of whom had received prior chemotherapy or radiotherapy) had demonstrated no improvements in survival times or symptoms. Pauling, when contacted for comment, could only reiterate his claims that the immune-enhancing properties of vitamin C therapy were compromised by the damage to the immune system caused by cytotoxic drugs. Confronted by this new study (the results of which were only ever published in abstract form), Pauling publicly released the news of the forthcoming positive results of Cameron's new trials of vitamin C at Vale of Leven and two other Scottish hospitals (Anon., 1983b; Tschetter *et al.*, 1983).

5.5 CAMERON'S CONTINUING RESEARCH

In July 1982, at Pauling's urging, Cameron had retired from his post as Senior Surgeon at Vale of Leven Hospital in order to accept appointment as Senior Research Professor and Medical Director at the Linus Pauling Institute. This had been discussed as far back as 1978, when Cameron and Pauling had been working together on *Cancer and Vitamin C*. Cameron had then put together a research programme for the Institute directed towards determining the 'modes of action of ascorbate in the treatment of human cancer, and . . . expedit[ing] its acceptance into routine clinical use'. It was an ambitious project, requiring the recruitment of a number of highly qualified scientists who would carry out research into immunology, biochemistry, virology, epidemiology, nutrition, animal experimentation, and clinical studies in relation to vitamin C.

Pauling had been particularly enthusiastic about the possibility of establishing a cancer clinic at the Institute under Cameron's direction, but Cameron himself felt that such a clinic could not exist on its own without extensive local hospital back-up facilities which he did not see to be forthcoming. His own preference was for the extension of the Scottish-based computer-recorded patient monitoring system he recently had established with the assistance of those clinicians who had previously assisted his vitamin C research – Drs. Allan Campbell and Leslie Moffat – and which was based on cancer patient attendance at three large general hospitals, including Vale of Leven. This 'sophisticated records system', he argued, was flexible enough to include patients from other hospital systems. Over the years it would build up invaluable information about the relative progress of very large numbers of test patients and 'exactly comparable controls', and so establish the benefits of vitamin C to cancer patients. Cameron's preference for this method was strengthened by the negative outcome of the first Mayo

Clinic trial. As he put it to the 1980 Sao Paulo Conference on vitamin C:

> Unlike Professor Pauling's hairless mice all suffering from basically the same tumor, the spectrum and behaviour of human cancer is very wide and beset with inconsistency of outcome . . . Also, unlike the hairless mice, it is just not possible to isolate dying human cancer patients in cages, feed them controlled diets, and dispassionately await the outcome, although this would appear to be the type of bizarre experiment that some of our critics seem to demand. (Cameron, 1982)

Cameron had managed to set up his monitoring system with an initial grant from the American-based National Foundation for Cancer Research, a private research foundation which organized its money-raising activities around the controversial work of the aging Albert Szent-Gyorgyi, the discoverer of vitamin C. Pauling vigorously opposed accepting this grant on the grounds that the fund-raising activities of the Foundation were suspect and that he did not want the Pauling name or Cameron's research to be associated with it, but even more because he viewed the Foundation competitively. Nevertheless, Cameron accepted a research grant from the Foundation. This, together with further modest grants from IBM and the Argyll and Clyde Health Board (Scotland), and a contribution from the Linus Pauling Institute, financed his growing data bank on ascorbate-treated patients and comparable controls.

From 1978 until the time he left the Vale of Leven Hospital in 1982, Cameron accumulated data on 2800 cancer patients, some 350 of whom received supplemental ascorbate as a supportive measure in the latter stages of their illness. As well, all ascorbate-treated patients and a sample proportion of the controls had their plasma and leucocyte ascorbate levels monitored monthly in order to gain more information about ascorbate metabolism in cancer patients and to test for compliance.

It was as well that Cameron brought his clinical data with him to the Institute. The ambitious research programme he had envisaged faded away before the financial realities of the hard-pressed Institute, which was struggling to survive the combined impact of the Robinson affair and the first Mayo Clinic trial. Under the terms of the out-of-court settlement, Robinson received $575,000, an amount considerably less than the alleged $25 million suit he had brought against the Institute. But the Institute had had to pay out more than $250,000 in legal fees as well, almost depleting its shoestring budget. It was, as Pauling himself put it, a 'hand-to-mouth' existence.

The hard economic fact was that the Institute's image as a Pauling and Vitamin C Institute no longer attracted the same degree of small-donor support which had been its mainstay during the late-seventies. In part, this was attributable to the economic recession of the 80s, and to the fact that the sixties-inspired support for alternative medicine and alternative lifestyles was losing its impetus. This was all too evident in the laetrile campaign. The attempts of its hardcore proponents to challenge legally the negative results of the Moertel-led uncontrolled trial were ineffectual, and popular support for the controversial drug withered away before the impact of the 'closed book' policy of the cancer establishment. Some hard choices had to be made at the Institute. In the end, under Zuckerkandl's direction, its research programme was weighted towards the more conventional area of molecular biology.

In an attempt to get NCI support for his clinical research, Cameron reversed his previous ethical rejection of randomised controlled double-blind trials on the grounds that he would direct the proposed trial and would not himself be involved in the actual clinical practice. But his grant applications were unsuccessful, and his clinical research was reduced to the analysis of the data he had brought with him to the Institute.

With the part-time assistance of a biostatistician, whose primary responsibility lay with the NCI-funded mouse experiments, Cameron analysed these data according to standard statistical methods. Following standard practice, he removed all patients who died within two weeks of first hospital attendance, and all patients whose illness had been followed-up for less than six months. This left a total of 1826 cancer patients who had been randomly allocated to either physicians who used supplemental ascorbate or physicians who did not. Of these, 296 had received ascorbate in the latter stage of their illness, while the remaining 1532 patients had received no nutritional supplements of any kind. The study, Cameron claimed, was 'effectively randomized, was completely prospective, but was not conducted blind'.

Analysis showed that the group given supplemental ascorbate survived significantly longer than the control group. The probability that the longer survival times were due to pure chance was calculated as less than one in 10,000. The median overall survival time had been increased from 180 to 343 days in those receiving ascorbate, as measured from the first day of hospital attendance to the date of death. In the sub-group of 218 patients suffering from incurable colon cancer, the results were even better, with an increase from 163 to 625 days median survival time.

Cameron considered these results to be 'highly significant' and to 'prove the value of supplemental ascorbate beyond doubt.' The next step was their publication in a mainstream medical journal. The paper was initially rejected by *Cancer Research* in 1981 on the grounds that the manuscript submitted contained serious methodological problems, a criticism that Cameron, who was unused to working with computerized systems, conceded. Cameron next submitted a revised study, as described above, to the *Lancet*. In mid-December 1984, he received word that it had been rejected again, this time on the grounds that it should go to one of the specialist journals. The *Lancet* editor assured Cameron that he was not denying the interest of the observations; the problem was that the journal had too many articles to publish them all (Monro to Cameron, 5 December 1984). Cameron now decided on the bold move of submitting the manuscript to the *New England Journal of Medicine*, which, he and Pauling had recently learned, was about to publish the results of the second Mayo Clinic trial of vitamin C. This he did, at the end of 1984 (Cameron *et al.*, 1984).

6 The Second Mayo Clinic Trial: A 'Conspiracy to Suppress the Truth'?

Vitamin C Therapy for Cancer Patients is Challenged Again:
Second Study at Mayo Clinic Fails to Confirm Benefit Claimed by Linus Pauling
> *The Wall Street Journal*, 17 January 1985 (Bishop, 1985)

Vitamin C Shown Ineffective Against Cancer; Pauling Disputes Results, Moertel Defends
> *Oncology Times*, March, 1985 (Stockwell, 1985)

Some time ago I wrote to you, asking for information about the process by which this fraudulent paper came to be accepted for publication in your journal. You have not answered my letter.

I hope that you will do me the courtesy of answering my letter. Your continued failure to do so would indicate that you also are involved in this conspiracy to suppress the truth.
> Letter from Linus Pauling to Dr Arnold Relman,
> Editor of the *New England Journal of Medicine*, 29 April 1985.

In October 1984, Pauling reopened his correspondence with Moertel. He had heard a number of reports to the effect that the second Mayo Clinic trial had been concluded and that publication of the results was imminent in the *New England Journal of Medicine*. Pauling asked if Moertel would send him a copy of the manuscript a few weeks before publication, so that he might have time to prepare for the reporters:

> I pledge that I would not make any public use of the information in the proofsheets or manuscript until the date of publication. This procedure is, of course, usually followed by scientists as a courtesy to one another. (19 October 1984)

On 30 November Moertel confirmed in a letter to Pauling that the paper had indeed been submitted to the *New England Journal of Medicine*. He undertook to make certain that a true copy of the manuscript would be in Pauling's hands a short time before publication date. But it was the press who got the pre-publication copies first, three days before Pauling received his on the actual date of publication – 17 January 1985. Feelings ran high at the Institute, with Pauling and Cameron besieged by reporters. Pauling was outraged by what he construed (and denounced in the media) as Moertel's 'unprofessional' conduct in deliberately withholding the paper from him and making it impossible for him to comment on a study he had not seen. By the time Cameron managed to obtain a copy from a United Press International reporter (on 16 January), the news was already going stale. Moertel had appeared on all major TV networks to denounce vitamin C as 'worthless' in cancer treatment and the Pauling–Cameron studies as biased.

Pauling's subsequent television interview (with Moertel and himself in separate studios) did not go well, with Pauling looking, in Cameron's words, 'tired, old, and upset (as indeed he was)'. But within a few days, Pauling had rallied sufficiently to charge the Mayo Clinic publicly with issuing 'false and misleading' claims and to accuse the *New England Journal of Medicine* and the NCI of condoning a 'fraudulent' study (Linus Pauling Institute, 1985b; Anderson, 1985). This was followed by media reports of possible suits by Pauling against all three bodies and the individuals concerned.

6.1   THE SECOND MAYO CLINIC TRIAL

What particularly rankled with Pauling was that the negative results of this second Mayo Clinic trial of vitamin C were officially endorsed in an accompanying guest editorial by Dr Robert E. Wittes, Associate Director of the Cancer Therapy Evaluation Program of the NCI. Such a legitimating guest editorial was the standard practice of the *New England Journal of Medicine* in the case of potentially contentious or significant papers; but from Pauling's point of view it compounded the 'misrepresentations' of the Mayo Clinic paper and implicated the NCI in the 'fraud'. Wittes hailed the trial as 'definitive' and claimed: 'It is difficult to find fault with the design or execution of this study. Ascorbic acid was given in the same daily dose and by the same route advocated by Cameron and Pauling.' The clear implication was that the study therefore constituted a replication and a refutation of Cameron's Vale of Leven trials. Wittes endorsed and reiterated the charge by the Mayo Clinic team in their published report that the 'apparently positive results' reported by Cameron were the result of case selection bias rather than treatment effectiveness. On this basis Wittes argued that 'additional controlled trials . . . do not appear warranted'. He concluded by congratulating the Mayo Clinic team on a study 'that actually helps physicians with clinical decisions'.

Wittes tried hard to cushion the blow. Pauling was 'one of the most versatile scientific minds of the twentieth century', with a 'legendary reputation for being right about all sorts of things'. Unfortunately he was wrong about the clinical efficacy of vitamin C for colorectal cancer. Vitamin C was an 'interesting molecule' with some notable *in vitro* and *in vivo* anti-carcinogenic and cytotoxic properties; but its immediate research should be confined to the laboratory.

> We may be sorry that the results were negative, but should nonetheless be grateful that at least the trial was methodologically sound and therefore definitive. (Wittes, 1985)

The tone of the study report by Moertel and his co-researchers was less conciliatory. They stressed that their randomised, double-blind trial of 'Vitamin C versus Placebo in the Treatment of Patients with Advanced Cancer who Have Had no Prior Chemotherapy', had been carried out in 'ideal' conditions. Their patients were in very good general condition, with minimal symptoms, and none had received any previous treatment with cytotoxic drugs. The Mayo Clinic team had elected to study patients with advanced cancer of the large bowel because this was the most frequent tumour type in the Cameron–Pauling studies and one for which Cameron claimed a striking improvement in survival with vitamin C therapy. This choice of cancer type, they emphasized, also satisfied the ethical criteria of the Mayo Clinic researchers:

> We felt ethically justified in studying this group of patients without first offering cytotoxic drugs because in our opinion there is no known form of chemotherapy for colorectal cancer that has been demonstrated to produce substantive palliative benefit or extension of survival.

The trial methodology, as they carefully reported it, scrupulously followed the standard randomized double-blind procedure. Patients participating in the trial with their informed consent had been randomly allocated to receive either 10g of vitamin C daily or placebo (lactose) in the form of twenty identical opaque gelatin capsules. Patients recorded their daily tablet intake and neither they nor attending physicians and staff were aware of their actual drug assignment. Patients were randomly checked for compliance by means of urinary assays, and all were re-evaluated at regular eight-weekly intervals for signs of disease progression. Therapy (vitamin C or placebo) was continued for as long as the patient was able to take oral medications or until there was evidence of 'marked progression of the malignant disease'. Progression was defined as 'an increase of more than 50 per cent in the product of the perpendicular diameters of any area of known malignant disease, if any new areas of malignant disease appeared, if there was substantial worsening of symptoms or performance status, or if there was a loss of body weight of 10 per cent or more.' At the closure of the study, the code had been broken and the results statistically analysed by the standard methods.

'In spite of this seemingly ideal setting', the trial had demonstrated that:

> vitamin C performed no better than a dummy medication. No patient had measurable tumour shrinkage, the malignant disease in patients taking vitamin C progressed just as rapidly as in those taking placebo, and patients lived just as long on sugar pills as on high-dose vitamin C. Surprisingly, and perhaps by chance, there were more long-term survivors receiving placebo than vitamin C.

This effectively undercut Pauling's criticism of the first Mayo Clinic trial. These were patients who 'presumably would have had their protective mechanisms as intact as possible in the presence of incurable cancer'. 'On the basis of this and our previous randomized study', the abstract of the paper now unequivocally asserted,

> it can be concluded that high-dose vitamin C therapy is not effective against advanced malignant disease regardless of whether the patient has had any prior chemotherapy.

Once again the Mayo Clinic researchers emphasized the methodological inadequacies of the Cameron–Pauling studies and linked these with Pauling's ethical inadequacies. Unlike their own methodologically sound clinical trials, the 'retrospective comparison between selected study patients and historical control patients' carried out by Cameron and Pauling had not protected against bias:

> [W]e are left with the inevitable conclusion that the apparent positive results of Cameron and Pauling were the product of case selection bias rather than treatment effectiveness. . . .
>   Whether one is dealing with the treatment of the common cold or of cancer, and whether one is dealing with a benign vitamin or a highly toxic chemotherapy program, it would seem to serve the interest of

the patient better for public advocacy of a proposed treatment to be withheld until that treatment had been proved effective by definitive studies of sound scientific design. (Moertel *et al.*, 1985)

6.2 THE PAULING–CAMERON CRITICISMS

Despite Wittes' official reassurance, Pauling and Cameron had, as Pauling dryly noted, 'no difficulty' in finding fault with the methodology of this seemingly conclusive second trial. They immediately and unequivocally rejected it as 'deviating grossly' from Cameron's experimental procedure, and therefore as not constituting a replication and refutation of the Vale of Leven trials. Within twenty-four hours of their first perusal of the paper, they and staff at the Linus Pauling Institute had identified what they construed as three major 'flaws' in the methodological design of the study. Their criticisms, which emerged over the next few days in press releases and interviews and in the course of the indefatigable Pauling's correspondence with other leading figures in the now deepening dispute, were not new. They had all been rehearsed before in the contexts of the earlier Sloan–Kettering pilot trial by Dr Charles Young and of the first Mayo Clinic trial. They may be summarized as follows (Richards, 1986):

(i) *Controls*: Out of 100 patients with colorectal cancer participating in the trial with informed consent, only 11 patients (and each on only one occasion) were checked for compliance by means of a 24-hour urine sample for analysis of ascorbate content. Of these, 6 were controls taking placebo. One of the controls was found to excrete well over 550mg per 24 hours, while the remaining five were found to excrcte 'negligible' amounts of 550mg or less (the lower figures were not furnished in the publication). Excreted vitamin C for healthy individuals ingesting a balanced diet has been established as around 30mg per 24 hours, while the value for cancer patients not supplementing with vitamin C is around 0 to 10mg. Thus at least 2 out of 6 of assayed controls excreted vitamin C in amounts one or two orders of magnitude above normal. According to Pauling and Cameron, these amounts are not negligible, and they mean that these controls were in fact ingesting significant amounts of vitamin C – around one or more grams per day. Pauling and Cameron therefore concluded that the Mayo team ignored readily available information which should have made them suspect that their study was problematical: a proportion of the controls was clearly medicating with the substance under evaluation.

This was Cameron's 'personal main criticism' of the trial. As we saw, he had published this same criticism of the first Mayo Clinic trial, and emphasized the need for consistent monitoring of patient compliance. His own patients at Vale of Leven Hospital were routinely tested every month for ascorbate levels by means of a blood test, which Cameron regarded as more reliable than urine analysis and had instituted as part of his programme for the investigation of the physiological role of ascorbate in cancer patients. Even Wittes acknowledged in his editorial that if more patients had been checked for compliance, 'surreptitious ingestion of this easily obtainable vitamin among the control patients might have been excluded with somewhat more confidence' (Wittes, 1985).

(ii) *Duration of Administration*: This was Pauling's immediate and major criticism of the second Mayo study. As we saw, in his very first letter to Moertel in 1977, Pauling had stressed the need for cancer patients to continue their oral ingestion of vitamin C 'for an indefinite time', citing the case of the truck driver whose cancer had recurred when his dosage was temporarily discontinued. 'The cancer', he had warned Moertel, 'may return if the ascorbate is stopped'. But in the second Mayo study, medication with vitamin C or placebo was discontinued immediately tumour progression became apparent. Administration of vitamin C was thus continued for a median time of only two and a half months, whereas, in the Cameron–Pauling studies, ascorbate was administered from the onset of the experiment until death (or, indeed, for a few long-term survivors, up to the present time). According to Pauling and Cameron, the Mayo study therefore measured the impact of vitamin C on reappearance of progression and the impact of vitamin C administration *during this interval only* on life-span, and found no positive impact. Pauling and Cameron have conceded that if the controls had been convincing, and if the existence of a rebound effect upon sudden withdrawal of supplemental vitamin C did not create an additional complication, *this much* might have been reasonably demonstrated for the case of colorectal cancer. But, they argue, it would not be enough to refute the Cameron–Pauling findings. In their studies vitamin C was administered from onset of treatment throughout life, so the effect observed was not only related to the question of whether or not tumour progression sets in, but also to the rate of tumour growth thereafter, *under continued administration of vitamin C*, and to any general health factors that might contribute to the patient's capacity to resist death from the presence of tumours.

(iii) *The Rebound Effect*: This was the criticism that Pauling had earlier made of Dr Charles Young's pilot study at Sloan–Kettering in 1976. As he then pointed out to Young, abrupt discontinuation of high intakes of vitamin C produces a 'rebound effect', with marked depletion of circulating ascorbate to well below normal levels. This effect had been known since

1973, and in their publications Pauling and Cameron had warned patients of its possible dangers (Cameron and Pauling, 1979b). They believe that the resultant temporary immuno-depression may induce an acceleration of tumour growth. The Mayo Clinic team either ignored or were unaware of this possibility. Medication was abruptly discontinued for those patients who showed signs of tumour progression, thus inducing the rebound effect in those taking vitamin C. According to Pauling and Cameron, the study, as it does not take this factor into account, is not a refutation of their findings. They have gone so far as to claim that the combination of the rebound effect and the subsequent administration of highly toxic chemotherapy may well have shortened the life-span of patients so treated in the Mayo study.

As far as Pauling was concerned, these 'flaws' in the design of a study which was supposed to test the validity of Cameron's Vale of Leven work added up to 'fraud and deliberate misrepresentation'. 'I have never seen him so upset', wrote Cameron. 'He regards this whole affair as a personal attack on his integrity' (personal communication, 4 March 1985). The issue of personal integrity and credibility aside, a further cause for Pauling's concern was the impact that Moertel's media coup and the adverse publicity it had engendered might have on the fund-raising activities of the Institute, already financially hard hit by the Robinson affair.

Pauling's litigious gestures (although by no means unprecedented in his long and controversial career) are best interpreted as a measure of his frustration that, after thirteen years of effort, he and Cameron had succeeded in making so little impact on their opponents' comprehension of their views on the role of vitamin C in cancer treatment. As Cameron once again carefully articulated their position: they had never at any time claimed that vitamin C could *stop* tumour progression, except for a very few fortunate patients. What they had claimed, on the basis of the Vale of Leven studies, was that, for the great majority of patients, they could *slow* tumour progression, improve their quality of life, and slightly, but significantly, prolong survival times (Cameron, 1985). From their point of view it was therefore 'quite illogical', if not suspect, for the Mayo Clinic researchers to have stopped vitamin C or placebo treatment the moment the patients seemed to get worse and (as had happened for half of the patients in the study) to substitute the highly toxic 5-fluorouracil which the researchers themselves held to be of no value in the treatment of colorectal cancer.

As Cameron and Pauling structured the situation, in spite of their repeated attempts to explicate the theoretical and clinical differences between the administration and evaluation of vitamin C and conventional chemotherapeutic drugs, the Mayo Clinic oncologists had tested vitamin C as they would test any cytotoxic drug which is administered for short periods of time, and whose therapeutic impact is measured primarily in terms of tumour shrinkage. They had made no effort to evaluate vitamin C within the framework established by Cameron and Pauling, and had ignored or were unaware of available information on the physiology of vitamin C which could have been taken into account in the design of their study.

Pauling now came to regard this apparent lack of understanding – and, in particular, the representation of the second Mayo Clinic study as a replication and refutation of the Vale of Leven trials – as wilful and malicious. He was convinced that Moertel had withheld the paper from him until the very day of publication because Moertel 'knew that it was a scurrilous piece of writing and that Dr Cameron and I would recognize at once that it was . . . and the paper wouldn't have been published the way it is'. Furthermore, he claimed that in their presentation of their results, the Mayo Clinic authors had tried to conceal the fact that their study was not a replication of Cameron's work. They had not explicitly stated that their investigation differed significantly from Cameron's in that the duration of vitamin C ingestion was 'only two and a half months. . . it's pretty well hidden in the paper'. Not even Cameron on a first quick reading had picked up this crucial point, and this confirmed Pauling's suspicion of deliberate suppression and misrepresentation. In Pauling's freely expressed opinion, physicians (who could make much more money in medical practice) were much more likely than scientists (who had high ethical principles) to commit fraud when faced with the hard job of being a scientific investigator. All of the recent cases of scientific fraud reported in the newspapers, as Pauling frequently pointed out, had in fact been committed by young medical researchers who were not trained in the scientific method, not by scientists (Pauling, 1986). As well, it bordered on the 'unethical' for the *New England Journal of Medicine* to have published the Mayo study without extending to himself and Cameron the usual courtesy among scientists of letting them see an advance copy of a paper purporting to be a replication of their own work (Horwitz, 1985). On the day of publication of the second Mayo study, Pauling told Institute staff at a hastily convened seminar:

> Well, we can ask why did they carry out such a study? I think that the reason is clear. Dr Moertel has carried out fifteen or twenty studies of new cancer drugs . . . where they collect some cancer patients and get them to sign a consent form . . . give them the new drug, and this is pretty dangerous, of course, the drug may have pretty bad side effects; it may not be much good anyway, and so if the patient begins to deteriorate, they take him off the drug. That's the proper thing to

do. So Dr Moertel doesn't realize that vitamin C is a nutrient . . . a food (laughs); he thinks it's a drug. So that explains that. But what explains their carrying out this study of this sort and trying to pass it off as a replication of Dr Cameron's work? I don't know the answer to that. (Linus Pauling Institute, 1985a)

He set himself to find out.

6.3 PLOYS AND TACTICS

Within a few days, while Pauling struggled to counteract the adverse publicity as the newspaper reports began to flood into the Institute, he had fired off letters to Relman of the *New England Journal of Medicine*, to DeVita and Wittes of the NCI, and to Moertel and his five co-authors at the Mayo Clinic. To each of them he represented his view that the trial was not a replication of Cameron's studies and therefore could not be considered to be a refutation of their claims. From Relman, he demanded copies of the referees' reports and a published 'statement of correction and retraction and apology' for the 'misrepresentations' of the Mayo Clinic report, arguing that the issue was too serious and too damaging to himself, Cameron and the Institute, and to the tens of thousands of cancer patients who now took vitamin C, to be handled by the usual letter to the editor (Pauling to Relman, 21 January 1985). He lambasted Moertel for his failure to get the preprint copy of the trial paper to him in time for Pauling to deal with the demands of the media. And he queried Moertel and each of the authors of the Mayo Clinic study as to whether they knew that the way they did their study did not correspond with Cameron's Vale of Leven trials. Pauling also requested further information about the trial from each author on the grounds that, while the study did not demonstrate the inefficacy of vitamin C, it could provide useful information about the effects of the rebound effect in cancer patients and he wished to analyse this. Pauling also, surely tongue-in-cheek, offered to visit the Mayo Clinic to give a seminar talk on the subject of 'Vitamin C and Cancer'. This was politely rejected by a Mayo Clinic administrator on the ground that it would not be possible to arrange a 'suitable audience' for him. From DeVita, Pauling demanded a copy of the Mayo Clinic trial protocol, his assurance that the NCI had not been wittingly involved in this 'misrepresentation', and his intervention in this 'fiasco'; and from Wittes he wanted another editorial, 'correcting' his previous one on the basis of the information that Pauling had now provided.

He made no headway with any of his repeated demands and requests. Relman summarily declined to publish the 'retraction, correction and apology' demanded by Pauling, and insisted that he should challenge the conclusions of Moertel and Wittes through the usual medium of a letter in the correspondence section of the *Journal* (Relman to Pauling, 28 January 1985). Pauling thereupon responded with two letters, one dealing with his objections to the Mayo Clinic study, the other addressing the 'misrepresentations' of Wittes' editorial. 'Because of the sensitiveness of this situation', he wrote Relman in a covering letter, ' . . . the two letters are to be published together, exactly as written by me, with no changes of any sort' (Pauling to Relman, 8 February 1985). When Relman declined to publish two letters from the same author at the same time, and suggested that Pauling should combine his criticisms of both papers in the one letter which should not exceed 40 typed double-spaced lines (that is, about 500 words), Pauling refused to cooperate on the grounds that he was writing about 'two different matters' which he did not want to confuse with one another. He resubmitted both letters (shortened to the correct length), requesting that they be published in sequential issues of the *New England Journal of Medicine*, along with the other relevant letters that Relman had received (Pauling to Relman, 19 March 1985). By this stage Pauling had been sent copies of at least five letters critical of the trial, by other scientists, that had been submitted to the *Journal* for publication.

Pauling's attempt to involve DeVita in his negotiations with Relman and Moertel also failed. For Pauling, DeVita summarized the orthodox point of view that the second Mayo Clinic trial had met the conventional ethical and methodological standards for clinical trials. It had been peer reviewed and published in a fine journal, and the proper place to dispute it was in that journal. He reminded Pauling that the NCI had tested vitamin C because of Pauling and his personal reputation, not because they had believed his and Cameron's methodology to be valid. For all DeVita could tell now, two trials later, there was no detectable effect of vitamin C as an agent for treatment of cancer under conventional clinical circumstances as detailed in the trials (DeVita to Pauling, 7 February 1985). Pauling next demanded an NCI-sponsored retrial: 'a proper test of the thesis that vitamin C in high doses, utilized in the proper way, has value to cancer patients . . . a trial in which the protocol used by Dr Cameron is followed, rather than by some quite different protocol' (Pauling to de Vita, 19 February 1985). DeVita refused to yield. Pauling, being Pauling, did not give up. He continued to write DeVita regularly, keeping him up to date with the course of the ongoing dispute, and pressuring him for a new trial, or, alternatively, for a comprehensive programme of research into the relationship between vitamin C and cancer. Pauling even took his case to the National Cancer Advisory Board, but without success. The Board reviewed the controversy, but was of the opinion that it should not intervene in a 'complex scientific issue' of this kind (Chairman, NCAB, to Pauling, 31 May 1985).

Meanwhile, Pauling maintained a correspondence with Wittes, trying to get him to reverse his opinion and to agree that the trial could or should have been done differently. The central issue here was Wittes' insistence that it was 'completely implausible' that administration of vitamin C past the point of demonstrable tumour enlargement could have any beneficial effect for the patient (Wittes to Pauling, 24 January 1985). For Pauling's benefit, Wittes carried out a personal review of the published case reports of the Vale of Leven trials (Pauling to Wittes, 7 February 1985; Wittes to Pauling, 27 February 1985). Wittes could not find any example in Cameron's case reports in which a patient had experienced tumour enlargement and then regression during vitamin C therapy. If he had been able to find such instances they would suggest that continuation of vitamin C past the point of tumour progression might well be justifiable, in which case Wittes might also have regarded the Mayo study as flawed for not having continued treatment. As it was, he could not. Nor could Wittes accept Pauling's argument about the rebound effect. How could the rebound effect, he rhetorically queried Pauling, possibly explain loss of tumour control if vitamin C was not stopped until tumour control was already lost?

In vain Pauling represented his and Cameron's view that

> the rate of progression of a growing malignant tumour probably is determined to a significant extent by the natural resistance of the patient, especially the effectiveness of the immune system, and that the rate of progression might accordingly have increased, through the rebound effect, when the high-dose vitamin C was stopped. The survival time of the vitamin C patients might well have been greater if the vitamin C had not been stopped. You are right in saying that the Mayo Clinic paper reports that the disease had already progressed before the vitamin C was stopped. You are not right in suggesting that the rebound effect is not operating. The rebound effect would increase the rate of disease progression before death, and accordingly change the survival times.

Pauling also suggested that non-compliance (as indicated by the results of the random urinary sampling) might account for the failure of the Mayo Clinic patients to have demonstrated any initial response to vitamin C therapy such as Cameron had repeatedly recorded. They had to take twenty capsules a day, whereas it was easier for Cameron's patients to take their vitamin C in the form of a syrup as described in their publications. Another possibility was that Cameron had been able to closely observe and record the initial progress of his patients who were all hospitalized, whereas the Mayo Clinic patients, who were all ambulatory, had not been examined during the first month of vitamin C ingestion.

In any case, the real point at issue was that the Mayo Clinic investigators

> should not then have described their investigation as a check on Dr Cameron's work, because Dr Cameron continued to give vitamin C. I object strongly to your having written that 'It is difficult to find fault with the design or execution of this study. Ascorbic acid was given in the same daily dose and by the same route advocated by Cameron and Pauling'. You failed to mention that the Mayo Clinic patients stopped the vitamin C, whereas Cameron's patients continued to receive it, so that your editorial article compounded the misrepresentation in the Mayo Clinic article . . . (Pauling to Wittes, 4 March 1985)

But not even a flattering visit from Pauling, for whom Wittes professed a good deal of personal admiration, could get Wittes to change his mind. In the face of Pauling's representations, he readily enough conceded that the second Mayo Clinic trial did not constitute a strict replication of the Vale of Leven studies but said on interview that this 'didn't matter', that Pauling's criticisms were 'not important'. He remained adamant that the methodology of the Mayo Clinic trial was quite proper; that it had satisfactorily demonstrated the inefficacy of vitamin C for colorectal cancer; and that further trials were not necessary (personal interview with Wittes, NCI, 28 October 1986).

The Mayo Clinic authors, Moertel and his co-researchers, confronted with Pauling's public accusations of 'fraud', simply retreated into silence and refused to answer Pauling's continuing letters. Moertel confined himself to issuing the odd counteracting statement when pressed by the media to respond to Pauling's charges:

> The Mayo study is solid and we have no apologies whatsoever. Our patients were taken off the treatment when their conditions showed no improvements; in fact, they were worsening. It would have been morally and ethically repugnant to keep patients on a programme they were getting worse under. (Mayo Clinic, 1985)

High hopes were raised at the Linus Pauling Institute when Pauling and Cameron, along with the Mayo Clinic researchers and the Director and other officials of the NCI, were summoned to go to Washington DC on 25 March to appear before a Congressional Subcommittee on Investigations and Oversight (Committee on Science and Technology) that was holding hearings on the role of nutrition in cancer and wished to investigate the latest Mayo Clinic trial (possibly, as Moertel alleged, as a result of representations that Pauling had made). But although Cameron and Pauling prepared lengthy statements and held themselves in readiness to attend, this investigation failed to take place after being twice rescheduled because of Moertel's inability to attend (Staff Director to Pauling, 12 October 1985).

By April, Pauling was losing patience with his failure to persuade his orthodox critics of the 'flaws' in the Mayo Clinic study. Initially he and the Institute had taken some legal advice on the possibility of filing a class action law suit against the NCI, the Mayo Clinic and the *New England Journal of Medicine* on behalf of the cancer patients in the United States, or, alternatively, of filing a libel suit against those whom Pauling regarded as guilty of deliberate and malicious misrepresentation. But they had been dissuaded from either course of action because of the associated costs and the extreme unlikelihood of making their charges stick. The attorney had vividly stated the case as he saw it:

> The next thing [the judge] is going to say to me is, 'Look, I am an educated man and I wouldn't presume to decide between Linus Pauling and the Mayo Clinic. Here is a Nobel prize-winning biochemist and here are 15 doctors from the world's leading something and one tells me yes and the other tells me no, and how the hell am I going to decide? I don't know anything about biochemistry.' So he will say, 'Look Mr. [Attorney], you make a very interesting and persuasive argument, but on the other hand Mr.—— over here makes a very persuasive argument and I mean isn't this a question for scientists to decide? The history of science for a thousand years is that someone comes up with an idea, the establishment ridicules him, then 50 years later they find he was right and he becomes a saint. That's just life, and Pauling is in the great tradition of outcasts.' That's if I had a good judge. The worst is if I had a bad judge. He'd say, 'Look, Pauling is not a doctor – these guys are doctors; that's enough for me.' That could happen. (Linus Pauling Institute, 1985c)

There was the further danger that legal action might alienate erstwhile supporters. One indignant subscriber to the Linus Pauling Institute summed up his reaction to media reports of the proposed law suit by scrawling the following message (which was carefully preserved in Pauling's files) across the Institute's latest mailout leaflet:

> Are you guys whacked out? I respect Dr Pauling but you don't settle medical controversies by suing a medical journal. You criticize, present your own data and fight it out with your peers, not in a court of law – the last place to look for scientific truth.

Nevertheless, Pauling was convinced that something must be done. None of his efforts had been able to counteract the damaging effects of Moertel's media coup. Subscriptions to the Institute were down. Newspapers that had previously carried the Institute's advertisements, such as the *Wall Street Journal*, had given prominent coverage to Moertel's claims, while Pauling's counterclaims were only minimally reported. He was kept busy writing letters of rebuttal which were then buried in the correspondence columns. Pauling even resorted to writing personal letters to disaffected subscribers to the Institute. At the same time, his protracted negotiations with Relman were delaying publication of his criticisms of the trial in the *New England Journal of Medicine*. He was beginning to despair of trying to make his professional critics understand or take note of these. 'The main point', he carefully reiterated to Wittes,

> which I have tried to make clear to you, is that vitamin C should be put in a category different from that in which drugs are put, especially the anti-cancer drugs. I am discouraged that I have had so little success in getting you and other people in the National Cancer Institute to understand this point. . . . Vitamin C is not a cure for cancer, nor is it a specific cure for any one kind of cancer. As Dr Cameron and I have pointed out repeatedly, it serves to strengthen the body's natural protective mechanisms, especially the immune mechanisms. . . . I am sorry that I have had to give up my hope that you would see that it is possible to find fault with the Mayo Clinic study, in that, as you yourself pointed out to me, the Mayo Clinic study was made on the basis of a protocol that is quite proper for a new anti-cancer drug. It is, however, completely inappropriate for a study of vitamin C. (Pauling to Wittes, 27 June 1985)

The strategy Pauling seems to have decided upon at this point was consistent with the legal advice he had received: that, rather than file a costly and potentially losing suit against his opponents, he should try to provoke them into a newsworthy public debate. If Pauling, for instance, were to appear on television and say:

> 'This is the worst offence to science since Galileo was excommunicated. Look at these people; they pretend to be scientists, they don't even know how to do an experiment, and they took it away from them after two and a half months', and you dress it up a little bit and you make a presentation and you accuse the Mayo Clinic and the National Institutes of Health of falsifying. You are just as immune as they are. Right? So now you have called them quacks and you have called them frauds and phonies and, all right, now what do they do?

They are above the fray. But, I'm telling you, if you would set up that campaign right the reporters will run to them and say 'Linus Pauling says you are a quack, what do you say?' 'I say he's a quack'.   (Linus Pauling Institute, 1985c)

Pauling would have needed little persuasion to such tactics or coaching in them. He had already publicly branded the second Mayo Clinic trial as 'fraudulent'. He now stepped up the provocation, developing a slide presentation of his version of events which he used to illustrate his many invited public lectures on the vitamin C and cancer controversy, and which alleged in bold type:

THE MAYO ARTICLE IS MISLEADING AND DISHONEST. IT MIGHT BE DESCRIBED AS FRAUDULENT. IT PURPORTED TO BE A REPETITION OF DR CAMERON'S STUDY, BUT IT WAS GREATLY DIFFERENT, IN A WAY THAT THE MAYO CLINIC INVESTIGATORS SUCCEEDED IN HIDING FROM THE READERS OF THEIR PAPER.

Pauling even addressed the armed forces at Washington DC in April on the topic of the 'flaws' in the Mayo Clinic trials, an invitation and topic of which he was careful to inform DeVita.

Apart from this public campaign, Pauling and his research associate, Dr Zelek Herman, had been working on a reanalysis of the Mayo Clinic raw data which, as they had not received the information requested from the authors, they were forced to extrapolate from the published staircase Kaplan-Meier diagrams of disease progression and survival times which had accompanied the article. Their reanalysis of these data purported to indicate a statistically significant increased death rate among the patients whose vitamin C was abruptly terminated. Pauling and Herman also reported that there was statistical indication that the subsequent administration of chemotherapy had exacerbated the damaging effect of vitamin C withdrawal. Pauling seized on the opportunity this reanalysis presented to turn the ethical tables on his Mayo Clinic opponents. 'We have recognized', stated the paper,

the desirability of getting more information about the seriousness of the rebound effect for cancer patients, but have felt that for ethical reasons no study of this effect could be carried out; no ethical inves-tigator, knowing the possible serious damage to the cancer patients in the subpopulation exposed to this effect, would agree to carry out such an investigation. Now, however, some important information has been made available through a randomized double-blind trial . . . that was carried out for another purpose by investigators at the Mayo Clinic who were ignorant about the rebound effect and did not recognize the possible danger to their 51 high-dose vitamin C patients of suddenly stopping the intake of vitamin C.

The great increase in recent years in the number of cancer patients taking vitamin C in high doses (10 to 30g per day) as an adjunct to appropriate conventional therapy requires that every opportunity to obtain more information about this possible danger be grasped. Since ethical considerations will probably prohibit any other randomized double-blind study of the rebound effect from being carried out in cancer patients, it is in our opinion important that the Mayo Clinic study be analyzed as thoroughly as possible. (Pauling and Herman, 1985)

Pauling now submitted this provocative analysis to the *New England Journal of Medicine* under the title: 'An analysis of a randomized double-blind study of the effects of giving vitamin C to patients with advanced colorectal cancer and then stopping the vitamin C and administering chemotherapy'. In his covering letter, Pauling informed Relman that he had, according to his own ethical standards, sent copies of this paper to the six Mayo Clinic investigators, asking for their comments and suggestions which, if they indicated the need for any significant changes, he would use to revise his manuscript. With the justification of keeping with Relman's practice of not contacting Pauling before his acceptance of the two Mayo Clinic papers, Pauling requested that Relman have no contact with the Mayo Clinic authors about his (Pauling's) manuscript (Pauling to Relman, 17 April 1985).

When this elaborate ploy failed to elicit any response from the Mayo Clinic authors, Pauling informed them in separate letters sent off by registered mail that he took this as evidence that they were 'involved in a conspiracy to suppress the truth'. In a letter to Relman (also dispatched by registered mail), he pulled no punches in repeating the same charge:

Three months ago I wrote to each of the six Mayo Clinic authors of their paper published on 17 January 1985 in The *New England Journal of Medicine*, asking some questions about the paper. Not one of the six answered my letter.

I have now written them again, pointing out that this fact is evidence that they are involved in a conspiracy to suppress the truth.

Some time ago I wrote to you, asking for information about the process by which this fraudulent paper came to be accepted for publication in your journal. You have not answered my letter.

I hope that you will do me the courtesy of answering my letter. Your continued failure to do so would indicate that you also are

involved in this conspiracy to suppress the truth. (Pauling to Relman,
29 April 1985)

This intemperate letter, if it was intended to incite Relman to public
or private debate, had the reverse effect. Relman now joined the Mayo
Clinic authors in refusing to answer Pauling's continuing communications. And, contrary to the usual policy of the *New England Journal
of Medicine* of publishing letters around six weeks after the relevant
article had appeared, Pauling's and other letters critical of the Mayo
Clinic trial remained unpublished, although Relman published a letter
highly critical of 'alternative' cancer treatments (Markman, 1985).

A professional forum being denied him, Pauling typically found his
own forum for the public dissemination of his views. He had been
working on the manuscript of a popular book, *How to Live Longer and
Feel Better*. This, when published by Freeman early in 1986, became the
major vehicle for his criticisms of the two Mayo Clinic trials and his
charges of 'fraud', 'suppression' and 'misrepresentation'. In his book
Pauling broadened the message of his earlier best-selling *Vitamin C and
the Common Cold*, advising the public to substitute 'proper intakes' of
the safe and inexpensive vitamins and other nutrients of orthomolecular
medicine for the harmful and costly drugs of 'organized medicine'. He
peppered the text with his attacks on the latter:

> The medical profession and the powerful medical institutions and
> enterprises in this country have taken to calling themselves the health
> profession, health centers, and health companies. This is a misnomer
> for what is really the sickness industry.

But on the whole Pauling recounted his encounters with organized medicine with a certain humour and tolerance. He projected the optimistic
view that his message was getting through and that the 'great popular
interest in improved nutrition is now having an influence on the medical
establishment'.

All tolerance and humour vanished, however, when it came to the
'Mayo Clinic fraud'. This was denounced as the 'most recent and the
most outrageous action by organized medicine against the new science
of nutrition and the well-being of the American people'. Moertel and his
collaborators, wrote Pauling,

> deliberately misrepresented their investigation . . . as a repetition and
> check on the work of Dr Cameron . . . They concluded that high doses
> of vitamin C have no value for patients with advanced cancer. In fact
> (although they suppressed this information), they supplied vitamin C

to the patients in a way completely different from that followed by Cameron. . . .

The National Cancer Institute was also a victim of the Mayo Clinic fraud. Its officers were misled into thinking that the Mayo Clinic had repeated Cameron's work. By making a public statement to this effect, they loaned their authority to this bogus effort and compounded its error.

The Mayo Clinic doctors have refused to discuss this matter with me. I conclude that they are not scientists, devoted to the search for the truth. I surmise that they are so ashamed of themselves that they would prefer that the matter be forgotten. The Mayo Clinic used to have a great reputation. This episode indicates to me that it is no longer deserved.   (Pauling, 1986)

6.4   THE PUBLICATION GAME

Cameron, meanwhile, pursued a different strategy. He had not joined Pauling, publicly or privately, in his charges of fraud and deliberate misrepresentation, and dissociated himself from what he saw as Pauling's 'over-reaction' and especially his litigious threats. His own privately expressed view of the matter was: 'Personally, I think we are dealing with a bunch of fools rather than a bunch of knaves'. He charged the Mayo Clinic authors with 'carelessness' in failing to research the background of the subject and 'incompetence' in their conduct of the investigation. He too argued the need for a new trial, a trial which he emphasized 'must not be carried out by vitamin C enthusiasts nor by bigots, but by fair-minded physicians, and conducted not in secrecy but in open cooperation using a mutually agreed protocol' (Cameron, 1985; Cameron to DeVita, 6 March 1985).

But Cameron's real hopes remained pinned on the publication of his manuscript in the *New England Journal of Medicine*. This, hopefully with a neutral accompanying editorial by Relman saying 'this question is still open and a final proper study must be performed', was to be Cameron's answer to this 'travesty' of a study. Acting on Relman's earlier telephoned advice that it would strengthen his argument, Cameron had revised his own manuscript to take account of the results of the second Mayo Clinic trial and re-submitted it to the *New England Journal of Medicine* on the day after the Mayo Clinic paper had been published. Because of this telephone call, and rather to Pauling's amusement, Cameron initially persisted in viewing Relman as a 'rather strange and unusual ally on our side'. He remained optimistic that Relman might publish his paper and was careful to refrain from any action that might jeopardize this desirable outcome:

It is a great pity that the whole matter has become so political. I think that in fairness they really have to accept my manuscript, having already published a study that is so severely flawed. (personal communication, 18 April 1985)

As the months went by, Cameron received no word from Relman. Nor did Pauling's nor any other letters about the trial appear in the pages of the *New England Journal of Medicine*. The irrepressible Pauling continued to write Relman at regular monthly intervals, pressing for publication of his letters and of his and Herman's reanalysis of the second Mayo Clinic trial:

Publication of the Mayo Clinic article has done and continues to do damage not only to me and to the Linus Pauling Institute of Science and Medicine but also to many patients with cancer, who have stopped taking vitamin C, as a supplement to appropriate conventional therapy, or whose physicians have stopped it, or who have been persuaded not to commence taking it. I have for some months counted on the publication of the several Letters to the Editor as an action that would, at least in part, rectify this situation. (Pauling to Relman, 12 August 1985)

But Relman remained silent, even when Pauling shifted to a more conciliatory mode and his charges of 'conspiracy to suppress the truth' gave way to persuasion in the form of the very positive results of the Institute's by-now-concluded NCI-funded study of the incidence of spontaneous mammary cancer in mice (Pauling *et al.*, 1985). These were published in the August number of the *Proceedings of the National Academy of Sciences*, and Pauling dispatched a copy of the paper to Relman, drawing to his attention the 'very large protective effect of high-dose vitamin C' that the study demonstrated. 'I think that this is the most carefully conducted study of nutrition in relation to cancer in animals that has ever been carried out', Pauling wrote persuasively but without effect (Pauling to Relman, 25 January 1986). He next tried to enlist the intervention of the President of the Massachusetts Medical Society (publishers of the *New England Journal of Medicine*) and of John C. Bailar, editor of the *Harvard Medical News Letter*. But the letters continued unpublished, while Pauling continued as obdurate that they be published by Relman in the *Journal*. He rejected the suggestion that he should withdraw the letters and publish them elsewhere, stubbornly insisting: 'It seems to me that it is the duty of Dr Relman to take action on these two letters' (Pauling to Dr Alexander Rich, 25 January 1986).

Nevertheless, Pauling's next move (in March 1986) was to make what he regarded as the considerable concession of withdrawing one of the

contentious letters (that dealing with Wittes' editorial) in order to comply
with Relman's conditions and so, as he put it, 'expedite [Relman's]
consideration of the publication' of the other letter dealing with the
Mayo Clinic article (Pauling to Relman, 8 March 1986). Relman did
not respond to this overture, but the tension eased a little, when, the
following month, the *New England Journal of Medicine* published a lengthy
article by a National Institutes of Health researcher on 'New Concepts
in the Biology and Biochemistry of Ascorbic Acid'. This article made
fleeting but even-handed reference to the ongoing vitamin C and cancer
controversy:

> It has been suggested that ascorbic acid is helpful in treating patients
> with several kinds of cancer. However, a recent study showed that
> ascorbic acid was ineffective in the treatment of colon carcinomas
> in patients who had not previously received chemotherapy. Since
> colon carcinomas are resistant to every known therapy, the failure of
> ascorbic acid in this instance may not preclude its possible beneficial
> effects in other forms of cancer. . . . [A]scorbic acid may yet have
> some role in the prevention or treatment of cancer. (Levine, 1986)

But this olive branch, if indeed it was intended as such, did not resolve
the continuing problem of the still unpublished letters. And Cameron
had now learned (some fourteen months after its submission) that his
paper had been rejected by the *Journal*. He was informed by Relman
that the editors and referees had all agreed that his data were 'provocative' but not interpretable because of 'flaws' in the study design,
the major problem being the lack of proper randomization. If Cameron
were prepared to revise his paper in the light of the reviewers' comments,
to retitle it as a 'preliminary study', and to present his conclusions
more tentatively as speculations rather than truths, he might resubmit.
Relman promised a fair re-review and a very prompt final decision
(Relman to Cameron, 12 March 1986). On contacting Relman for clarification, Cameron was 'horrified' to discover that Relman's letter had
been precipitated by the threat of legal action by a firm of attorneys
representing the Linus Pauling Institute. Although he agreed that the
delay in refereeing his manuscript had indeed been 'extraordinary',
Cameron immediately dissociated himself from any such implied action,
revised the manuscript as suggested and resubmitted it with a courteous
covering letter to Relman (Cameron to Relman, 12 May 1986).

While Pauling's letters remained unanswered, Cameron's revised
manuscript now became the centre of a prolonged and increasingly
aggressive ball game between himself and the *New England Journal of
Medicine*. For the next year the manuscript bounced back and forth,
while Relman and editorial staff bent over backwards to ensure its

'fair' refereeing by successive teams of 'expert' reviewers, and a grimly determined Cameron revised it three more times in an effort to meet their objections. In the end, as he, the referees, and editorial staff agreed (although, predictably, not for the same reasons), it was futile to continue the game. None of his many revisions, nor any of the new information Cameron could pull out of the computer, could meet the *Journal's* stringently enforced criteria for an adequately designed and controlled clinical trial of vitamin C. As far as Cameron was concerned, none of the reviewers' criticisms had presented any 'insuperable objection' to publication. He now angrily concluded that the *Journal's* rejection had been motivated by 'political concerns' rather than 'scientific inadequacies', and he announced his 'reluctant conversion' to Pauling's conspiracy theory:

> If you people have any conscience at all, you must be uncomfortably aware that you had a duty and an obligation (to the American public if not to me) to publish our manuscript as a counterbalance to the much-publicized Mayo Clinic study, which you surely must know by now to have been so seriously flawed as to be unbelievable. And you compound that genuine mistake by publishing a facetious supportive Editorial and suppressing all critical correspondence and manuscripts including my own.
>
> In my long, pleasant and productive association with Linus Pauling, we have had one matter of constant disagreement. Dr Pauling, like many of the American public, sincerely believes that the medical profession is waging some kind of monstrous conspiracy to maintain its prestige, its power, and its fee-earning capacity at the expense of the public. I have argued vehemently with him that this is not so, and that our profession may well be too conservative and slow to accept new ideas, but is always motivated by the highest ethics and ideals. This latest episode makes me wonder whether it is I who have been overly naive these many years.   (Cameron to Salzman, 4 May 1987)

By mid 1987 it was more than two years since the *New England Journal of Medicine* had published the second Mayo Clinic trial of vitamin C, and it had been sitting without apparent decision on Pauling's letter and his and Herman's manuscript of their reanalysis of the Mayo Clinic trial for almost as long. The only opportunity Pauling had been given for a detailed presentation of his criticisms of the trial in the professional literature had come about in the previous year, after the journal *Nutrition Reviews* had published a report headed 'Ascorbic Acid does not cure Cancer' and which stated:

> The Mayo Clinic group then carried out a new study that duplicated the experimental conditions of Cameron and Pauling, except that the

investigation was a prospective, randomized, double-blind study. . . .
This study lays to rest the ghost of the theory that megadoses of
ascorbic acid will cure advanced cancer. (Anon., 1985b)

When the ever-vigilant Pauling wrote to protest this interpretation of the
Mayo Clinic study and of his and Cameron's claims, the journal (which is
not in the mainstream of clinical medicine or cancer research) published a
special report on the controversy. This reproduced Pauling's criticisms,
followed by Moertel's invited rebuttal of these, and expressed the pious
hope that 'this exchange of views, plus the published record, will clarify
and perhaps settle the controversy'.

Given its history, and the calibre of its protagonists, this was, perhaps,
a little optimistic on the part of the editor. Moertel summarily dismissed
Pauling's primary criticism of the trial on the grounds that 'actual duration of treatment made no difference whatsoever. Whether patients were
continued on treatment for 1 month, 3 months, 6 months, or 12 months,
high-dose vitamin C never performed any better than sugar pills.' Nor
did any patient show any symptom of 'withdrawal scurvy' as charged by
Pauling: 'Survival distributions measured from the last dose of vitamin C
or the last dose of placebo completely overlap.' Moertel also strongly
disputed the charge of non-compliance and surreptitious ingestion of
vitamin C by the controls in the study, arguing that their random urine
tests had demonstrated a 'remarkable compliance record in our patients'.
At the same time, he gave his opponents a hearty serve back:

> We would agree that such careful monitoring of compliance is essen-
> tial for the validity of any study requiring active patient cooperation.
> It is notable that the publications of Cameron and Pauling presented
> no evidence regarding the compliance of their treated patients. Since
> their control data were derived from history reviews, any monitoring
> of their untreated patients would have been impossible. (Moertel,
> 1986a)

Following on this public crossing of swords, Pauling had written
Moertel, yet again requesting the original data of the Mayo Clinic trial,
and suggesting that they should collaborate on a reanalysis of the data
and attempt to resolve their differences. 'I have been concerned', he
wrote,

> about the possibility that many cancer patients who might benefit by
> receiving high-dose vitamin C as an adjunct to appropriate conven-
> tional therapy are being deprived of this benefit because of a general
> misunderstanding about the significance of the existing evidence, in
> particular a possible misunderstanding about the interpretation of

results that you and your associates reported in the *New England Journal of Medicine* . . . I am accordingly writing to you to make the suggestion that you and I collaborate on an effort to clarify this situation.

You have made many contributions to cancer therapy, and I am well known as a scientist, with a generally good reputation. I think that a statement to which both you and I subscribed would have much value.

The sting in the tail of this proposal (a copy of which Pauling thoughtfully mailed to DeVita of the National Cancer Institute), was Pauling's concluding reminder to Moertel:

I am sure that you saw the editorial in the *New York Times* for 28 July 1985, based on the report of a committee of the National Academy of Sciences. The last sentence in the editorial is 'A scientist who denies legitimate inquirers access to the data frustrates the validation process of science'. (Pauling to Moertel, 7 January 1987)

This piece of provocation had the effect of finally extracting a letter from Moertel, but not the hoped-for trial data. Moertel, in his turn, wrote to remind Pauling that he had accused the Mayo Clinic team on public media of having committed fraud, which was a criminal offence. Pauling had also announced his intention to bring suit against Moertel and his co-authors. As a scientist, Moertel found this all very saddening, but in the circumstances, and following legal advice, he must refuse Pauling's request for collaboration and the data (Moertel to Pauling, 27 January 1987).

In August 1987, all else having failed, Pauling resorted to legal pressure to force the *New England Journal of Medicine* to a decision about the publication of his letter and his and Herman's manuscript. A communication from a prominent firm of New York lawyers served to remind Relman that, although the *Journal* had decided a long time ago not to publish the manuscript, he had never written to Pauling to explain why. He finally informed Pauling that his manuscript could not be considered for three reasons. (1) The paper was not an original research report but a reanalysis of data already published in the *Journal*, and would therefore have to be seen by the authors of the original report before a decision could be made to publish it. Pauling's insistence that there be no communication with the Mayo Clinic researchers placed the *Journal* under unacceptable constraints. (2) There was a basic flaw in the logic of the manuscript. Even if the statistical analysis had been valid (and this was disputed by the statistical referee as described), there was no convincing reason to conclude that stopping vitamin C made the cancers worse. Many of the patients in the study had continued on vitamin C for more than two months, and Pauling and Herman had cited no evidence to show that the ones who died in the 2 to 5 month period had all stopped vitamin C. Further, they had presented no evidence that the rebound effect plus cytotoxic chemotherapy could cause a longer-term putative increase in deaths. It was just as logical, wrote Relman, to suggest that such an increase in mortality was due to a delayed toxic effect of the vitamin C. (3) The statistical analysis was invalid. With such small samples, the actual small differences in the numbers of deaths could only be significant if each point in the Kaplan-Meier curves was treated as an independent data point, which they, of course, were not. (Not having any access to the raw data of the trial, Pauling and Herman, it will be recalled, had extrapolated the data from the published Kaplan-Meier diagrams.)

As for Pauling's letter to the editor, Relman and his colleagues required some revisions before they would be willing to consider publication. Pauling should make it clear that: the duration of administration of vitamin C in the Mayo Clinic study was for the *median* time of 2.5 months (range 1 day to 25.5 months); that vitamin C had not been arbitrarily stopped but was continued until the patient could no longer tolerate the dose or until there was objective evidence of marked progression of the cancer; and that there was no statistically significant difference between the mortality curves for the first twelve months, and that the difference after that time favoured the placebo. If Pauling were to rewrite his letter making these points, it would 'probably' be published. He was, of course, free to express any opinions he wished, but he was not free to misrepresent the Mayo Clinic study, nor to state conclusions based on invalid reasoning (Relman to Pauling, 4 September 1987).

Pauling's reaction to what Cameron described as this 'incredible' letter was to inform his lawyers that he and Herman, having considered the enclosed referee's report, thought that their paper should not be published in its original form. Their paper had been based on the assumption that the patients in the Mayo Clinic study had died in the same order in which they were taken off the vitamin C or placebo. Their conclusions would be more reliable if they had detailed information about the individual patients, but Moertel had refused to give them this information. They had done the best they could on the basis of the figures in the Mayo Clinic paper, but clearly they needed more data.

Pauling also, to the astonishment of Cameron and Herman, revised his original letter to the editor, interpolating the three statements required by Relman, and this was forwarded to the *New England Journal of Medicine* by Pauling's lawyers in October 1987. But, this revised letter has never been published.

Nor has Cameron been able to secure the publication of his much-revised manuscript in any of the mainstream medical journals to which it has been submitted. The list of rejections now includes *Cancer Research*, the *American Journal of Epidemiology*, the *Journal of the Royal College of Surgeons of Edinburgh*, and the *British Medical Journal*. The consistently stated reason for rejection has been that the study was not prospectively randomized, and therefore that uncontrolled biases were inherent in the trial design. Cameron has reacted angrily against what he discerns as the 'current fetish with randomization' and the 'blind bigotry and prejudice surrounding us on all sides':

> [C]an the [editors] not see that we were simply reporting a very significant observation, that one very large group of incurable cancer patients, given ascorbate, lived very significantly longer than an even larger group not given ascorbate? This increase in survival time, to say nothing of enhanced quality of life and freedom from iatrogenic side-effects, is very much greater than could have been achieved by any form of chemotherapy known, or Interferon, or Interleukin-2, or monoclonal antibodies, or hyperthermia, or any of the other currently fashionable modalities. Against that broad achievement, nit-picking comments about 'start dates' and 'selection bias' are surely trivial and irrelevant.   (personal communication, 17 November 1987)

6.5   CLOSING THE CONTROVERSY

Another major setback for Pauling and Cameron appears to be looming in the form of the previously referred to and still unconcluded Report on Unorthodox Cancer Treatments which is being prepared by the Health and Life Sciences Division of the Office of Technology Assessment (see 2.6). In mid-1988, Cameron was informed by a contact that the physician who had been sub-contracted to write the section on vitamin C was preparing a 'pretty damning report':

> This was all news to us. We had never heard of this [Yetiv] and he had not contacted us. I found him, a 30 year-old MD, working in the Emergency Room of Sequoia Hospital here in Redwood City. He condescended to visit us the next week after his report had been submitted . . . , and proceeded to lecture Pauling and me on statistics, his worship of the Mayo Clinic's infallibility, while admitting that he had never treated a single cancer patient in his life. His accusation, presumably in his report, was that my advocacy of vitamin C was criminal in that patients under my care were being denied conventional treatment. I pointed out to this surgical adolescent that I had been operating on cancer patients most of my professional life, and that blanket chemotherapy was not carried out in my country. I doubt

if this youth had ever read a bloody word we have ever written, and yet his judgements are now enroute to Congress as a contracted 'expert'. . . . I am still soldiering on 'bloody but unbowed' . . . I have not given up hope.   (personal communication, 15 June 1988)

Dr Jack Z. Yetiv (who has a medical degree and a Ph.D. in pharmacology – the study of drugs) is the author of *Popular Nutritional Practices: A Scientific Appraisal* (Yetiv, 1986). He is also a contributing editor to *Nutrition Forum*, the leading popular journal devoted to the exposure of nutritional quackery, and is identified as a prominent 'quackbuster' by the alternative network. In his book, Yetiv offered a 'scientific appraisal' of the Vale of Leven trials (citing Victor Herbert's criticism of such uncontrolled trials) and of the two 'carefully performed scientific studies' carried out at the Mayo Clinic. Yetiv's account does not acknowledge the Pauling-Cameron criticisms of the second Mayo Clinic trial, and, as evidence of the 'potential toxicity' and 'careless use' of vitamin C megadose, he cited an anecdotal case report of kidney failure in an elderly man who had been given a vitamin C infusion for an atherosclerotic condition. Yetiv's book endorsed the now-established party line of the vitamin C 'non-believers': that vitamin C might play some preventative role, but that 'current evidence clearly suggests that vitamin C has no role in the treatment of cancer' (Yetiv, 1986).

Despite its confidential status, the preliminary draft of the as yet unreleased OTA Report on Unorthodox Cancer Treatments has been widely circulated throughout the alternative network and has become the focus of a fierce controversy in its own right. In a replay of a by now familiar scenario, it has provoked senatorial interventions, public denunciations by the NHF, appeals to Congress to 'save OTA from bias and the influence of Sloan–Kettering', charges of 'suppression' by OTA of contract reports sympathetic to alternative treatments, of 'dishonesty' and 'negative bias' of OTA staff, of 'shoddy' research on the adverse effects of alternative therapies, and countercharges by OTA staff of the 'lack of objectivity' of certain contracted researchers and their 'selectively positive' treatment of the data on unorthodox therapies.

This contentious OTA draft report encapsulates the all-too-familiar interpretative difficulties of therapeutic evaluation and the inherently political nature of the process. Vitamin C features prominently as the unorthodox cancer treatment which has undergone the most complete orthodox testing. But there is no discussion in the draft report of Pauling's and Cameron's criticisms of the second Mayo Clinic trial. Instead, coverage is given to the third and little-known multi-centre randomized clinical trial which, according to one of the investigators (who was also involved in the first two Mayo Clinic trials), was undertaken to forestall criticism of possible bias in the two single-centre Mayo Clinic trials (see 5.4). According to this same Mayo Clinic informant, analysis of the study was never completed because the early results were unpromising, consistent with the results of the two Mayo Clinic studies. The draft report cites this investigator's belief that the vitamin C question had been laid to rest and that it was not therefore important to complete and publish full details of this study.

Although the OTA draft report makes the point that the Pauling-Cameron claims of improved quality of life were not adequately tested in the Mayo Clinic trials, it concurs with orthodox opinion that *three* randomized clinical trials have failed to confirm the claims of improved survival made by Cameron and Pauling. According to the report, the evidence produced by these three randomized trials would be more than sufficient to quell interest in an orthodox anti-cancer drug, and there is general consensus amongst orthodox researchers that the case for high dose vitamin C as a cancer treatment is considered closed. It is the extensive continued use of vitamin C by unorthodox physicians in the United States and Mexico, after what appears to be valid evidence suggesting no benefit, that now unequivocally places vitamin C in the unorthodox camp.

In response to enquiries about vitamin C, the National Cancer Institute issues a prepared statement. This gives details of the two NCI-sponsored trials of vitamin C at the Mayo Clinic, and claims that 'although vitamin C has no effect as a cancer treatment', the NCI is currently sponsoring studies to determine whether dietary or supplementary vitamin C might have some role in cancer prevention (NCI, 1988).

The American Cancer Society has not as yet placed high-dose vitamin C on its Unproven Methods List. But it has made a move in this direction by citing the negative results of the two Mayo Clinic trials of high-dose vitamin C in connection with its condemnation of 'Metabolic Cancer Therapy' on the grounds of 'no evidence of objective benefit' (ACS, 1987). This therapy purportedly includes a minimum of 15g per day of vitamin C, along with laetrile and various other vitamins and 'enzymes'. The ACS Statements on Unproven Methods are currently in the process of revision, and the ACS will not make any statement on its intentions with respect to vitamin C. But upon enquiry about the status of vitamin C as a cancer treatment, the ACS provides copies of the two negative Mayo Clinic studies.

Moertel himself has no doubts about the matter. As a result of the 'definitive and believable answers' of the Mayo Clinic trials, 'the vitamin C issue is dead' (Moertel, 1989).

Part III
The Politics of Therapeutic Evaluation

What motivates Dr Pauling, 84 last month, to be in there fighting tooth and claw? Is it vanity and hurt pride? Perhaps some of it; after all we all have our self-respect. Is it for publicity and honor? I do not think so. I have known him a long time now, and I am convinced his main motivation is humanitarian, as with his other great interest in the Peace Movement.

What motivates me? I do not know. It is certainly not for publicity, awards, financial reward etc. It is a small country surgeon with one blazing idea and a life-long desire to do something useful about the cancer problem. Sounds too romantic to be true, perhaps, but that is how I think of myself, with all due modesty and conceit.

More interesting, what motivates Moertel and his cronies?. . . . Normally we might have received a letter something like this:

'Hi guys
We think your ideas sheer codswallop and utter garbage, but, because of public interest, we have been contracted by the NCI to test them.
Here's what we plan to do. Any comments now to save later misunderstandings?
We'll look at the matter as fairly and honestly as we can, but frankly we expect to find nothing.
We'll keep you posted how things are going, and let you see our results ahead of publication.
        Sincerely, etc.'

But instead this wall of impenetrable silence and the hostility in the publication and especially in the Press Release and media appearances. Why?
                    Ewan Cameron, personal communication, 4 March 1985.

169

7 The Social Shaping of the Vitamin C and Cancer Controversy

Cancer is not a simple 'military' situation with a simple decisive answer. It is a complex multifactorial behaviour problem requiring a political solution.

To treat cancer intelligently demands a rethink of our whole therapeutic philosophy. We should abandon our futile and illogical policy of trying to kill cancer cells. Instead we should endeavour to understand the cause of their discontent and seek a compromise solution. If we are prepared to accept that cancer cells *too* have a right to survive, we could be well on our way to a negotiated peace and an end to the cellular rebellion.   (Cameron, March, 1972)

Pauling asserted that the analogy with chemotherapy reflected a profound misconception about the use of Vitamin C in treating cancer. 'Vitamin C is not a drug, that is the mistake made by Dr Moertel and his associates,' said Dr Pauling.   (Horwitz, 1985)

The claim that a life-extending treatment for a disease must be given until the day the patient dies is a bit unusual.   (Moertel, 1986a)

The remainder of this book is an analysis of the vitamin C and cancer controversy in its social and institutional contexts. The goal of this analysis is to explore the implications of this exceptionally well-documented case study for our understanding of the social shaping of the evaluation and implementation of medical therapies and technologies.

The foregoing account has permitted us to follow the development of the controversy from initial conflict to pending closure. For all Cameron's and Pauling's expressed optimism and Pauling's continuing efforts to reopen the debate, right now it seems most likely that they have lost the battle over vitamin C as an adjuvant treatment for cancer. Orthodox medicine is in the process of closing the controversy by foreclosing any future trials of vitamin C megadose for cancer, and by refusing Pauling and Cameron a professional forum for their criticisms and claims. Orthodoxy will concede a limited preventative role for vitamin C but not a curative one.

As far as Pauling's Mayo Clinic opponents are concerned, they have definitively disproved the efficacy of vitamin C as a cancer treatment. In their view they have scrupulously obeyed the rules and won the conflict by fair means. Although they did not agree with Pauling's criticism of their first trial and thought the scientific basis of his criticism 'obscure', they went to the length of carrying out another trial which was specifically designed to test his claim that high-dose vitamin C is effective therapy for advanced cancer in patients who have had no prior chemotherapy. They believe that they have now conclusively demonstrated that high-dose vitamin C is not effective against advanced malignant disease, irrespective of whether the patient has had prior chemotherapy or not. As they see it, Pauling must now admit his scientific defeat and assume his ethical responsibilities to cancer patients by refraining from promoting an ineffective cancer treatment.

Their stand is officially backed by the NCI, whose senior personnel DeVita and Wittes confirmed that the second Mayo Clinic trial met all the conventional ethical and methodological standards for clinical trials and that its negative results are 'definitive'. The NCI has therefore, quite legitimately in their view, refused to sponsor any further trials of vitamin C. Relman and editorial staff of the *New England Journal of Medicine* did their best to ensure the standard fair and equitable editorial and peer review of all the relevant papers and reports. Indeed, it might be argued that they bent the rules in Cameron's favour by giving his manuscript such repeated access to the reviewing process. As for Pauling's letters and manuscript, the problem there was Pauling's intransigence and refusal to conform with journal policy, not to mention his gratuitously abusive public statements and private letters and his litigious threats. These latter have both 'saddened' and appalled Pauling's orthodox critics and opponents. His charges of 'fraud' and 'conspiracy' and threats to resort to the law courts are perceived to be totally out of place in scientific debate, and a serious violation of the standard ethical norms. Pauling's opponents and critics believe that the only appropriate response to such ethical violation from such an eminent scientific figure is to reassert the norms of science, to retreat to their own higher moral ground and to refuse all communication and scientific cooperation with the transgressor. Thus the refusal of Moertel and the Mayo Clinic investigators to give Pauling access to the raw trial data may be perceived, from their point of view, as a proper and ethically justifiable decision.

Yet, as the foregoing account makes explicit, the orthodox disproof of the efficacy of vitamin C as a cancer treatment has been achieved only by disregarding the theoretical framework and the associated clinical and evaluative practices of their alternative opponents. In the second and 'definitive' clinical trial, the Mayo Clinic oncologists tested vitamin C as they would test any conventional cytotoxic drug which is administered for short periods of time and whose therapeutic impact is measured primarily in terms of tumour shrinkage. In other words, their methodology was determined by their own theoretical and professional perspectives on how a chemotherapeutic drug should be administered and tested. They did not administer and evaluate vitamin C within the exact framework established by Cameron and Pauling, but administered and assessed it within their own professionally-endorsed framework of expertise. Within this framework, as they rightly claim, vitamin C does not work. It is not an effective chemotherapeutic drug. The problem is that Pauling and Cameron have never claimed it to be. This is the crux of their critique of the second Mayo Clinic trial and their categorical rejection of it as constituting a replication and refutation of Cameron's Vale of Leven studies. So Pauling and Cameron are right also, within their own terms, in their contention that the Mayo Clinic oncologists have not disproved their claims. As they see it, ethical norms have been violated by the intransigence of their orthodox opponents, their public and professional misrepresentation of their work as replicating and definitively refuting Cameron's Vale of Leven studies, their refusal to reopen negotiations or to allow Pauling and Cameron a professional platform for their views, and their withholding of the raw trial data. It is these misrepresentations and unethical actions by their opponents that have provoked Pauling's charges of 'fraud' and forced him to resort to threats of litigation in his attempt to have his own views heard.

If the orthodox claim of the inefficacy of vitamin C as a cancer treatment prevails, then it will do so, *not* because of the unambiguous falsification of the Pauling–Cameron claims, as the standard view of medical science would have it. Nor will the orthodox claim prevail as the result of agreement or consensus brought about by the disinterested application of the impersonal rules of experimental procedure in the form of the randomized controlled clinical trial, as the reformers and critics of medicine urge. Rather, *social and political means will have been crucial in closing the controversy.*

I do not mean by this to suggest that we must subscribe to Pauling's conspiracy theory and charges of fraud and misrepresentation. We have no more reason to doubt the scientific integrity and good faith of Pauling's opponents than we have to doubt the integrity and good faith of Pauling and Cameron. Rather, I am trying to show that the process of therapeutic evaluation is *inherently* a social and political process, and that the idea of neutral appraisal is a myth. Judgements about experimental findings are inextricably, *necessarily*, bound up with the professional and wider social values and interests of those who are carrying out the evaluation. This applies as much to the judgements of Pauling and Cameron as to those of their orthodox opponents. The foregoing detailed reconstruction of the vitamin C and cancer controversy demonstrates the constant merging and interaction of the theoretical arguments and clinical evidence of the vitamin C 'believers' and 'non-believers' with a whole array of what are generally thought of as 'non-scientific' or social activities.

7.1 THE SOCIAL NEGOTIATION OF THE EFFICACY OF VITAMIN C AS A CANCER TREATMENT

The old ideal of science as the achievement of great men thinking their great thoughts in splendid isolation dies hard. But the reality is that fact-making in science is a collective enterprise. As study after study has shown, in order to establish the 'truth' of a claim and make it resistant to criticism and dissent, that is, to turn it into a 'fact', a complex network of allies who participate in the construction and defence of the claim is necessary. Allies are enrolled through becoming convinced that it is in their interests to participate in these fact-making processes (Latour, 1987). This is not necessarily a conscious or purposive process on the part of the individuals concerned. They may be drawn into fact-making negotiations when their own claim is incorporated into other claims, or becomes a resource for other claim makers.

It is important to understand, as Barry Barnes has emphasized, that this process of collective scientific construction is not to be compared with the way in which brickbuilders construct a house 'with each brick checked for shape and soundness and then permanently cemented into the structure of the house' (Barnes, 1985). Scientific claims are constantly being re-evaluated and renegotiated. Their applications are open-ended and always revisable by other users. The scientific 'bricks' and the 'house' they support are constantly changing. The history of the vitamin C controversy has provided a vivid illustration of the complex and subtle negotiations and claim modifications that typically go on among allies and their critics.

The great majority of these negotiations, as we have seen, go on behind the scenes, out of sight and out of earshot of the audience. What is presented on stage in the form of the published paper, is the carefully scripted, cleaned-up, thoroughly rehearsed and polished product. Only occasionally, when the scenery collapses, the actors forget their lines, or the stage management goes awry, does the audience catch a glimpse of the flurry and chaos of off-stage action. We, who have been standing in the wings, have been privileged observers of the processes by which the efficacy of vitamin C as a treatment for cancer has been socially negotiated and rejected. We can no more believe that what we have watched take shape is a natural event, or has been determined by nature, than we can sustain the illusion that what we see on stage is real life.

As the narrative history of the controversy makes clear, letter writing has been one of the major means of these behind-the-scenes fact-making negotiations among the disputants. By their letters, they sought to initiate and forge alliances, attempted to break up opposing coalitions, persuaded, coerced, or simply wore down, foot-dragging grant-giving bodies, recalcitrant editors and referees, and doggedly pursued or needled and provoked opponents. Letters were used to enhance the credibility of the writer and to undermine that of his critics. They were a vehicle for rhetoric, invective, threats, persuasion, and morale raising. By their tone they conveyed tacit as well as explicit information. Letters were also a means of negotiating the construction and publication of formal papers. These, as other historical and sociological studies have found, are thereby revealed not to be straightforward and unproblematic reports of observations and experimental results, but carefully crafted, persuasive arguments designed to gloss over inconsistencies and weaknesses, and to present the claims of the authors in the best possible light (Latour and Woolgar, 1979; Mulkay and Gilbert, 1982; Rudwick, 1985).

As the study of their correspondence has shown, the little-known Cameron was able to attract the famous Pauling's attention by attaching his PHI/ascorbate hypothesis to Pauling's well-publicized interest in furthering the anti-cancer potential of vitamin C. By linking his thesis into Pauling's struggle to establish the orthomolecular programme, Cameron gained a powerful ally who would act as referee for grants, assist with the publication of results, lend his name and authority to publications, and, generally, mobilize resources and support for Cameron's research. In return, Cameron proffered the essential experimental findings and the promise of further systematic clinical research of vitamin C that Pauling was finding hard to obtain in the United States. But in order to retain the more powerful Pauling as an ally, Cameron had to 'translate' (Latour, 1987) his primary interest in PHI as the potential 'cure' for cancer into Pauling's interest in furthering the theoretical and clinical rationale for vitamin C therapy. To this end, Cameron stressed the closeness of their theoretical approaches, and he adopted Pauling's orthomolecular terminology and the orthomolecular medical framework for the presentation of his work. He thus acquiesced in the theoretical and clinical displacement of PHI by vitamin C.

Cameron's translation of his cancer claims into Pauling's interests extended even to politics and ideology. In the early stages of his collaboration with Pauling, Cameron, as we saw, neatly summed up the crucial distinctions between vitamin C therapy and conventional cytotoxic therapy in political terms that could be guaranteed to appeal to the famous anti-war activist. It is a measure of its attractiveness to Pauling and of its potential appeal to a large and more radical sector of the alternative health movement, that Cameron's peaceful coexistence and disarmament metaphor, with all its ideological and political overtones, was later incorporated into the popular presentation of his and Pauling's claims. In their book, *Cancer and Vitamin C*, they argued that cancer cells were not 'foreign invaders' with some fundamental difference in origin and metabolism from normal body cells that was capable of chemotherapeutic exploitation. Where conventional cytotoxic treatment sought to destroy the cancer cells in the hope of effecting a cure, their 'alternative strategy' was to focus on the control of their invasiveness, to 'disarm malignant cells and render them non-invasive' (Cameron and Pauling, 1979b).

Initially, Pauling attempted to use Cameron's promising pilot data as a means of enrolling American clinicians and the NCI in the clinical evaluation and research of vitamin C. But Pauling's failure to interest American clinicians and grant-giving bodies in vitamin C meant that Cameron and his Scottish-based studies became indispensable to Pauling's struggle to establish the anti-cancer potential of vitamin C as a central element in the orthomolecular research programme. From this point of view, it was in Pauling's interest to lend his name to Cameron's research, to promote its publication and enhance its credibility. The prestigious Pauling certification enabled Cameron to interest Scottish physicians, institutions and grant-giving bodies in his research, and so to get on with the crucial clinical evaluation of vitamin C as a cancer therapy. When Cameron was confronted by his early failure to achieve a measurable response to vitamin C treatment in terminal cancer patients and began to cast about for alternative hypotheses, it was Pauling who kept him on course and set the goal of the 'ten-per cent' response and its recognition and evaluation. When Cameron had achieved this Pauling-set goal, was rewarded with a research grant from the Linus Pauling Institute, and wanted to use it to investigate the relation of ascorbic acid to PHI, Pauling advised him to 'leave the biochemistry to the biochemists' and redirected him to his essential 'clinical studies of ascorbic acid in relation to cancer' (Chapter 4.5).

The subsequent organization of the fund-raising activities of the faltering Linus Pauling Institute around Cameron's Vale of Leven trial results linked the viability of the Institute with the credibility of the Vale of Leven trials. With this consolidation of the Pauling-Cameron alliance (which led eventually to the physical relocation of Cameron and his work to the Linus Pauling Institute), both scientists worked in tandem to refine their methodology and strengthen the credibility and professional medical impact of Cameron's experimental results. At the same time, as they had done from the beginning of their collaboration, they sought to augment and intermesh their vitamin C claims with other claims and to mobilize more allies and supporters. In the process, their original claims were subtly modified.

The most prominent and best-documented instance of this was the long-deliberated and very conscious decision by Cameron late in 1973 to 'shift their ground a little' as part of his strategy of promoting vitamin C as a standard supportive measure to reinforce established methods of cancer treatment. It will be recalled that he hoped to defuse the expected criticisms and opposition of conventional oncologists by this means. Vitamin C was therefore offered as 'supportive care' that would strengthen the intrinsic defence mechanisms of the patient and so bring about 'striking improvement' in the response to standard forms of treatment. In order to promote this non-threatening image, Cameron moved the initial PHI/ascorbate hypothesis off centre stage and gave greater theoretical prominence to the role of ascorbate in stimulating the immune system and generally enhancing resistance to cancer (Cameron and Pauling, 1974). Later, he and Pauling were able to reinforce this claim by linking it with research on the low lymphocyte ascorbate content of cancer patients (see section 4.7; Cameron *et al.*, 1979). But this supporting evidence was not available at the time they made this subtle theoretical shift. It was a strategy prompted by their essentially *social* need to present and publish the experimental findings in such a way as to placate a potentially hostile audience of conventional oncologists. This same strategy had the additional advantage, as Cameron was well aware, of allying vitamin C therapy with the interests and purposes of the orthodox immunotherapists, who, around the same time, were also attempting to promote immunotherapy as part of a combination treatment for cancer (Currie, 1972).

These subtle modifications in the selection and emphasis of available theoretical arguments for the presentation of Pauling's and Cameron's claims are typical of the interpretative flexibility of scientists' findings (Collins, 1985; Pinch, 1986). This interpretative flexibility is also illustrated by the way in which Cameron was able to 'tinker towards success' (Knorr-Cetina, 1979), and produce for Pauling the necessary 'ten-per cent response' in the face of the difficulties he initially experienced in evaluating vitamin C's effectiveness for terminal cancer patients. He managed this largely by drawing a crucial distinction between the evaluation of cytotoxic chemotherapy and vitamin C therapy. As Cameron represented it, the clinical evaluation of a treatment which controls or palliates rather than cures cancer necessarily entailed the drawing of finer discriminations in patient response than that of conventional methods. When the predicted and claimed majority response of retardation of tumour growth proved 'almost impossible' to measure, Cameron shifted his emphasis from tumour size to the palliation of cancer symptoms and survival times. As we saw, after time and experience had tempered his initial 'over-enthusiastic phase', Cameron carefully modulated his experimental findings and their presentation around the deliberately modest claim that he could 'lighten varying shades of grey', rather than produce the 'dramatic contrasts in black and white' that he argued his conventional colleagues had been taught to look for in their evaluation of cancer treatments. This was also consistent with his strategy of not promoting vitamin C as a cancer treatment in its own right, but as an adjunctive to established methods of treatment.

By no means should this strategic manipulation and presentation of Cameron's and Pauling's theoretical and experimental claims be understood as an index of their lack of scientific rigour or as constituting a reason for the outright rejection of their work. It should be understood, rather, as a typical manifestation of normal science in the making. Scientists routinely transform their raw research as they prepare and write it up for public presentation. They may re-evaluate and reconstruct what happened at the laboratory bench or in the clinic many times in an effort to get it into the form which will best satisfy the collective criteria of judgement of their peers (Latour and Woolgar, 1979; Barnes, 1985).

7.2 MORE NEGOTIATIONS: THE SOCIAL CHARACTER OF THE PUBLICATION PROCESS

This typical process of transformation and scrutiny is formalized in the reviewing process when papers are reassessed and re-evaluated by referees, who are supposed to be specially selected for their expert and detailed knowledge of the topic involved. These are the accredited gatekeepers: they filter the new claims through the accepted knowledge of the community that adjudicates that field. This formal process of refereeing is also a highly social one. Senior scientists with high professional standing such as Pauling usually have fewer refereeing difficulties than their juniors. They are themselves the accredited experts, standard setters and adjudicators, and in certain instances their status enables them to bypass the normal reviewing process. Pauling's high scientific ranking as a member of the National Academy of Sciences thus entitled him to publication in the Academy's journal, the *PNAS*, without formal refereeing.

The social character of the publication process was borne out when the Editorial Board of the *PNAS*, confronted by the Pauling–Cameron hypothesis paper which they did not want to publish and by the additional complication of the eminence of one of its authors, changed the rules in mid-play in order to reject it. The stated reason for their rejection was the essentially social one: that a paper advocating therapeutic procedures in such an 'emotive' area as cancer should be put through the filter of the normal medical reviewing process. As Pauling's enquiries revealed, this requirement of reviewing by the relevant specialty had never been enforced for other theoretical papers. The unstated concern of the Editorial Board clearly was that a hypothesis published in the prestigious *PNAS* and endorsed by the Pauling name would impact on professional practices in cancer treatment.

The means by which Pauling was able to override this sudden and arbitrary imposition of professional medical vetting of the hypothesis is equally revealing of the socially mediated character of the reviewing process: the publicity provoked an offer, *sight unseen*, of publication from *Oncology*, on the basis of Pauling's reputation and the enthusiasm of the editor for vitamin C therapy. The adverse publicity and Pauling's reputation were also crucial to Pauling's continuing negotiations with the *PNAS* Editorial Board, whereby he successfully forced an expression of 'regret' from the Academy, the softening and redefinition of its revised editorial policy, and a formal invitation to revise and resubmit the contentious paper. Pauling's insider and privileged status as past Chairman of the Editorial Board and his prominent membership of an extended scientific network are symbolized by the first name terms with which he and the successive Chairmen of the Board addressed one another. A succinct 'Dear Bob' or 'Dear Linus' at the beginning of a letter negotiating publication or editorial policy, summons up a whole set of underlying social relations which inevitably enter into and influence the outcome of these negotiations.

Again, none of this should be construed as unusual or as somehow transgressing the bounds of 'normal' science. Trust and personal warrant play a much greater part in fact-making negotiations within science than is often realized. The idealized image of science, where every statement is scrutinized and judged with equal care irrespective of its source, is not borne out in scientific practice. Claims made by outsiders or marginal figures usually do not count; they are seldom taken seriously and may be readily dismissed without scrutiny; if they are to be accepted they must be rigorously and independently checked out by an insider. The assertions of qualified scientists, on the other hand, are almost invariably taken seriously and often trusted to be correct simply because of the reputation of the scientist making the claim (Barnes, 1985; Pinch, 1986). In Pauling's case, both sets of forces came into play: while he was an eminent and trusted insider in the scientific community, he was generally perceived as marginal to or outside the medical community.

On each occasion of successful publication achieved by the alternatives, it was Pauling's eminence and networking that carried the day. Pauling's name and intervention conjured up openings in scientific journals, rearranged printing queues, and bulldozed over the 'severe exceptions' and 'strongly negative' comments of critical and quibbling referees. Pauling's scientific status and networking skills were also significant factors in the negotiation of the publication of the correspondence between the disputing parties following on the first Mayo Clinic trials. A review of the relevant correspondence strikingly bears out the previous point: that published material represents only the tip of the iceberg of the negotiations between the parties concerned. The publication of the first letter of 'correction' from Creagan and Moertel that sparked off the exchange of hostilities in the *New England Journal of Medicine* was negotiated by letters and telephone calls among Pauling, Moertel, Relman and Arthur Sackler, editor of the *International Medical Tribune*. The publication of Pauling's response involved prolonged negotiations, twelve letters in all, between Pauling and Relman (see section 5.1).

However, in spite of repeated efforts by Cameron and himself, on only two occasions did Pauling manage to breach the barriers and obtain publication of a vitamin C paper in orthodox medical journals: the 'hypothesis paper' in *Oncology*, in the instance noted above, and once in *Cancer Research*, when Pauling, before the first Mayo Clinic trial was underway, was invited by the editor to submit a review article on vitamin C and cancer (Cameron *et al.*, 1979). In this latter case, against their intentions, Pauling and Cameron were obliged to confine their paper to the theoretical case for vitamin C therapy.

At no stage, for all Pauling's formidable clout and networking resources, did they attain publication of Cameron's clinical results in a medical journal. This meant that the only discussion of the Vale of Leven trial results in the standard medical literature was that as represented by their opponents in the highly negative contexts of the published reports of the two Mayo Clinic trials, in the published exchanges that followed, and in orthodox reviews of the literature. Not even with the deployment of legal representation and its implicit threat of legal action, was Pauling able to negotiate the publication of his criticisms of the second Mayo Clinic trial in the form acceptable to him (nor, as it has turned out, in the form imposed on him) in the *New England Journal of Medicine*. His orthodox opponents, on the other hand, were twice granted publication of their negative results in this most prestigious and powerful of medical journals. Far from experiencing publication difficulties, these qualified insiders and their vitamin C claims were given the additional certification of an authoritative guest editorial by the NCI.

Publication and the diffusion of research claims is crucial to the fact-making process in science. The lack of positive exposure of Cameron's trial results and Pauling's criticisms of the second Mayo Clinic trial severely delimited the diffusion of the Pauling–Cameron claims and the enrolling of potential allies within orthodox medicine. It is not difficult to see that the debate might have followed a different course, had, for example, the alternatives been able to publish their initial claims in the *New England Journal of Medicine*.

7.3 FACT-MAKING AND THE MEDIA, WITH A LAW SUIT ON THE SIDE

Contrary to the standard view of science, informal or 'non-scientific' publication via newspaper reports, popular publications, or the television interview or appearance, also plays an important part in the fact-making process. When formal publication is difficult or denied, the media becomes the primary means of communicating the claims to the public and indirectly to the relevant specialty, research area, or funding body. Through media exposure of the claims, the public or certain sections of it may be enrolled in the dispute, and may contest or attempt to influence research priorities and funding and even the interpretation of data (Goodell, 1987). But even where formal publication is assured, the venue of the press conference or press release to announce research results, to urge greater funding for the relevant specialty or research area, and so on, has become a common part of science.

Just how effective and powerful the media can be in generating support for experimental therapies will become clear in the discussion of interferon (see section 8.3). But the media also played a significant part in the shaping of the vitamin C and cancer debate. Both sides in the controversy made conspicuous use of the media in the promotion of their claims and their negotiation of what is to count as an effective evaluation of vitamin C as a cancer treatment.

Without the vehicle of the media, Pauling would not have been able to promote vitamin C into a leading alternative treatment for cancer and organize it onto the orthodox medical agenda. The favourable and wide-spread publicity given to Cameron's early Vale of Leven results was crucial to the adoption of vitamin C megadose as a cancer treatment by the alternative network, to the success of the Linus Pauling Institute's fund-raising programme, and to Pauling's campaign for an NCI-funded trial of vitamin C and orthodox recognition of vitamin C as a potential cancer treatment. The balance swung back the other way with the adverse publicity generated by the Robinson affair and the two negative Mayo Clinic trials.

The media was also an important source of information for the disputants. It is notable that while Pauling's authority was sufficient to keep the Robinson affair out of American scientific and medical journals (but, significantly, not out of the leading British science journal, *Nature*), it was the media that acquainted the American scientific and medical communities with Robinson's allegations over the mouse experiments. In his turn, Pauling picked up vital clues about the course of the first Mayo Clinic trial and the Moertel-led laetrile trial from newspaper reports and reporters. And it was from a United Press International reporter that Pauling and Cameron managed to obtain their first viewing of the report on the second Mayo Clinic trial.

Both parties to the dispute also utilized the media to voice their criticisms of their opponents and their research procedures and results. The importance of the media to the disputants and to the course of the dispute is epitomized in Moertel's media coup and Pauling's and Cameron's outraged reactions on the occasion of the second Mayo Clinic trial. Deprived of the essential copy of the preprint of the paper which was made freely available to the media, the alternatives were thoroughly disadvantaged by their inability to comment on a study they had not seen. Having lost the initial media grab, Pauling's attempts to retrieve the situation were frustrated by the lack of media interest in his detailed criticisms of the trial. He could recapture media interest only by escalating his charges to 'fraud' and threats of legal action.

Media jousting by disputants in scientific controversy is attended by all the problems of misrepresentation, oversimplification, and exaggeration that the three-minute television grab, or the reporter's note book or ruthlessly edited tape imposes on the disputants and the debate. There have been any number of such instances in the vitamin C and cancer debate. Headlines such as 'Pauling Wrong on Vitamin C for Cancer', or 'Pauling Backs Laetrile', proved very difficult to correct or counteract, and all played their part in shaping the course of the dispute. As well, Pauling's lawyer-inspired tactic of using the media to provoke his opponents to a newsworthy public debate with the possibility of a law suit on the side was a dangerous one with a tendency to rebound on Pauling, and it failed to come off. His opponents, having won the current round of media jousting hands down, could afford to sit tight and largely disengage from the trading of insults and hostilities. They had the satisfaction of deflecting Pauling's shafts back at him by publicly deploring his behaviour and using his media threats of litigation to deny him the data from the second Mayo Clinic trial.

7.4   THE IMPORTANCE OF RHETORIC

As these exchanges also illustrate, the tone adopted and the rhetoric employed by the disputants were significant elements in their formal and informal negotiations. Rhetoric such as 'highly speculative' and 'extraordinary survival increase', employed in the wake of the first Mayo Clinic trial by Moertel and Creagan in referring to the claims of their opponents, all played their part in denigrating the arguments and casting doubt on the integrity and credibility of the Pauling-Cameron team. This implication of cooking the books prepared the ground for their explicit charge after the second Mayo Clinic trial that Cameron and Pauling had obtained this 'extraordinary' increase by 'case selection bias' rather than by treatment effectiveness.

Later, in the course of their published dispute over the results of the Moertel-led laetrile trial, Pauling was described by Moertel as taking 'venerable dramatic licence' with the evidence and making an 'obviously fallacious' claim. The innuendo of the following statement in the published report of the second Mayo Clinic trial needs but little elaboration: 'Surprisingly, and perhaps by chance, there were more long-term survivors receiving placebo than vitamin C'. The 'perhaps by chance' interpolation here may be translated as: 'We cannot demonstrate a statistically significant difference in survival times'. By such rhetorical means, disputants are able to make imputations that their own standards of evidence might not directly support, such as this suggestion that vitamin C ingestion actually decreased the survival times of the patients. Pauling's counter-rhetoric of 'misrepresentation', 'misleading', 'fraudulent', 'unethical', 'dishonest', 'most recent and most outrageous action by organized medicine against the new science of nutrition and the well-being of the American people', serves the same purpose. It is also a rallying call to the alternative network for their support in the dispute. Similarly, Moertel's rhetoric consistently invoked professional solidarity against the inroads of the alternatives, who were depicted as not behaving rationally or responsibly, and thereby endangering professional ethics and standards.

Another rhetorical ploy adopted by the Mayo Clinic team was their trivialization of their opponents' criticisms and claims and even of their institutional affiliations. Pauling's criticism of the first Mayo Clinic trial, a criticism that was crucial to defending the credibility of his and Cameron's claims, was represented as 'valid but scientifically trivial' and 'minor quibbling' by Moertel and Creagan. Just how seriously the disputants themselves regard such rhetorical ploys is evidenced by Pauling's interchange with Moertel over Moertel's published reference in *Oncology Times* in 1981 to Vale of Leven Hospital as a 'little' hospital (see section 5.3). This was, admittedly, not nearly as damaging as Victor Herbert's previously published description of Vale of Leven as a 'nursing home in the Scottish Highlands' (see section 3.6). But Pauling took Moertel's single adjective seriously enough to take time out from his attempt to extract the raw data of the laetrile trial from Moertel in order to carry out some bed counting at nearby Stanford University Hospital and so defend his claim that Vale of Leven was a 'large' hospital. More important, in warning Moertel that he considered his description of Vale of Leven as a 'little' hospital to have been used 'for the purpose of derogation', Pauling implied his readiness to resort to litigation and the full force of the law. Rhetoric thus plays a very significant role in the negotiation of knowledge claims, as the disputants themselves clearly recognize.

7.5 THE RHETORICAL DEPLOYMENT AND MALLEABILITY OF ETHICAL CLAIMS

One of the most important uses of rhetoric in the vitamin C controversy has been in the promotion and public presentation of the conflicting ethical positions of the disputants. Ethical reasons, based upon their opposed interpretation of the phenomena, have been consistently deployed by both sides in these negotiations over what is to count as a competent evaluation of the efficacy of vitamin C.

Thus, for some time, the orthodox successfully resisted the claims advanced by Pauling and Cameron by invoking the necessity for randomized double-blind testing procedures. The alternatives responded by gradually refining their experimental procedures and pressing for orthodox recognition of their renewed claims in the form of research funding and/or testing. When what was to be the definitive controlled experiment was finally carried out by the Moertel team in 1979, it was rejected by Pauling and Cameron on the grounds that it was not a replication of Cameron's trial and therefore had no bearing on the validity of their findings. The Moertel team, in accounting for their inability to satisfy the methodological requirements of their opponents, claimed that they did not consider it 'conscionable' to withhold accredited treatments of 'known value' in order to duplicate the experimental conditions and fully test the claims of Pauling and Cameron. Their published rhetoric, which is reproduced for the reader's scrutiny, also implied that Pauling was violating ethical norms by capitalizing on the cachet of a famous scientific name in order to lend credibility to an unproven method of cancer management:

> Overshadowing such minor quibbling is the major obligation that both we and Dr Pauling must assume to cancer patients and the general public. On the basis of claims derived from speculation and non-randomized studies endorsed by the Pauling name, megadoses of vitamin C are being used by thousands of patients with cancer,

and such treatment has been embraced by the metabolic-therapy cults. (Moertel and Creagan, 1980)

Pauling's implied irresponsibility and association with marginal and suspect medical 'cults' were thereby contrasted with the impeccable scientific and ethical credentials of the orthodox, who would themselves withhold any cancer treatment 'unless it has been proved to be of value by properly designed scientific study'.

On their side, Pauling and Cameron defined ethical behaviour in terms consistent with their claims for the efficacy of vitamin C. They defended their decision not to employ the standard randomized controlled clinical trial methodology by pointing to the ethical problems associated with the withholding of vitamin C in otherwise hopeless situations where they were convinced it was of value, 'merely', as Cameron stated, 'for the sake of obtaining observations of dubious significance for statistical comparison' (Cameron and Campbell, 1974). Their definition of ethical behaviour also involved the public dissemination of their theoretical and experimental claims for the value of vitamin C as adjunctive therapy for cancer. Thus in the terms of their own knowledge claims, they *were* behaving responsibly, and it was their opponents who were exhibiting irresponsible behaviour by failing to test their claims and by issuing 'false and misleading' counterclaims which might induce cancer patients to discontinue their vitamin C.

Subsequent events demonstrated the malleability of these largely rhetorical claims. As we saw, in 1982, after Cameron had relocated to the Linus Pauling Institute which was facing hard times in the wake of the first Mayo Clinic trial and the Robinson affair, he reversed his previous ethical objection to randomized controlled trials in an attempt to get NCI support for his clinical research. His ostensible reason for this ethical reversal was that he would be directing the proposed trial and would not himself be involved in the actual clinical practice (5.5). His orthodox rivals underwent an earlier about-face and demonstrated even greater ethical flexibility when, confronted by the publicity and political leverage Pauling had managed to recruit to his cause, they were forced in 1979 to undertake a new trial involving patients who had not had prior chemotherapy. Thus, within the space of *six months* they had to modify their ethical stance to the point where they apparently *did* consider it conscionable to withhold oncologic therapy of 'known value' in order to further their claim of the inefficacy of vitamin C in cancer treatment. By the time of the writing up of the results of the second Mayo trial (late 1984), the investigators were able to state:

We felt ethically justified in studying this group of patients without first offering cytotoxic drugs because in our opinion there is

no known form of chemotherapy for colorectal cancer that has been
demonstrated to produce substantive palliative benefit or extension
of survival. (Moertel *et al.*, 1985)

Yet, having found vitamin C ineffective according to their own criteria,
the investigators fell back onto treatment of more than half the patients
in the study with the powerful cytotoxic drug 5-fluorouracil, which they
themselves, on the basis of the same criteria, held to be of no value in
the treatment of colorectal cancer. Moertel subsequently defended this
decision to withdraw vitamin C (which was described in the study as
'relatively nontoxic' and 'benign') or placebo, and to substitute the highly
toxic and ineffective fluorouracil, on ethical grounds. It would have been
'morally and ethically repugnant', claimed Moertel, to keep patients on
vitamin C when they were getting worse (see section 6.3).

The indefinite malleability of ethical claims and their interaction with
methodological procedures and knowledge claims is illustrated yet again
by Pauling's provocative introduction to his and Herman's reinterpretation of the second Mayo Clinic trial. Here, it will be recalled, Pauling
amusingly turned the ethical tables on his opponents by alleging that 'no
ethical investigator', knowing the possible serious danger to his patients
from the rebound effect, would have designed and carried out such a
trial. It was therefore important to analyze the trial and the effect of
the rebound effect on cancer patients as thoroughly as possible, because
'ethical considerations' would probably prohibit the future replication of
the study (see section 6.3).

7.6   THE CENTRALITY OF METHOD TALK:
ITS RHETORICAL AND POLITICAL FUNCTIONS

As this review of the history of the debate makes clear, most of the
conflict has centred around the issue of what constitutes a competent
evaluation of the effectiveness of vitamin C as a cancer treatment. Judgements of methodological competency are inextricable from the opposing
beliefs of the disputants. The 'believers' who are committed to the efficacy of vitamin C claim that a 'competent' experiment is one that exactly
replicates Cameron's procedures and reliably detects this phenomenon,
while those that fail to do so are judged to have been 'incompetently'
performed. Conversely, the 'non-believers' committed to the opposite
view judge that Cameron's Vale of Leven experiments that indicated
the efficacy of vitamin C were not competent experiments. Their own
criteria of methodological competency are determined by their pre-
conceptions of how an effective and reliable chemotherapeutic agent
should be administered and evaluated. Their two consequent negative

and 'definitive' assessments of vitamin C have led the Mayo Clinic investigators to the 'inevitable conclusion' that Cameron's 'apparent positive results' were the product of 'case selection bias' rather than treatment effectiveness; while these same Mayo Clinic trials have been denounced as 'misleading', 'flawed' and 'fraudulent' by Pauling for their failure to replicate Cameron's methodology and results. At the same time, Pauling has sought to turn these 'flawed' trials and their negative results to alternative advantage: the first Mayo Clinic trial was evidence of his claim that cytotoxic chemotherapy so weakened the immune system as to negate the benefits of vitamin C, while the second trial confirmed the deleterious effects of the rebound effect in terminal cancer patients.

Both sides therefore can effectively justify their positions and procedures with a defensible argument based on their opposing beliefs. Both sides have impugned the methodology of their opponents, and brought rhetorical, ethical and other resources to the defence of their own procedures. All this contradicts the standard view that experimental results, provided the experiments are competently carried out, must compel the rational assent of scientists. In practice, as the history of the vitamin C dispute strikingly exemplifies, all experiments are always open to criticism and revision. The judgment of 'competence' or replication of procedures and results is flexible and negotiable. With the interpretative and other resources available to them, both sides to the dispute could continue indefinitely to resist the experimental procedures and claims of their opponents. Indeed, as Collins insists, 'it is difficult to see how scientific debate could be brought to a close or scientific opinion formed without the intrusion of interests, tactics and devices which are not normally thought of as being constitutive of scientific knowledge' (Collins, 1982). Other sociological studies of scientific controversies have abundantly demonstrated that whether the conflict is over the existence of quarks or high fluxes of gravitational radiation, or over the detection of solar neutrinos, neither nature nor disinterested logic nor the impersonal criteria of the experimental method determines the judgements made by scientists (Shapin, 1982; Pickering, 1984; Collins, 1985; Pinch, 1986).

In particular, these and other post-Kuhnian studies have undermined the old ideal of a single efficacious method that offers a reliable guide to the objective 'truths' of nature. Enough has been said already to indicate that all methods are context-dependent, each scientific field, in Kuhnian terms, having its own self-contained and unique method or methods, inextricable from the contents and dynamics of its existing paradigm or research tradition. These method(s) are not permanently set in concrete, but, as previously emphasized, there is a constant, subtle, ongoing revision and negotiation of the elements of the paradigm, so that its method(s), inextricable from the paradigm, are also in flux. Further, as has also been stressed, fact-making is essentially a collective or social process. The paradigm or tradition within which routine problem solving and negotiation takes place is socially embodied and socially sustained. It is the activities of *persons*, not disembodied ideas or theories, that constitute a research tradition. Above all, it is the social and political life of the field that sustains the subtly altering tradition or socio-cognitive domain within which knowledge-making and knowledge-breaking manoeuvres are contained. A method or research procedure which is bound to a particular paradigm cannot therefore be dissociated from the political and social structure of the specialist community that embodies and sustains that paradigm (Schuster, 1984; Schuster and Yeo, 1986).

This has been compellingly demonstrated by Cameron's presentation strategy and its failure to transfer successfully to the American context. The presentation of vitamin C as adjuvant therapy which would enhance established modes of treatment was developed within and was appropriate to the context of conventional Scottish methods of cancer treatment where surgery and radiotherapy were the established therapies. It was quite inappropriate to the American medical context where cytotoxic chemotherapy had become the norm in conventional cancer treatment. It is worthwhile briefly to retrace the trajectory of the debate surrounding the first Mayo Clinic trial in order to bring to the fore the professional and social interests that underlay the previously analysed deployment of ethical and other rhetorical devices on this occasion.

When Pauling, through his discussions and exchanges with NCI officials as the first Mayo Clinic trial got under way, was alerted to these national differences in cancer practices and their possible implications for any American replication of Cameron's Vale of Leven work, he summarily reshaped his and Cameron's claims to the American context. Pauling now insisted in his correspondence with Moertel that a proper trial of vitamin C could only be carried out on patients with intact immune systems who had not received chemotherapy. But, against Pauling's repeated representations, Moertel persisted in perceiving vitamin C's most valuable potential as adjuvant treatment, as, indeed, Pauling and Cameron had previously represented it, *not* as a substitute for conventional treatment. As we saw, Moertel initially was willing to interpret Cameron's claim of increased survival in preterminal patients in terms compatible with his own American-based professional interests and experience: as the possible restoration of immune processes that had been depressed by the various modalities of cancer therapy to which the patients had been previously exposed, including, he presumed, the cytotoxic drugs. The trial protocol for vitamin C was therefore designed in accordance with this professionally acceptable interpretation. When Pauling and Cameron informed him that cytotoxic chemotherapy was not usually administered in Scotland, Moertel, in his turn, invoked conventional American professional practices and pointed to the difficulty of selecting patients who had not been routinely exposed to chemotherapy.

In their published report of the negative results of the first Mayo Clinic trial and the heated exchanges that followed, Moertel and his co-researchers subsequently deployed this same professionally-based argument to defend their trial design and to undercut Pauling's allegation that their results were 'misleading' and invalid. They opposed what they termed Pauling's 'highly speculative' claim that prior chemotherapy had prevented their patients from achieving the 'extraordinary survival increase' claimed by Cameron and Pauling, by arguing that their Mayo Clinic patients were well beyond any acute immuno-suppressive effects of cytotoxic therapy when they entered the study. As we saw, they presented no evidence of this, but relied instead upon their socially-derived and ethically-laden counterclaim: that the administration of chemotherapy was routine treatment for cancer patients in the United States, and high-dose vitamin C, if it was incompatible with such treatment, was therefore useless for American cancer patients. In other words, his orthodox American opponents attempted to close the debate and discount Pauling's claims, not, as the standard view of science would have it, by setting up a new trial designed to disprove his specific claim of immune system impairment, but rather by seeking to foreclose any further trials of vitamin C; and they did this by the essentially social means of invoking conventional American professional practices and their contingent ethical values. In order to reopen the debate, Pauling also resorted to social means: the personal and public criticism and the high-ranking political pressure he was able to mobilize and place on the NCI. In this way, Pauling was able to overturn the professionally-based objections of his orthodox opponents, who were then forced to modify *both the context and content* of their counterclaim of the impossibility of withholding professionally accredited treatments of 'known value': that is, in order to repeat the trial with patients who had not had prior chemotherapy or radiotherapy, conventional American professional practices, experimental procedures, and the claims of existing efficacious treatments on which they were based, had to be suspended or changed.

The second Mayo Clinic trial is an even more powerful illustration of the context dependence and political nature of method discourse. More than enough has been said to locate the conflict over its design and interpretation in the radically different ideological, theoretical, and professional contexts of the orthodox 'cure' by the 'killing' of cancer cells and the alternative strategy of 'control' by their 'disarmament'. Cameron's peaceful coexistence and disarmament metaphor, which he consciously counterposed to the militaristic metaphors of conventional cancer treatment, encapsulates and illuminates these important contextual distinctions between the 'believers' and 'non-believers'. There is no need further to labour the point that the methodology of the second Mayo Clinic trial was dependent upon the theoretical framework and professional practices of its orthodox designers. *Within this context*, its defenders could extol its design as faultless and hail it as the 'definitive' test of vitamin C, while, from the perspective of the alternatives, who stood *outside this context*, its methodology was hopelessly flawed. Vitamin C could only be made to work as a cancer treatment in the way claimed by Pauling and Cameron if its orthodox assessors were willing and able to administer and assess it in accordance with its alternative theoretical and methodological framework, that is, to continue its administration 'indefinitely' and to shift their evaluative focus from tumour shrinkage to survival times, the palliation of cancer symptoms, and the general quality of life. Their inability to evaluate vitamin C within its alternative context is a particularly striking instance of the sociological thesis that experimental design 'cannot be divorced from the commitments of the communities that frame and evaluate experiments' (Shapin, 1982; Collins and Shapin, 1989). And, once again contrary to the standard view, Pauling's opponents did not respond to his criticisms of the second trial by attempting to disprove them by a retrial in which vitamin C dose is continued 'indefinitely', but have effectively closed the debate by refusing a retrial and by blocking publication of his criticisms in the professional literature. Yet again these orthodox moves have been defended, not by disproving Pauling's specific claims, but by drawing upon a rhetorical ensemble of ethical and methodological criticisms.

Recent work in the history and sociology of science suggests that debates or discourses about scientific methods function primarily as 'rhetorical resources for use in those negotiations and struggles over the framing and evaluation of knowledge claims that go on at all levels of scientific activity, from the laboratory bench, through published texts, to disciplinary debate and its necessarily associated micro-politics of groups and institutions' (Richards and Schuster, 1989). To reiterate, such deployments of method discourses are highly flexible and context dependent. Scientists may give different accounts in different argumentative contexts, sometimes even contradicting themselves or offering contradictory interpretations of their own methods, depending upon the contingent context and the aims of debate and deployment. John Schuster has argued that method discourses should be treated as 'myths' that systematically mask processes of social construction and control. They serve rhetorical and political purposes and are resources in the power struggles within and between specialist communities and wider social forces (Schuster, 1984; Schuster and Yeo, 1986). In the case of the vitamin C and cancer controversy, the myth of the 'properly designed' or 'definitive' clinical trial and the objective therapeutic evaluation it supposedly entails have been mobilized by the orthodox or 'non-believers' to validate their assumption of the role of disinterested adjudicator in the determination of what is or is not a correct and effective cancer treatment. They have thereby successfully legitimized their foreclosure of any future trials of vitamin C and thus the political closure of the debate in their favour.

8 Comparative Analysis of the Controversy: Vitamin C, 5-Fluorouracil and Interferon

In 1978 it must be concluded that there is no chemotherapy approach to gastro-intestinal carcinoma valuable enough to justify application as standard clinical treatment. By no means, however, should this conclusion imply that these efforts should be abandoned. Patients . . . and their families have a compelling need for a basis of hope. If such hope is not offered, they will quickly seek it from the hands of quacks and charlatans.

Dr Charles Moertel, *New England Journal of Medicine* (Moertel, 1978b)

Where does one get a programme to tell the quacks and the charlatans from the legitimate medical profession?. . . . If there is no clinical justification for these agents, why do we use them?

Dr Joseph C. Fitzgerald, Response to Moertel, *New England Journal of Medicine* (Fitzgerald, 1979)

If there's the slightest possibility that [interferon] might prove helpful to future cancer patients, we feel that every effort must be made to check it out. The exciting promise of a new family of natural substances with anti-viral and anti-tumor activity demands nothing less than a full-dress, prompt, carefully planned and carefully controlled clinical trial.

Dr S. B. Gusberg, National President, American Cancer Society (Anon., 1980a)

I never thought Interferon was a magic bullet for cancer treatment, but you've got to go for broke.

Frank Rauscher, Former Director of the NCI, Senior Vice-President of the American Cancer Society (Sun, 1981)

Whether you are talking of mummy dust or crocodile dung, or whether you are talking of laetrile or vitamin C . . . you are talking about things that are really not scientifically derived. It's sort of like the Holy Water of Lourdes. . . . Our hope for cancer has to be in scientifically-based treatment . . .

Dr Charles Moertel (Moertel, 1989)

In the previous chapter, I gave a detailed sociological account of the processes by which vitamin C was actively constructed as a putative cancer treatment by Pauling and Cameron, and evaluated and found ineffective by their orthodox opponents. I have shown that we cannot account for the orthodox consensus on the inefficacy of vitamin C as a cancer treatment in terms of the disinterested and rational processes generally attributed to the application of the experimental method to the evaluation of medical therapies. Clinical trials, no matter how rigorously they are organized and conducted, do not give unproblematic direct access to nature or reality. There is no neutral, 'objective', or value-free way of engaging in them. I have argued that the methodology or protocol of the clinical trial is bound to the research tradition or paradigm of the specialist community that embodies and sustains that paradigm, and cannot be dissociated from the political and social structure of that community. It is the accepted knowledge of the community, together with the vested interests and social objectives that it embodies, that adjudicates the 'truth' or 'falsity' of therapeutic claims. Reality or nature is filtered through that knowledge and its sustaining interests and social objectives.

Thus far we have followed the processes and recovered the sociological factors which explain *how* the knowledge claim of the effectiveness of vitamin C as a cancer treatment became 'false'. Our sociological analysis is not yet complete. We now must go on to show *why* this particular judgement was made. We must display the connections between the judgement it has rendered and the interests and social concerns of the adjudicating community, that is, of the vitamin C 'non-believers' (Shapin, 1982). We must also be able to demonstrate that we are not merely offering a sociology of error or of pseudoscience, but that the processes and connections we uncover are applicable to accepted or 'true' knowledge as well as to rejected or 'false' knowledge. To this end, as explained previously, the history of the vitamin C controversy will be compared with those of the 'successful' conventional cancer treatments, 5-fluorouracil and interferon.

8.1 5-FLUOROURACIL: 'THE BREAKTHROUGH THAT NEVER WAS' AS CONVENTIONAL CANCER TREATMENT

5-Fluorouracil (5-FU or fluorouracil), conventionally employed in the adjuvant treatment of colorectal cancer, is a fluorinated pyramidine, an antimetabolite that exerts its cytotoxic effects by inhibiting DNA synthesis in the cell. It was developed in 1957 and approved for marketing by the FDA on the basis of results from non-randomized, uncontrolled clinical trials. Initially the patent was held jointly by Roche and the American Cancer Society. In 1970, in the wake of the regulatory tightening of the Kefauver-Harris Amendments which demanded evidence of efficacy as well as safety, 5-FU was reviewed by the National Academy of Sciences and found to be 'effective' for the palliative management of cancer of the colon or rectum. In 1978, as the initial patent expired, the FDA approved an injectable form of 5-FU, marketed by Roche, concluding that the drug was 'safe and effective' (Petersen and Markle, 1981; Moss, 1980).

As indicated in Chapter 1, 5-fluorouracil is an extremely toxic substance. It is available only on prescription, and carries the FDA-imposed 'warning' that it must be administered in a hospital or clinic under expert medical supervision and constant monitoring of its toxic side effects, which have been previously detailed (1.1).

Since the early seventies, Charles Moertel has been a leading and persistent critic of 5-FU as standard therapy for gastro-intestinal cancer. Moertel's criticisms of 5-FU consist of the familiar mix of methodological and ethical rhetoric with knowledge claims of its inefficacy and toxicity. Thus, in 1974, Moertel argued on methodological grounds against the accepted ethical procedure of first administering the standard treatment of 5-FU to patients with gastro-intestinal cancer before their admission to phase II trials designed to evaluate the effectiveness of new cancer treatments. A major criticism on this occasion was that prior therapy with cytotoxic drugs might damage immuno-competence and 'could significantly influence the patients' responses to a new agent'.

> To insist on 5-FU as standard therapy for advanced gastrointestinal cancer offers precious little to today's patient and is a distinct disservice to tomorrow's patient.
>
> If we are to make any progress in the treatment of this resistant group of neoplasms, it must be through the development of new treatment modalities. To test a new agent or approach in only the 5-FU failure or the patient who is disabled and passing into the terminal stages of his disease, is to play a losing game. Negative results must be anticipated even with regimens of considerable therapeutic activity (Moertel *et al.*, 1974).

Yet, as we saw, Moertel and his co-researchers subsequently denied this possibility in relation to the negative results obtained in their first trial of vitamin C and defended their experimental design on ethical and professional grounds.

In 1976, in the *Journal of the American Medical Association (JAMA)* Moertel slammed 5-fluorouracil as the 'breakthrough that never was'. He condemned the previously published uncontrolled trial that claimed to demonstrate 5-FU's 'significant improvement of five-year cure rate' for patients with colorectal cancer and the accompanying 'endorsing editorial' in *JAMA*, cited the 'uniformly negative' results of five concurrently controlled randomized trials 'involving more than 1,700 patients', and denounced 5-fluorouracil as 'worthless':

> . . . one can hope that the good judgment of the American physician will dissuade him from treating thousands of post-operative colon cancer patients with this toxic drug in the misinformed belief that it will provide them with therapeutic benefit. (Moertel, 1976)

Again, in pursuing his case against 5-fluorouracil, Moertel in a 1978 paper in the *New England Journal of Medicine*, assessed the conventional chemotherapeutic treatment of gastrointestinal cancer and concluded that such chemotherapy was not only costly and caused deleterious toxic effects, but was all but ineffective. 5–Fluorouracil, even when administered in 'almost ideal regimens', produced objective response (that is, a reduction of more than 50 per cent in tumour size) in only 15 to 20 per cent of patients, and this was usually only partial, very transient, and frequently illusionary:

> This minor gain for a small minority of patients is probably more than counterbalanced by the deleterious influence of toxicity for other patients and by the cost and inconvenience experienced by all patients. There is no solid evidence that treatment with fluorinated pyrimadines contributes to the overall survival of patients with gastrointestinal cancer regardless of the stage of the disease at which they are applied. . . . In 1978 it must be concluded that there is no chemotherapy approach to gastrointestinal carcinoma valuable enough to justify application as standard clinical treatment. (Moertel, 1978b)

Inevitably, the alternatives, who monitored Moertel's anti-fluorouracil campaign with considerable interest, seized upon and approved of his conclusion. In such a situation, Pauling and Cameron represented their own ethical position as follows:

> We would interpret this conclusion as sound reason for not subjecting patients to the misery, trouble, and expense of chemotherapy. (Cameron and Pauling, 1979b)

Yet in the face of his own devastating critique, Moertel made it clear that he would not discourage patients with gastrointestinal cancer from entering clinical research programmes 'of sound scientific design' for the continuing evaluation of conventional chemotherapy, including 5-fluorouracil:

> By no means, however, should this conclusion imply that these efforts should be abandoned. Patients with advanced gastrointestinal cancer and their families have a compelling need for a basis of hope. If such hope is not offered, they will quickly seek it from the hands of quacks and charlatans. Enough progress has been made in chemotherapy of gastrointestinal cancer so that realistic hope can be generated by entry of these patients into well designed clinical research studies (Moertel, 1978b).

Moertel's recommendation provoked contradictory ethical and professional objections from two physician readers of the *New England Journal of Medicine*. The first, a privately-practising oncologist, strongly rejected Moertel's 'mandate that all patients with advanced colorectal cancer . . . be treated in a research setting', and defended the 'right' of such patients who did not want to take part in clinical trials to treatment with existing chemotherapy based on 'unbiased information presented to them by a medical oncologist'. 'Forcing all patients desiring treatment to participate in research protocols', rhetorically declared this oncologist critic, 'is a denial of basic human rights' (Cohen, 1979). Moertel's other professional critic demanded to know,

> Where does one get a programme to tell the quacks and the charlatans from the legitimate medical profession?. . . . If there is no clinical justification for these agents, why do we use them? They have associative morbidity, mortality and cost. We should stop deceiving the patients and face up to reality. To do less is to be a charlatan or a quack.   (Fitzgerald, 1979)

In a lengthy response, Moertel rejected both criticisms and strenuously defended the continuing clinical research of 5-FU. To place the withholding of ineffective cytotoxic drugs under the category of denial of human rights, he sarcastically told his oncologist critic, 'strains even the most liberal political philosophy'. Nor is the oncologist abandoning patients whose condition is one for which no effective chemotherapeutic treatment exists, if he 'fails to descend upon [them] with routine 5-fluorouracil' and either offers them entry into a clinical-research programme, or, if they reject this option, the 'best-proved' measures of symptomatic and supportive care. On the other hand, his second critic, whom Moertel identified as a 'cardiologist' (and thus, by implication, as venturing outside his area of expertise), was guilty of the medical sin of 'extreme therapeutic nihilism regarding all chemotherapy approaches'. Moertel spelt out for the benefit of this outsider the various 'unequivocal evidence', 'solid documentation', and 'strongly suggestive evidence' of extended life span and substantial palliation for a number of cancers treated by chemotherapy (although not, he conceded, the gastrointestinal cancers). He 'stood firm' with his conviction that 'routine' chemotherapy offered 'little of substantive value to the patients with gastrointestinal cancer today, but that realistic hope can be offered by entry of this patient into a well designed and thoughtfully conducted clinical research program' (Moertel, 1979).

Yet, shortly after making these claims with respect to 5-fluorouracil, Moertel, in confronting Pauling and Cameron after the first Mayo Clinic trial, reversed them with respect to vitamin C. In this different argumentative context, it was 'not conscionable to withhold oncologic therapy of known value' in order to duplicate the experimental conditions and test the claims of Pauling and Cameron.

These interchanges and inconsistencies indicate the selective deployment of ethical arguments and rhetoric in the defence of orthodox knowledge claims and methodologies and the rejection of alternative ones, even where the orthodox claims and methods are themselves the subject of internal dissension and criticism within medicine.

A similar selectivity prevails in the invocation of canonical scientific methodological criteria for the evaluation of alternative claims. Thus, as has been stressed, the randomized double-blind test pressed upon Pauling and Cameron is neither universally accepted nor applied within medicine. The majority of cytotoxic drugs currently in use, including 5-fluorouracil, have been professionally accepted and become conventional cancer treatments *without* prior evaluation by randomized controlled trials (Geehan and Freireich, 1974; McKinlay, 1981; Buyse *et al.*, 1984).

The previous reconstruction of the vitamin C controversy has also pointed up the fact that the Moertel-led trial of laetrile, which it was argued 'had to pick its way through a minefield of formidable [ethical] obstacles' was neither randomized and controlled nor blind. Nevertheless, its conclusion, 'Laetrile doesn't work', was hailed as 'decisive', and its methodology editorially defended as a 'triumph of pragmatism over principle' by Relman in the *New England Journal of Medicine*. It was this self-same Relman who consistently rejected Cameron's manuscript on the grounds of lack of proper randomization, but who, in this different argumentative context, found sound reason for Moertel's failure to randomize the laetrile trial. As we saw, Relman, on this occasion, turned the persistent orthodox criticism of Cameron's Vale of Leven trials on its head, and authoritatively asserted that the lack of concurrent controls in the laetrile trial was 'partially offset by the fact that all patients were in the advanced stages of a disease known to be almost uniformly and rapidly fatal', and that 'any objective responses in tumour size or apparent prolongation of survival could be identified by comparison with historical controls' (see section 5.3). It will be recalled that this was precisely the argument used by Cameron in his early correspondence with Pauling when he decided against the need for a controlled clinical trial of vitamin C, and it was subsequently deployed by Pauling and Cameron in their published comparisons of vitamin C-treated and untreated patients.

Within this same context of the laetrile trial, Moertel, who had consistently represented the Vale of Leven trials and all other such historically controlled trials (including 5-fluorouracil) as open to bias and misinterpretation, also, when challenged by Pauling, found sound ethical reason for not carrying out a trial involving the use of controls given either no treatment or standard cancer therapy: given such negative results, it would be 'unconscionable human experimentation' to carry out such a trial (5.3).

On the other hand, Moertel and his co-researchers do not perceive their continuing accumulation of negative or equivocal data from subsequent controlled clinical trials of fluorouracil-containing chemotherapy to be ethically or methodologically problematic (Gastrointestinal Tumor Study Group, 1984; DeCosse, 1984; Cullinan *et al.*, 1985; O'Connell *et al.*, 1985). Some fourteen years after Moertel denounced 5-fluorouracil as the 'breakthrough that never was', there is still no question of the abandonment of this orthodox line of research. Nor, in spite of all the rhetoric, has the failure to produce uncontroversial evidence of the benefits of this toxic treatment led to any demonstrable modification of orthodox professional practices. Undeterred by their conspicuous lack of success, Moertel and other researchers continue to tinker with the model, trying different combinations and different routes and durations of administration, and may yet tinker towards success. Their clinical trials continue alongside the routine clinical practices that they criticize and call into question.

'We Still Don't Know' declared a recent meta-analysis of all published randomized, controlled, clinical trials on adjuvant therapy for colorectal cancer carried out by several prominent biostatisticians (Buyse *et al.*, 1988). An accompanying editorial endorsed their study as providing 'little justification for the routine use of adjuvant chemotherapy for colonic cancer' (Levin and O'Connell, 1988). It cited the 'small magnitude of putative benefits and the possibility that these results could be wiped out by failure to include any negative unpublished trials in the meta-analysis', and the further possibility that in combination chemotherapy with 5-fluorouracil and other agents 'apparent survival gains may be diminished in time by the delayed onset of [chemotherapy]-induced leukaemia'. Nevertheless, all of these analysts, guest-editors and biostatisticians alike, found sufficient reason to urge the large-scale testing of 5-fluorouracil-containing regimens. Their rationale for this is that previous trials, with an average size of about 400 patients, were 'inadequate' to detect small, yet medically worthwhile, treatment benefits: 'Trials much larger than those published up to now are needed' (Buyse *et al*. 1988).

8.2   THE ADJUDICATING COMMUNITY: THE PROFESSION OF MEDICINE

Sociologists of medicine, in attempting to come to grips with such seeming inconsistences and irrationalities, have generally invoked professional factors. Thus Eliot Freidson, whose work has been extremely influential, emphasizes that medicine is primarily a practising or consulting profession, rather than a scholarly or learned scientific one. Freidson has drawn a sharp distinction between the body of scientific knowledge possessed by the profession and the knowledge used in applying that knowledge to work situations:

> As opposed to the medical knowledge which is medicine as such, there are the practices which grow up in the course of applying that knowledge to concrete patients in concrete social settings. The 'pure' medical knowledge is transmuted, even debased in the course of application. Indeed, in the course of application knowledge cannot remain pure but must instead become socially organized as practice. (Freidson, 1970)

General professional knowledge, as distinct from medical knowledge, is 'concretized' by professional practices and customs. It may at times be suspended by the individual judgement of the consultant or clinician. Or, because of the practitioner's 'moral commitment to intervention', medical intervention may occur even where there is no knowledge of the illness or its treatment. This, for Freidson, constitutes the 'problem' of professional medical knowledge: it is above all applied knowledge, and, according to Freidson, medicine, unlike theoretical physics, is not neutral. Its professional knowledge is value-laden – dogmatic, biased, distorted – and its efficacy and reliability are suspect: 'it is a creation of the profession itself, expressing the commitments and perceptions of a special occupational class', and as such cannot properly be a guide for social policy. Nevertheless, in spite of Freidson's own interpretation of illness as primarily socially defined, he proceeds to argue that medicine's basic knowledge of the course of illness and the procedures most likely to cure or alleviate the effects of illness is 'pure' ('theoretical, scientific, objective, systematic') in the sense that 'methods of applying it to practical reality are distinct and separate from it' (Freidson, 1970). Even in his most recent writings, Freidson maintains this distinction between 'formal knowledge' and its 'institutional transformation' for professional purposes (Freidson, 1986).

On the face of it, Friedson's analysis goes some way towards explaining the seemingly irrational and contradictory nature of medicine which its many critics have explored and deplored. What might seem cognitively irrational may be seen to be professionally rational. Methodological procedures and theoretical assumptions may be invoked or suspended, and risk assessments and ethical values varied to suit professional vested interests. The underlying cognitive content of medicine remains unaffected by these professional practices.

But Freidson manages this rigid demarcation of the cognitive from the practical aspects of medicine only by explicitly exempting from his analysis (and from the profession!) 'medical men and medical work to be found in the highly visible prestigious teaching and research institutions of medicine'. He limits his analysis to the practising members of the profession, the clinicians. 'The former are the formal spokesmen, the leaders and sometimes the models of the profession. The latter *are* the profession' (Freidson, 1970).

Yet, even in the most prestigious teaching and research institutions of medicine, such as the Mayo Clinic, professional practices typically impinge on cognitive content or knowledge claims. An explicit instance of this is Moertel's professionally evoked concern with giving hope to patients and keeping them out of the hands of quacks and charlatans as sufficient reason for finding some credibility in and pursuing what he otherwise argued to be ineffective and highly toxic conventional lines of clinical research. It must be understood that Moertel is here restating a standard professional argument that is embodied in oncology textbooks. The cancer authority Victor Richards, for example, in his widely used text of the seventies, *Cancer, the Wayward Cell: Its Origins, Nature, and Treatment*, acknowledged the ineffectiveness of chemotherapy for solid tumours, but argued that chemotherapy 'serves an extremely valuable role in keeping patients oriented toward proper medical therapy' and away from 'cancer quackery' (Richards, 1978; Moss, 1980). Similarly, the substitution of 5-fluorouracil for vitamin C in the second Mayo Clinic trial may be interpreted as the professionally-motivated preference for the treatment which is professionally controlled and administered, and fits the established theoretical framework, even though it is argued to be toxic and ineffective.

As this study and other sociological case studies of scientific knowledge have demonstrated over and over again, the social practices of scientists and other professionals shape knowledge claims as well as their application (Collins and Pinch, 1982). In the case of medicine, it cannot be over-emphasized that the production of medical knowledge is necessarily bound up with and is subordinate to the production of medical care, which is the basis of its economic viability. *It is on the basis of selling medical care* that the production and distribution of medical knowledge is ensured (Jamous and Peloille, 1970; Sadler, 1978). We cannot, therefore, arrive at a coherent and comprehensive explanation of therapeutic claims within medicine without recognizing the inevitable intrusion of professional practices and interests on the construction and evaluation of these claims.

The theoretical distinction that Freidson and other sociologists of medicine maintain between 'pure' and 'applied' medical knowledge is thoroughly artificial and cannot be sustained in practice. It is contradicted, moreover, by other aspects of Freidson's valuable analysis of the profession of medicine. In particular, Freidson has emphasized that the hallmark of a profession is its control or socially-recognized authority over the determination and assessment of the knowledge used in its work:

> What is critical for the status of medicine and any other profession is its ultimate control over its own work. . . . Control need not be total – what is essential is control over the determination and evaluation of the technical knowledge used in the work. (Freidson, 1970)

Freidson's insight offers the key to the way in which we might best understand medicine and interpret the events and contradictions that this study has revealed. By focusing on medicine's sources of power and authority and the ways in which it uses them, we may see how medicine's ultimate control over its own knowledge, its 'cognitive authority', is crucial to the maintenance of the professional status and social power of its practitioners. It is this socially recognized authority to speak and act in medical matters – above all, to determine what counts as *legitimate* medical knowledge – that is central to medicine's privileged and powerful position in society (Johnson, 1972; Jamous and Peloille, 1970; Larson, 1979).

A good working definition of 'cognitive authority' has been offered by the sociologist of science Thomas Gieryn:

> Cognitive authority is legitimate power to promulgate and disseminate knowledge that is accepted as truthful and reliable. A variety of resources typically accompany cognitive authority: money and time to create truth, and access to institutionalized means for spreading it (e.g., systems of education). (Gieryn, 1983)

In their pursuit of social authority and its material and symbolic resources and rewards, professionals compete with non-professionals and with one another for cognitive authority. We must understand that the social power of the medical profession is inseparable from its cognitive authority. A threat to the cognitive authority of the profession is a threat to its social standing and, above all, to its economic base, to its marketing of medical care, and must be forcefully resisted by the profession.

In western societies, the institution of medicine has grown more powerful and prestigious through asserting its cognitive authority over an expanding domain of knowledge claims. Areas of life, such as birth and death, that were once treated as social or cultural events, have been thoroughly medicalized and become the province of medical expertise and technological intervention. Medicine's successful assertion of cognitive authority in these and other domains ultimately resides in its interlinked claims of possessing the requisite craft training and a scientifically-based, and, therefore, 'truthful and reliable' knowledge of illness and its treatment (Sadler, 1978). The profession, in asserting its cognitive authority, thus lays great stress on the essential worth and uniqueness of its professional knowledge. It regards itself as the repository and guardian of specialized skills and objectively-based knowledge, and it enlists the aid of the state in maintaining its control over who does what and to whom. At the same time, the profession forcefully resists the intrusion of the state on the evaluation of its knowledge and the regulation of its practice. The familiar slogans of 'freedom to prescribe', the 'sacredness' of the doctor-patient relationship, and 'self-regulation', symbolize the profession's need to protect its socially conferred monopoly over the evaluation and application of medical knowledge and hence its cognitive and social authority. Individuals or sectors of society may contest the truth and reliability of its knowledge, or proffer alternative versions of medical knowledge, but only the profession of medicine can serve as the final court of appeal in settling disputes over what is to count as *legitimate* medical knowledge.

The medical profession's control over what is to count as medical knowledge, its cognitive authority, is clearly political in nature. All knowledge is measured against the yardstick of that which is professionally endorsed; it is evaluated by members of the profession; and innovations are only acceptable to the extent that they do not threaten the existing power position of the profession within society, or the dominant groups within the profession (Johnson, 1972).

As we saw, vitamin C was tested and found wanting in this way. Oncologists made no attempt to evaluate vitamin C within the framework established by Pauling and Cameron, but evaluated it within their own professionally-endorsed framework of expertise. To take the argument further, the professional expertise of oncologists does not lend itself to the evaluation of cancer treatments that are readily available and may be self-administered. They have developed their expertise in dealing with highly toxic drugs that are inaccessible to the general public, and whose administration they entirely control. Nor, it may be argued, is it in their professional interest to extend their expertise to a treatment that amounts to self-medication and is designed to make this expertise redundant.

Oncologists have not disproved the 'truth' of Pauling's and Cameron's claims for vitamin C, but they have most certainly rejected them. They are not deemed to be 'scientific'. Moertel, in his most recent pronouncements on the matter, lumped vitamin C together with laetrile, mummy dust and crocodile dung. He likened such 'really not scientifically derived' treatments to the Holy Water of Lourdes, and rhetorically proclaimed that our hope for cancer has to be in 'scientifically-based treatment' (Moertel, 1989). Moertel's science/non-science distinction between the 'legitimate' experimental cancer treatments, such as the 5-fluorouracil that he continues to work with, and the discounted vitamin C, cannot be shown to fit any consistently applied scientific criteria or methodological recipe. In analysing Pauling's and Cameron's construction of a theoretical and experimental rationale for vitamin C in the previous chapter, I have been at some pains to show that 'nothing unscientific is happening' (Collins and Pinch, 1979). Vitamin C is no less scientific than 5-fluorouracil. The real problem with vitamin C is that it fundamentally threatens the cognitive and social authority of oncologists, whereas, although its effectiveness is disputed within the profession, 5-fluorouracil does not. Vitamin C challenges accepted oncological theory and practice; it does not fit easily into the established cancer research tradition or paradigm; it is freely available over the counter and does not require a professional's prescription or intervention for its administration; it draws its support primarily from outside the medical profession and stands in competition and conflict with it. It threatens to take the treatment of cancer out of the hands of the professionals, the experts, and into the hands of non-professionals, even into the hands of patients, who are the major consumers of medical knowledge and its application as medical care.

We may best understand the medical demarcation of vitamin C from legitimate 'scientifically-based' cancer therapies as a manifestation of professional policing or 'boundary work'. Such policing is an integral part of the maintenance of the profession's control over its own work, and of its dominance of the medical market place. In the United States, as we saw, this essential ongoing defence of professional vested interests in orthodox cancer treatments is largely assumed by the American Cancer Society, which has been very successful in marginalizing and excluding unconventional cancer treatments. The allegation of 'pseudo-science', 'charlatanism' or 'quackery' does not require a disproof of the 'truth' of any specific observation, experiment or idea. It may be more usefully seen as an aspect of the rhetorical and organizational means by which oncologists and their allies seek to distinguish the domain of oncology and to discredit their competitors in the process of maintaining and extending the cognitive authority, funding, monetary rewards, and other interests and values of those associated with the orthodox research and treatment of cancer (Johnson, 1972; Gieryn, 1983; Wallis, 1985).

Apart from the overt tactics of the American Cancer Society, the very organization and structure of professionally endorsed cancer research and treatment functions to exclude unconventional treatments, and to reinforce the notion that there is a central core of correct and effective theory and practice. As Pauling's own experiences indicate, it is extremely difficult for those promoting marginal therapies to negotiate the complex pathways to official recognition, research funding, publication in professionally endorsed journals, and above all, to the formally constituted professional clinical trial.

Professional acceptance and accreditation of unconventional therapies hinges on their evaluation by professionally-endorsed assessors and by professionally-endorsed methods. Whether or not the medical profession actually engages in formal evaluative procedures (and all the evidence I have adduced goes to show that it does so only exceptionally), it is its assumption of this adjudicating role, backed by claims of expertise and objectivity, that empowers the profession of medicine in its confrontations with unorthodoxy. Without professional evaluation, unconventional cancer treatments may readily be dismissed as 'quackery' by their orthodox opponents, or relegated to marginal 'unproven' status. But orthodox evaluation entails the subjection of alternative claims to orthodox evaluators and orthodox methodology, to a situation where their opponents are also the adjudicators who determine the rules and make the judgements about what is, or what is not, an effective and appropriate treatment for cancer. As is clear, this is a situation which can only prevail so long as orthodox medical knowledge retains its special status of value-neutrality and objectivity. The current ground rules cast the orthodox expert in the role of privileged and unbiased arbiter of medical truth, and proponents of orthodoxy have a great deal invested in their promotion of this assumption. As I have previously stressed, the myth of the 'definitive' clinical trial and the neutral evaluation it supposedly entails is central to medicine's assertion of its adjudicating role. It is the major source of the tactical strength of the 'non-believers' in the vitamin C and cancer dispute; it legitimates their foreclosure of any future trials of vitamin C and thus the political closure of the debate in their favour; and it is constituted by the economic and political power of the coalition of institutional, professional, and business interests outlined in Chapter 3.

Nevertheless, for all its formidable professional power, it is essential to recognize that medicine's control over its own work is not absolute. In spite of its articulation with the wider social power of the state in establishing and maintaining its cognitive authority, the sources of power available to medicine have never been sufficient to impose on all consumers its own definition of truthful and reliable medical knowledge. Cognitive authority is never fixed or absolute. The boundaries of medicine are ambiguous, flexible, and constantly disputed and renegotiated. Not only is there the need for incessant boundary work around the margins, but there are also tensions within the system which consistently threaten its stability. A major tension stems from the conflict between consumer choice and medical authority. The medical profession is dependent upon the existence of a 'large, heterogeneous clientele, exercising effective demand'. This diverse clientele may include the state, business corporations, consumer pressure groups, and patients of different social classes and ethnic groups. It acts to destabilize and counterbalance the occupational control of the profession through the pressure of its different demands or choices of available services or therapies, for example, by channelling fees towards some professionals rather than others (Johnson, 1972).

Medicine is not a single 'community' of practitioners, all pursuing identical goals and sharing the same interests and values. Rather, medicine is characterized by its high degree of specialization and hierarchical fragmentation. This division of labour within the profession is manifested in the different skills and technical competences of its practitioners and specialists. These diverse technical abilities and competences have been acquired through lengthy processes of training and socialization and represent a considerable investment on the part of their possessors. They therefore represent diverse and potentially conflicting and competing vested social interests *within* the medical profession. In the area of cancer treatment and research, for instance, general practitioners or internists, radiotherapists, surgeons, medical oncologists, clinical researchers, biostatisticians, epidemiologists, and so on, compete with one another, as well as with non-professionals, for the demarcation of territory, the allocation of the privileges and responsibilities of expertise, the structuring of claims on resources, and, above all, for cognitive authority and its professional and social rewards. Boundary work, therefore, is not limited to demarcations of legitimate 'scientific' medicine from 'quackery', but is also used within medicine for the demarcation of specialties or of theoretical orientations or practices within them. At the periphery of conventional clinical medicine there are struggles with holism and orthomolecular medicine, and within the field of conventional cancer treatment and research there are controversies over 5-fluorouracil and other treatments, as various competing specialties attempt to dominate the field and impose the definition of truthful and reliable medical knowledge best suited to their own particular interests. Client choice and the pressures inherent in client diversity operate upon these ongoing competitive struggles within and around the boundaries of medicine.

It is easy to understand that in response to these pressures the general practitioners, who command less authority and fewer resources within the medical hierarchy, might, for instance, form alliances with holists, incorporating certain orthomolecular practices or theories into their orthodox practice, as indeed seems to have happened; while the more powerful specialist oncologists are better placed to resist such modifications in the producer-consumer relationship and to deploy their cognitive authority in warding off the orthomolecular threat and protecting their legitimate cytotoxic therapies.

In other words, the balance of power within medicine is not static, and consensus on treatment evaluations shifts and changes in response to these fluctuations. The vagaries of consumer choice and wider social interests can thereby introduce pressures towards diversity within the profession, and structure knowledge claims and judgements about experimental findings. This conception of medicine as the site of professional power struggles for cognitive authority and control thus allows us to understand how and why consumer pressures or market forces may also impinge on professional judgements of the efficacy or risks of therapies or technologies.

The following comparison between the very different research and funding careers of the non-patentable, cheap, and freely-available vitamin C and the expensive, high-technology 'wonder drug' interferon, is intended to make explicit these larger social influences on the processes of therapeutic evaluation.

8.3 INTERFERON: FROM 'PSEUDOSCIENCE' TO PROFESSIONALLY ACCREDITED CANCER TREATMENT

Interferon was first discovered in the late 1950s by the British virologist, Alick Isaacs, and his Swiss collaborator, Jean Lindenmann. It was represented as a naturally occurring therapeutic agent, an 'interfering protein' which inhibited viral infections. Initially, as Sandra Panem has documented in her account of the 'Interferon Crusade', interferon had a very low image – it eluded physical isolation and rigorous chemical definition – and the handful of virologists and biochemists engaged in its study were viewed disparagingly by the scientific establishment as 'phenomenologists and fringe scientists'. Interferon itself was dubbed 'imaginon' or 'misinterpreton' by its detractors (Panem, 1984; Edelhart and Lindenmann, 1981). Nevertheless, its anti-viral potential interested British drug companies enough for them to form a syndicate with the Medical Research Council for the investigation of interferon's commercial possibilities. The technical and economic difficulties of manufacturing industrial quantities of interferon proved insuperable, and industrial interest in the drug fell away by the mid-sixties (Yoxen, 1983; Laurence, 1983). What kept interferon on the research agenda was the discovery in 1967 that it had a 'modest' anti-tumour activity in mice. It was its potential as a cancer cure which led to the first real scientific interest in interferon, and to efforts to isolate and purify enough for clinical research in humans (Panem, 1984). However, its extreme scarcity and high cost remained significant drawbacks to its research.

Then in the mid-seventies, the possibility of its largescale production by recombinant-DNA techniques added a new dimension to its clinical and economic prospects. Interferon was taken up by the emerging biotechnology industry, and became the primary lure for trapping venture capital for newly established genetic engineering firms such as Genentech and Cetus. As well, the large pharmaceutical corporations, notably Hoffmann-La Roche, Schering-Plough and G. D. Searle, joined the young biotechnology firms, and many millions of dollars were invested in the race to genetically engineer and patent interferon. The whole exercise, as Panem's analysis makes explicit, was predicated on the assumption that interferon would be needed and used by the medical community as a cancer treatment, and on the huge commercial return this would engender. In 1980, it was estimated that interferon had a potential world market of around three billion dollars by the end of the decade, and that its use by American cancer patients alone would represent a market value of around $270 million per year (Anon., 1980b).

The medical community itself was divided over interferon. A core group of politically well-connected enthusiasts, notably Dr Matilde Krim of Sloan–Kettering (whose husband was a close associate of President Lyndon B. Johnson and treasurer of the Democratic National Committee), became its avid promoters. These were the 'interferonologists', and they successfully 'sold' interferon to the public, to government and to industry. Within medicine, they recruited support from immunotherapists who had been trying (without much success) to treat cancer by enhancing immunocompetence. Interferon's supposed mode of action was readily assimilable into their research programme. Predictably, however, there was a good deal of opposition to this trend from established oncologists, particularly those working with cytotoxic drugs (Barnes, 1987; Edelhart and Lindenmann, 1981). At the height of the interferon 'hype', a 'strong statement' in opposition to the interferon movement was officially released by the Board of Directors of the American Society of Clinical Oncologists, with Charles Moertel as President (Moertel, personal communication). In addition, on the basis of peer assessment from leading oncologists, the NCI and the ACS initially resisted the demands of the interferonologists for massive funding of interferon research. However, through their recruitment of media, politicians and industry to their cause, Krim and the interferonologists triumphed, and succeeded in marshalling huge public and private resources to interferon research and clinical testing. In January 1980, amidst intense publicity and to international applause, Biogen and Schering-Plough jointly announced the successful cloning of a human interferon gene. A few weeks later, interferon was on the cover of *Time* magazine, while Schering-Plough's stock rose by eight points. By October, to even more enthusiastic applause, Hoffmann-La Roche-backed Genentech had followed suit with its version of human interferon, and a wave of 'biomania' rippled across Wall Street and the burgeoning biotechnology industry (Teitelman, 1989). Between 1978 and 1981, the increase in government spending on interferon research greatly outpaced the overall rate of growth of funding of biomedical research in general (Panem, 1984). By 1981, the NCI and the ACS, both so reluctant to investigate vitamin C, were reported to have spent a combined total of $18 million on the purchase alone of interferon for clinical trials, at an estimated cost of $20,000 to $30,000 per patient, and the public and politicians were clamouring for an even greater investment (Sun, 1981a).

In the event, interferon did not turn out to be the much-touted cancer cure. It was finally admitted that the major cancers – breast, bowel and lung – did not respond to interferon treatment. However, in spite of these failures (which, we might note, had made vitamin C unworthy of further testing), the researchers persisted with further clinical trials in the face of the finding that interferon had deleterious side effects (Panem, 1984; Nethersell and Sikora, 1985; Krown, 1986; Sikora, 1986; Smyth *et al.*, 1987). Meanwhile, Hoffmann-La Roche and Schering-Plough engaged in a major legal battle over the patent rights to interferon production. Their competing claims on patent infringement were finally dropped in order to allow commercial production to go ahead. Agreeing to share the market, the pair decided to cross-license. In 1986, their two patented versions of alpha interferon (differing by only one amino acid) were approved by the FDA as treatment for a single, relatively limited form of cancer, hairy-cell leukaemia (of which there are about 500 to 1,000 cases in the USA each year), and went on sale in the USA (Jackson, 1985; Smith, 1986). In 1989, the FDA approved interferon's use for genital warts and Kaposi's sarcoma (the cancer associated with AIDS). The market for interferon is currently estimated at $100 million worldwide, with predicted expansion in three or four years to around $150 million for each of its patent holders: 'That's not a blockbuster', stated an industry analyst, 'but it is a nicely profitable drug' (Teitelman, 1989).

The really interesting question for our purposes is: *Why did vitamin C fail and interferon succeed in becoming an accepted cancer therapy?*

It is difficult to separate the two substances on the grounds of the status of the theoretical explanations of their putative anti-cancer effects. If the anti-viral, anti-tumoural mode of action of vitamin C is contentious, so is that of interferon. Although a number of hypotheses have been formulated and a great deal of money has been mobilized to its research, the production, mechanism of action, and biological role of interferon remain unclear. The picture is complicated by the existence of at least three kinds of interferon – alpha, beta and gamma – and at least fifteen different alpha sub-types (Sikora, 1986; Krown, 1986). In so far as therapeutic potential was concerned, it was initially argued that the interferons offered a 'unique therapeutic approach because they act not as toxins directly on the tumour cells, but through the immune system' (Newmark, 1981). The current consensus is that all types of interferon possess antiviral, immunomodulatory, and antiproliferative activities that may play a part in tumour control (Krown, 1986). As we saw, exactly the same claim was and is made by Pauling and Cameron for the mode of action of vitamin C. In fact, in what may be perceived as an attempt to capitalize on the interferon crusade, Pauling and others have linked the anti-viral, anti-tumoural properties of vitamin C with the cellular production of interferon, and argued for vitamin C on the basis of its cheapness and greater accessibility (Siegel, 1975; Cameron and Pauling, 1979b; Stone, 1980; Pauling, 1986).

The decision of the NCI and the ACS to fund interferon research so massively was made on the basis of comparable experimental evidence of its therapeutic potential to that presented by Pauling and Cameron for vitamin C: that is, anecdotal evidence, some non-randomised, historically-controlled clinical trials (very restricted ones in the case of interferon), animal studies, and *in vitro* evidence of anti-tumoural properties.

The preliminary clinical trials of interferon's anti-cancer efficacy were conducted around the same time as Ewan Cameron's early clinical research on vitamin C. Beginning in 1972, Dr Hans Strander, a Swedish physician at the Karolinska Institute in Stockholm, administered interferon to a number of children and young adults with osteogenic sarcoma, a rare but extremely malignant bone cancer for which conventional therapy gave predictably poor results. Like Cameron, Strander felt it was 'unethical' to deny any possibly beneficial treatment to his patients for the sake of carrying out a randomized concurrent trial (Panem, 1984). Also the number of patients with this form of cancer was limited, as was Strander's supply of interferon, which was laboriously produced by Dr Kari Cantell at a government-run laboratory in Helsinki. Like the early trials of vitamin C, Strander's clinical trial of interferon was therefore uncontrolled. Similarly, Strander subsequently drew on the Institute records in order to compare his interferon-treated patients (only thirty-four cases by 1979) with the medical histories of patients with osteosarcoma who had been treated by other means. On the basis of this comparison, Strander claimed a significantly improved disease-free survival for the interferon-treated patients (Strander, 1977, 1982; Culliton and Waterfall, 1979; Panem, 1984; Nethersell and Sikora, 1985).

Strander's experimental work, which, according to Panem, 'received media attention to a degree unwarranted by its level of scientific certainty', was pivotal in focusing medical and public interest on interferon. A panel of American physicians, appointed by DeVita of the NCI in 1975 to evaluate Strander's data, was highly critical of his methodology. Dr Arthur S. Levine, the oncologist who headed the panel, argued that Strander was 'comparing apples and oranges'. It was at his insistence that Strander pulled together some concurrent control data for patients being treated at other Swedish centres. Levine then alleged that Strander's claim of improved disease-free survival was not significant and could be accounted for by 'problems of diagnostic interpretation [and] inadvertent skew due to prognostic variables, selection, and demography of referral' (Panem, 1984; Nethersell and Sikora, 1985). The NCI-appointed panel concluded that interferon's experimental use for osteogenic sarcoma was 'premature'. Nevertheless, following on Strander's anecdotal reports of interferon's success at the International Workshop on Interferon in the Treatment of Cancer, organized by Mathilde Krim at the Rockefeller Institute in New York City in April 1975, the NCI by-passed the normal review channels and agreed to fund the first cancer clinical trial of interferon in the USA (Panem, 1984).

The Rockefeller Institute Workshop, which was supported in part by both the National Institutes of Health and the private sector and was well-attended by industrial, medical, and NCI representatives, is recognized as the turning point in generating support for interferon. But, as Krim herself observed, no new evidence of interferon's anti-cancer potential had occurred or was presented: 'It was consciousness raising' (Panem, 1984). Various influential philanthropists and patrons of cancer research, such as Mary Lasker, lent their support to Krim and lobbied hard for a special interferon programme. By 1978, the American Cancer Society had emerged as the leading proponent of the experimental use of interferon in cancer, with an initial investment of $2 million for the purchase of interferon for clinical trials. Frank J. Rauscher (ex-president of the NCI and Senior-Vice President of the ACS) is quoted by Panem as stating that he recommended such a heavy investment of ACS resources in interferon trials on the basis of information from cancer specialists in the U.S. that interferon may have had some effect in some forms of cancer 'in maybe eight to ten patients'.

Initially, a good deal of emphasis was placed by its promoters on the presumed non-toxic qualities of interferon. Rauscher, for instance, in hindsight, referred to the representations of researchers that interferon would be without the side-effects associated with the cytotoxic drugs (Sun, 1981a). In fact, as researchers reluctantly conceded, interferon when administered in clinical doses has toxic side effects similar to those of conventional chemotherapy: nausea, hair-loss, bone marrow depression, sudden high fever, lethargy, central nervous symptoms and weight loss. Initially it was argued that the contaminants present in the earlier, less pure preparations of interferon were responsible for these side effects (Newmark, 1981). It is currently concluded that the side effects of even the highly purified recombinant interferons are 'profound'. The most serious problems are severe neurotoxicity, which can lead to coma if the drug is continued, and life-threatening heart arrhythmias and myocardial infarction (Sikora, 1986; Krown, 1986; PDR, 1989).

According to Panem, interferon's side effects were first noted in 1977, but there was an initial coverup by the interferonologists, and several articles detailing the severe side-effects were suppressed. It was only in 1982, when the deaths from heart attacks of four interferon-treated patients at the Pasteur Institute in Paris became public and the French government suspended clinical trials of interferon, that the NCI finally issued an official warning on its toxic effects (Anon. 1982). Here, vitamin C compares more than favourably. The well-attested absence of such side-effects from vitamin C megadose in cancer patients had, as we saw, earlier led to the expectation that this aspect of its properties *alone* would attract attention to its clinical research.

Next there is the difference that, in spite of many negative trial outcomes, the clinical testing of interferon has become a growth industry in its own right. It is acknowledged by specialist reviewers of the literature that clinical trials with the interferons have, with a few exceptions, been 'disappointing'. The exceptions comprise a handful of rare cancers (most of which already respond to chemotherapy), where phase II trials and a very few phase III studies have indicated that interferon, as a single agent, 'may have a role'. Roche's and Schering-Plough's patented versions of recombinant interferon, Roferon A and Intron A, were approved for marketing for the treatment of hairy-cell leukaemia on the basis of historically controlled studies (PDR, 1989). According to the interferon experts, it remains to be seen whether interferon actually modifies the natural history of this cancer and that of Kaposi's sarcoma, and significantly improves survival times. Nevertheless, they are agreed that the interferons show 'considerable promise' and that much more clinical testing is warranted (Sikora, 1986; Krown, 1986; Wittes, personal interview, 1986; Smyth *et al.*, 1987).

Ironically for Pauling and the vitamin C believers, a 'major concern' of the interferonologists has been that premature negative conclusions about the lack of efficacy of interferon might result from inadequate testing under inappropriate circumstances. There have been suggestions that clinical trials with interferons and other biologicals that act to control tumour growth through the immune system should be designed 'considerably differently' from those for chemotherapeutic agents; for instance, that the best test of interferon's effectiveness might be on patients with low tumour burdens, or 'even in patients with minimal or no detectable disease who have not received chemotherapy or radiotherapy' (Herberman, 1985). Also, as with 5-fluorouracil, it is argued that there is evidence that the different routes of administration of interferon might affect treatment outcomes, and that this requires further investigation (Smyth *et al.*, 1987). This same argument for vitamin C was not accepted.

But above all, the interferon experts are united in their insistence that differences in biological activites exist among the different types and subtypes of interferon, and between the recombinant produced interferons and those produced by other means, and that the potential anti-cancer effects of all these different kinds of interferon have as yet to be ascertained. Along with this claim, they stress that there are indications that the different forms of interferon are synergistic with one another and with certain cytotoxic drugs, with other biologics, with radiation therapy, hyperthermia, and hormones. All these combinations and adjuvant potentials of interferon, it is claimed, merit formal evaluation in clinical trials (Sikora, 1986; Krown, 1986; Smyth *et al.*, 1987). This 'combined-modality integration' framework of interferon research has been heavily promoted by the pharmaceutical industry and by the NCI's newly formed $40 million Biological Response Modifiers Program, for which interferon was the prototype. With so many possible combinations and permutations, the search to find the 'true role' of the interferons in cancer treatment could well become 'an industry unto itself'. As new forms of interferon become available they are eagerly seized upon for testing, alone, in combination with one another, and with chemotherapeutic and other agents (Panem, 1984; Smith, 1986; Barnes, 1987). Interferon research is thus open-ended, unlike vitamin C research, and it has succeeded in so far as it has been successfully insinuated into existing practices.

On the basis of the foregoing analysis, it seems reasonable to conclude that the economic potential of interferon in cancer treatment, the huge sums invested in its research, the publicity it received, and the public and political expectations it aroused, have structured judgments about its efficacy in cancer treatment, so that interferon has not been rejected unequivocally, as vitamin C has been, but deemed to have a limited efficacy and to be worthy of further trials. Pauling's promotion of vitamin C on the grounds of its accessibility, cheapness and non-patentability has not advanced his cause.

There can be no doubt that as far as the pharmaceutical industry was concerned, interferon *had* to work. A 1982 survey of American corporate investment in interferon research and development reported the involvement of six multinational pharmaceutical corporations and a 'multitude' of small companies. The industry interest in the interferons was heightened by its perception of its aging product range (the patents on many of the traditional top-selling pharmaceuticals were running out, presenting the opportunity for generic firms to make and market cheap copies), tougher government regulation and threatened price freezes (Wyke, 1987). By 1983, the two major multinational competitors Schering-Plough and Hoffmann-La Roche were each spending approximately $40 million – that is, fifteen per cent of their respective research budgets – in order to begin production of a drug that, as of that date, had not been demonstrated to have important therapeutic benefits and was conceded to have severe side effects. Nevertheless, in confident anticipation of interferon's clearance by the FDA as a cancer treatment and of the cash flow to follow, Schering-Plough had already begun construction of a giant $106 million interferon factory in Ireland (Kenney, 1986). Events have borne out their confidence. Interferon may not have lived up to earlier predictions of its economic potential, but, as noted earlier, it is a 'nicely profitable' drug for its patent holders. And its combined modality promotion leaves open the prospect of its further profitability.

Nor can there be any doubt that the NCI found it politically and economically expedient to yield to public and Congressional enthusiasm for interferon research and to continue to find sufficient rationale for its continuation in the form of the Biological Response Modifiers Program. As Panem notes, by the late 1970s, the NCI's anti-viral programme was waning in the face of its poor returns and mounting Congressional criticism. The interferon crusade and the multiform nature of interferon provided the NCI with an opportunity to switch focus from the anti-viral properties of the substance to its anti-tumour potential as a regulator of the immune system. It utilized some of the Congressional grant for interferon research and trials to establish a comprehensive Biological Response Modifiers Program (BRMP). The mandate of the BRMP is to identify, develop, and bring to clinical trials potential therapeutic agents that may alter biological responses important in the biology of cancer growth and spreading (Oldham, 1982). The agents investigated in this programme include the interferons and interferon inducers, and the lymphokines, the best-known of which are the controversial interleukins whose history to date shows every sign of duplicating that of the interferons (Chase, 1986; Moertel, 1986b; DeVita and Roper, 1987; Wyke, 1987; Teitelman, 1989).

The establishment of the BRMP coincided with the scaling down of the NCI's funding for chemotherapeutic development (Barnes, 1987), and may be perceived as a tacit recognition of the limitations of the cytotoxic drugs that have for so long dominated cancer clinical research and treatment. BRMP directors and personnel have been careful to promote the biologicals as an 'additional modality for cancer therapy' that might be combined with other, more standard forms of therapy, and are reportedly encouraged by the increasing acceptance of the biologicals within and outside the NCI. In an unwitting, but far more successful, replication of Ewan Cameron's earlier strategy for vitamin C, they have emphasized the potential of the biologicals to enhance the effectiveness of the cytotoxics. By giving chemotherapy in combination with interferon or another biological that enhances bone marrow growth, it may be possible to give more of the cytotoxic than is currently possible, and so increase the chances that all cancer cells are completely destroyed (Barnes, 1987). We may suspect that it is this reassurance that it does not threaten existing treatments that has reconciled the oncologists to interferon and to the Biological Response Modifiers Program, whereas Pauling's insistence on the incompatability of vitamin C and conventional cytotoxic therapy could only be perceived as threatening to existing practices. The belated attempts by Pauling and Cameron to retrieve the situation by arguing that high-dose vitamin C does not interfere with the administration of chemotherapy and may protect the patients against its toxicity, have met with no such comparable response from the oncologists (Pauling, personal communication, 12 April 1989).

We may infer further reasons for the acceptability of interferon over vitamin C, in interferon's better conformity with the professional preference for treatments which are hospital- or clinic-based and entirely controlled and administered by the profession. Interferon, being a naturally occurring substance in the human body, may legitimately be considered part of the orthomolecular repertoire, and Pauling has claimed it as an 'orthomolecular substance' (Cameron and Pauling, 1979; Pauling, 1986). But to date its cost and general inaccessibility have kept it out of the hands of the unorthodox and firmly under the control of the profession. As marketed in the U.S., interferon is a prescription drug that is administered by subcutaneous or intramuscular injection and only 'under the guidance of a qualified physician'. Like the standard cytotoxics, its toxic side effects must be closely monitored by a battery of clinical tests (PDR, 1989). The FDA condemned earlier attempts to market interferon as a health food supplement (Yoxen, 1983).

Finally, we may note that interferon is assimilable to the militaristic metaphors that have characterized conventional cancer research. Matilde Krim led the way by dubbing interferon a 'kind of chemical Paul Revere'. As she reportedly explained to *Time* journalists: when a virus invades a cell, it takes over the cell's 'factory' and uses it to turn out carbon copies of the 'alien' virus which then invade other cells. Enter interferon, the body's Paul Revere. The initial invasion by the foreign virus triggers the production of interferon which assumes the role of intercellular messenger and travels to neighbouring cells to 'warn against viral invasion and stimulate the defence forces' (Anon., 1980c). Krim's patriotic interpretation of interferon's biological behaviour was given concrete expression by a *Time* artist, who depicted cannonball-like viruses bombarding anachronistic modern-day cell 'factories', with a pistol-brandishing Paul Revere galloping between them. Vitamin C's association with disarmament and peaceful coexistence was thus ideologically outmatched by Krim's astute appeal to patriotism and military preparedness.

In summation: On the basis of available theoretical arguments and clinical evidence of efficacy and toxicity, there was no reason why oncologists could not have done vitamin C research as well as or instead of interferon research. As I have stressed, vitamin C is *not* incompatible with the orthodox reductionist biomedical model, and it, rather than interferon, might have become the prototype of the NCI's Biological Response Modifiers Program. The research and therapeutic successes of interferon, and the failures of vitamin C, are only fully understandable in social and political terms: interferon 'made it' from pseudoscientific status to officially credited cancer treatment, where vitamin C did not, because the interferonologists could command more powerful rhetorical, economic and political resources than those available to vitamin C advocates, and because interferon was more compatible with professional vested interests than vitamin C. The therapeutic claims of the interferonologists thereby overrode the resistance of the oncologists, and a place was found for interferon alongside accepted treatment modalities.

Conclusion: Making and Creating Choices

In examining the effectiveness of alternative systems of medicine a number of specific points must be taken into account. It is not possible simply to embark on this task using the scientific methods that are current in medical science. . . . The Commission believes that the division between alternative and orthodox medicine is not – or is not principally – of a scientific nature, but owes its origins and its continued existence to both socio-political and scientific factors. This implies that the gap cannot be closed simply by making scientific recommendations.

> The Secretary for the Commission for Alternative
> Systems of Medicine, The Hague, 1981
> (The Commission for Alternative Systems of Medicine, 1981)

Some political leaders and medical spokesmen have misled the public as to what they will and can do. . . . [T]he FDA does not always enforce regulations equitably. In the area of anti-cancer drugs, the FDA has approved drugs for commercial distribution, and physicians have used these drugs, for types of cancer for which these drugs have no demonstrable benefit, and yet these are among the most toxic drugs on the market. These facts are obvious to ordinary people, and they wonder quite appropriately what, if anything, the FDA seal of approval means.

The quality of health care that people receive is rightly subject to political control, for the people who use it pay for it. The body politic usually delegates its power to define standards to expert groups, but there is no *a priori* reason why it cannot set and abide by its own standards. When the public perceives that the government or its experts (in this case the medical establishment) have failed to enforce standards of quality, it is reasonable for it to withdraw its mandate and revise it or cancel it entirely.

> Robert S. K. Young, Division of Oncology,
> Food and Drug Administration (Young, 1987).

We cannot refine the politics out of medicine. We are not faced with a choice between medicine *or* politics, but with the inescapable reality of medicine *as* politics. By this I do not mean that we can simply reduce medicine to politics, to arbitrary power as opposed to rational knowledge. Rather, I mean, as this study has made manifest, that medical rationality is a framework of thought and action interpenetrated by professional and socioeconomic interests and values. My intention is to expose the artificial and unrealistic separation of medical knowledge from its political context, from the social distribution of power.

Medical knowledge of disease and its treatment is the result of complex social interactions and negotiations. It is constrained by nature, by the reality of the human organism, but it is actively constructed or invented by social beings, by *people* who, whatever their intentions or efforts, can never entirely escape the values and interests of the institutions and the wider society in which they live and work. By their interpretations, actions and practices, they socially negotiate the 'truth' or 'falsity' of medical knowledge. There is no finite or absolute boundary that divides medicine from the society in which it is constructed and practised. There exist only the arbitrary barriers that are politically imposed and maintained by medicine's interest-serving and socially-credentialed claim to cognitive and social authority. Just as medicine pervades every aspect of society, so at every level of medical activity – from the researcher at the laboratory bench, at every step of the formally constituted clinical trial, through all the formal and informal interactions of publication and academic debate, to the diagnosis and treatment by the practitioner in the clinic, to the patient's response to the prescribed treatment – society intervenes. Medicine and society are mutually constitutive of one another.

The history of the vitamin C and cancer controversy is best understood as a political struggle concerning control over the determination and evaluation of cancer treatments. By means of his personal prestige, well-developed political and institutional skills and connections, and his alignment with holism and the health food lobby, Pauling succeeded not only in promoting vitamin C into a leading alternative treatment for cancer, but also in organizing it onto the orthodox medical agenda. He thus brought it into competition with conventional cancer treatments, and forced two professional evaluations of the Pauling–Cameron experimental claims via the professionally endorsed methodology. Both professionally conducted trials have been demonstrated to be problematic. They have not disproved the specific claims made by Pauling and Cameron. Nevertheless, through the assertion of its cognitive authority, backed by claims of objectivity and professional disinterest, and constituted by a powerful amalgam of institutional and professional interests, orthodox medicine appears to be in the process of foreclosing any future trials of vitamin C, thereby bringing about a political closure of the debate in its favour.

Comparative analysis of the controversy has borne out my further contention that therapeutic evaluation is inherently a social and political process and that the idea of neutral appraisal is a myth. The standards of objective assessment that apply in any particular evaluative context are determined by the internal and external politics of medicine. The research and therapeutic successes of 5-fluorouracil and interferon and the failures of vitamin C cannot be accounted for in terms of the disinterested and rational processes conventionally attributed to the evaluation of medical therapies. The orthodox medical assessments of these three putative cancer treatments have been shown to be riddled with inconsistencies and interpenetrated by professional and wider social interests. They can only fully be understood in social, political, and economic terms.

All this contradicts the conventional view of medical controversies: that the dispute may be objectively resolved and the bias, interests, prejudices, or whatever, of the disputants eliminated by the application of the scientific method to medicine in the form of the rigorously designed and properly applied clinical trial. As this study has demonstrated over and over again, the clinical trial, no matter how tightly it is organized and evaluated, can neither guarantee objectivity nor definitively resolve disputes over contentious therapies or technologies. The methodology or protocol of the clinical trial is tied to the research tradition or paradigm of the specialist community that embodies or sustains that paradigm, and is inextricable from the political and social structure of that community. Judgements about experimental findings are necessarily bound up with the professional values and interests of the adjudicating community, and, as the case of interferon has compellingly illustrated, they may be structured by wider social interests such as consumer choice or market forces. From this we may infer that the very notion of therapeutic efficacy is politically defined and defended, and that the practical success of a therapy is asserted and sustained by the power of the interests that sponsor and maintain it.

In other words, there is no way that the evaluation of therapies can be prised apart from the vested interests and social objectives that they embody. To think that better and better clinical trials and more and more scientific facts will solve the inherently political problem of therapeutic evaluation is naive. It is, above all, to endorse medicine's own self-interested representation of itself. The myth of neutral assessment is crucial to medicine's privileged and powerful adjudicating role and, while it prevails, medicine will assert it to protect its cognitive and social authority, to render opposition or competition ineffective or, if that is not possible, to coopt or subordinate it.

If the image of medicine I have conveyed is one wherein medicine lurches along, riven by internal professional power struggles, impelled this way and that by arbitrary economic and sociopolitical forces, and sustained by bodies of myth and rhetoric that are elaborated in response to major threats to its survival, then that is the image supported by this study.

OPTIONS AND PRESSURES FOR CHANGE

The contradictions between the expectations aroused by the myths and rhetoric of medicine and the reality of the arbitrariness of medical practice have engendered a large critical literature that has focused on improving and implementing the procedures of therapeutic evaluation. Most of this critical literature has fallen back on the standard invocation of methodological reform via the rigorously conducted clinical trial for the elimination of 'bias' from treatment assessments. Even those whose own studies support the view that medical theory and practice are shaped by socioeconomic and professional interests generally assume that medical knowledge can somehow be evaluated independently of those interests (Doyal with Pennell, 1979; McKinlay, 1981; Doyal and Doyal, 1984).

But, if they are to be effective, the critics and reformers of medicine will have to move beyond their hackneyed invocation of methodological reform to a better understanding of its inherent limitations. Their reliance on the reforming powers of the controlled clinical trial lends itself to the highly misleading idea that therapeutic efficacy can be definitively and universally established by natural law, that more precise knowledge, more widely disseminated, will lead naturally and inevitably to the adoption by all concerned of a consensual view of disease and its treatment.

This consensual ideal is contradicted by the critics' or reformers' own studies that have pointed up the significant financial, public and professional obstacles to the abandonment of professionally endorsed treatments, even if they are determined by clinical trial to be ineffective and to harm patients (McKinlay, 1981; Chalmers, 1974, 1981; Silverman, 1984). An even more fundamental problem is that it is based crucially on the fallacious view that rationality in medicine is purely a function of technical sophistication, in this case of the refinement and application of the clinical trial. But, to repeat the point I previously emphasized, medical rationality must be understood as a framework of thought and action interpenetrated by professional and socioeconomic interests and values, and these interests and values are embodied in the evaluative standards and methodological procedures adopted and imposed by medicine and its diverse professional practitioners.

On the face of it, the alternative critique and confrontation of the conventional assessment of alternative therapies would seem to offer the best possibilities for providing an appropriate understanding of the limitations of the clinical trial. But, with a few notable exceptions (Aakster, 1986), the scanty sociological literature on the evaluation of alternative or holistic medicine has been unable to provide this. While it acknowledges the difficulty of assessing treatments within such a different conceptual and practising framework, most of this literature also stresses the need for objective scientific validation of alternative therapies, usually via the controlled clinical trial, and suggests various ways in which this might be achieved (Rosch and Kearney, 1985; Patel, 1987a, b; Fulder, 1988).

This ultimate reliance on objective scientific assessment is shared by most alternative critics of 'establishment' medicine. The most representative and recent of such alternative critiques has been compiled by Robert Houston, an American science writer and longstanding champion of alternative medicine. Houston's *Repression and Reform in the Evaluation of Alternative Cancer Treatments* was commissioned by the newly-formed coalition of the most politically active of the dissident cancer groups, the Coalition for the Evaluation of Alternative Therapy. It offers a hard-hitting, if predictable, critique of what Houston condemns as the orthodox manipulation of the randomized controlled cancer trial and the 'bias' and the 'double standards' of the NCI, the FDA, and the ACS. As predictably, Houston's solution to the politics of treatment assessment is to fall back onto clinical studies of 'greater scientific validity and precision' which he equates with 'fairer evaluation' (Houston, 1987).

Houston's many suggestions for reform and safeguards against 'evaluator bias' in assessment methodology range from the involvement of the chief proponent scientist in the design of the protocol of the proposed trial and the exclusion of known opponents of alternative medicine from its formal clinical evaluation, to greater reliance on non-randomized trials and computerized data bases, and the shifting of evaluative criteria from tumour size and survival times to 'objective' measures of quality of life. Houston also puts forward a number of suggestions for legislative change that he perceives as necessary steps towards the implementation of the unbiased assessment and research of alternative cancer treatments. These include proposals for a specific budgetary allocation by Congress to the NCI for research into alternative treatments, limits to the authority of the FDA which has taken a 'particularly vengeful stance' towards alternative treatments and their practitioners, the liberalization of the 'efficacy' requirements of the Kefauver-Harris amendments of 1962, and legal changes permitting unpenalized access by patients and their doctors to 'unproven' treatments in the interests of their 'fair evaluation'. According to Houston, what was intended as a system to distinguish effective from ineffective treatments has become a 'system that recognizes mainly money and power as justification for approval, considerations rationally irrelevant to truth'. The crux of his critique and his proposed reform measures is that the scientific ideal of 'experimentation without prejudice' has not been symmetrically applied to alternative treatments and that the concept of evidence has been 'distorted self-servingly' by orthodox medicine:

Beyond the misuse of the concept of evidence, such dismissive policies are antiscientific in the fundamental sense that they involve rejection on social grounds that are extraneous to scientific concerns. (Houston, 1987)

Houston's recommendations, were they to be implemented, might bring about a measure of reform in the evaluation of alternative cancer treatments. A few 'unproven' remedies might even eventually win ortho-dox acceptance through their positive assessment via the methodological reforms that Houston envisages. But it would not be because this reformed methodology had eliminated evaluator bias and brought about 'greater scientific validity and precision, and hence, fairness', as Houston supposes. It would be, as this study has demonstrated, because of the renegotiation and reconstitution of the processes of therapeutic evaluation and the standards of objective assessment via the play of those forces such as money and power or professional self-interest that Houston condemns as 'rationally irrelevant to truth' and 'extraneous to scientific concerns'.

The methodological and associated legislative changes that he recom-mends could only be implemented through the exertion of continued political and economic pressure by the shifting coalition of 'freedom fighters', the holistic health movement, the health food lobby, and alternative practitioners and their patients. They could be expected to be resisted forcefully by oncologists, 'quackbusters', and their allies. But these pressures might be sufficient to win majority congressional support, as they did in the previously discussed case of the Proxmire Amendment (see section 2.7), and to bring about an overtly political solution to the dispute through the curtailing of the powers of the FDA, and through direct congressional pressure on the NCI. Or they might act primarily through legal challenges to state anti-quackery legislation, as in the case of laetrile, or in the recent case where the U.S. Court of Appeals overturned a $500,000 malpractice award against a physician convicted of using an unconventional cancer therapy on a patient who had signed an informed consent statement. In this latter case, in what has been hailed as a decision of wide significance by the alternative network, the Appeals Court ruled that there was no reason why a patient 'should not be allowed to make an informed decision to go outside currently approved medical methods in search of an unconventional treatment' (Chowka, 1988; Ladas, 1988; Houston, 1987). These counterbalancing economic, political, and legal pressures might exert their greatest effects through consumer resistance to cytotoxic treatments and growing prefer-ence for alternative cancer therapies, and so act to threaten the economic viability of conventional cancer treatments and their practitioners, to destabilize the existing power relations within medicine, and so reshape treatment assessments and practices. By any or all of these political and economic means, those alternative treatments that are most compatible with the medical model and medical professionalism and with the economic and larger social forces that sustain them, might be subsumed within conventional medicine. But it would require major changes in the structure and exercise of power and authority in society before medicine itself underwent any major and effective reforms.

That there will be some significant changes to current evaluative procedures and consequently to cancer therapies is inevitable. A major factor for change must be the multifaceted worldwide disillusionment with medicine. This extends from critiques of medicine's ineffectiveness and inability to deal with a disease pattern of chronic and degenerative illnesses, to its high costs, its bureaucratic indifference, and its iatrogenic outcomes. Besides those promoting alternative medical systems and the holistic health movement, the pressure groups in the area of medical politics include the consumer activists concerned with malpractice and informed consent issues, the feminist movement with its critique of patriarchal medicine, the environmentalist lobby, a variety of socialist groups seeking greater equality in health care and the elimination of the profit motive from medicine, and a massive self-help movement opposed to the increasing dependence on technological medicine. The popular disillusionment with medicine is manifested in the new health consciousness with its emphasis on the pursuit of individual lifestyle changes and the accompanying commercialization of health and fitness (Crawford, 1984; Turner, 1987; Coward, 1989). These changing social attitudes towards medicine, aided by political programmes aimed at shifting the responsibility for health care and the burden of costs back onto the consumer in a period of world economic recession, must be refracted in medical theory and practice.

In the United States, the escalating costs of conventional cancer treatment and health insurance are particularly potent factors for change in a context where an estimated 37 million Americans have no health insurance coverage. Many of these are children who are not covered by their parents' work-related insurance packages, and the childhood leukaemias have always been the mainstay of chemotherapeutic success. Many of the uninsured are those who fall into the category of not being able to afford the high cost of private insurance, but who earn too much to qualify for the federal-state health programme for the poor. These people can obtain access for themselves and their children to the expensive conventional cancer treatments only at the price of their impoverishment. Every year, the number of uninsured grows by an estimated million more (Rich, 1986; Mathiessen, 1989).

This grave threat to the medical care market has alerted the profession to the need for major reforms, even to the unprecedented extent of viewing favourably proposals for a national health insurance system and tolerating, in the name of cost-benefit analysis and finite public resources, the prospect of broader-based evaluative criteria for the assessment of technologies and therapies. Arnold Relman, in a recent editorial in the *New England Journal of Medicine*, assured his professional constituency that such proposals did not represent the 'socialization of health care', but were necessary to repair or replace 'our present disastrously inadequate health care financing system'. Relman himself favoured a 'comprehensive plan which includes improved technology assessment and malpractice reform as well as other reforms in medical practice' as the only way likely to achieve the goals of 'universal access, cost containment, and preservation of quality that everyone seems to want'. He exhorted the profession to 'make common cause with government and with the major private payers in seeking solutions to a pressing social problem that is not going to solve itself' (Relman, 1989).

If physicians do not accept the necessity of co-operating with the growing economic and social pressures for evaluative reform, as Relman urges, then it seems likely that government and the private health insurers, through their mutual interest in containing the costs of medical care, will do it for them. One recent government initiative has been the implementation of a controversial programme for the testing, approval, marketing and prescribing of cheaper generics as a substitute for expensive brand name drugs. Predictably, this has been strongly contested by some sections of the medical profession and the pharmaceutical industry on the grounds that the FDA-approved generic equivalents are not therapeutically equivalent to the innovator patented drugs (Horwitz, 1989b). In the private sector, insurance companies have responded to the spiralling costs of health care by targeting the more expensive diseases, notably cancer. As a way of reducing costs, insurers are attempting to reimburse only for those treatments that have been deemed effective by the FDA for particular conditions. A recent audit has indicated that half of the current chemotherapy uses by oncologists in the U.S. lack specific FDA approval, and insurance companies have been quick to capitalize on such widespread unlabeled and inappropriate uses of the anti-cancer cytotoxics and biologicals (Mortenson, 1988; Mannisto, 1988). Recently they have begun denying payment for investigational, experimental, and a variety of conventional cancer chemotherapy treatments, which they have reclassified as 'unconventional' (Anon., 1989a). These initiatives by government and big business constitute a serious challenge to the maintenance of medicine's traditional control over the evaluation and use of its own technical knowledge.

Another major pressure for change in evaluative standards and practices has occurred in the context of medical, regulatory, and community reactions to the perceived severity of the AIDS crisis.

These have demonstrated compellingly the potential for change through the impact of consumer pressure. This new infectious disease with its complex social, political, and cultural ramifications, its threatening epidemic proportions, its lack of an established medical specialty or institutional power base, and its initial 'life-style' model prior to the isolation of a putative causal agent (HIV), provided an unprecedented opportunity for the play of consumer power in its definition, treatment and prevention. The prominent role of consumer action in the American AIDS epidemic has been aided by a health polity geared to chronic degenerative disease rather than to infectious epidemics, the absence of any national coordinated programme for its research and containment, the prevailing political rhetoric of deregulation and competition, and, above all, the existence of a well-organized and politically active gay rights movement that provided a basis for the development of community-based strategies and tactics in negotiating and shaping health care responses to AIDS (Fee and Fox, 1988; Brandt, 1985).

It was the AIDS crisis and the associated consumer pressures (pressures, it should be noted, that meshed with those applied by the pharmaceutical industry which has consistently lobbied for a relaxation of the Kefauver-Harris amendments) that led to the recently implemented U.S. drug regulatory changes permitting the earlier release and marketing of 'promising' experimental drugs (see section 3.4). In 1987, the FDA broke new ground when it released the experimental AIDS drug azidothymidine (AZT) under the new TINDs guidelines. AIDS patients and their support and advocacy groups are determined upon a further relaxation of these guidelines, arguing that they are not giving AIDS patients fast enough access to new experimental drugs that might help their condition. They want an even faster 'parallel track' for the distribution and marketing of experimental AIDS drugs outside a clinical trial setting before they go through the conventional time-consuming Phase II trials that test their activity. Following mass demonstrations and intense political and bureaucratic lobbying by AIDS patients and activists, the 'parallel track' concept has been endorsed publicly by some Congressmen and by leading federal health bureaucrats, including Vincent DeVita and Samuel Broder, past and present directors of the NCI, Frank Young, commissioner of the FDA, and Anthony Fauci, chief of the National Institute for Allergies and Infectious Diseases, and, of course, by the pharmaceutical industry. This novel coalition of interested parties overrode the objections of some medical professionals and consumer groups that the proposed procedures would change the ground rules of medical research, clinical care markets, and health insurance, and jeopardize the conduct of more rigorous clinical trials. In particular, concerns were expressed by some scientists running clinical trials on AIDS drugs that the early distribution of experimental drugs outside the clinic would make it impossible to control the trial patients' medication and to interpret trial results, and would add to the growing problem of recruiting patients for trials. In response, the leader of a militant gay advocacy group reportedly told a congressional health subcommittee hearing that AIDS patients were not in awe of the 'strange and abstract god, clean data'. At the same time, and somewhat contradictorily, AIDS activists claimed that they were not contesting the need for randomized controlled trials, and that patients were more likely to comply with the researchers' requirements if they perceived the rules as fair. It was the FDA restrictions that were 'polluting' the trials, they argued, because patients, desperate for access to experimental drugs, lied about their medical history. At the same hearing, Fauci, who coordinates a national effort to test new AIDS drugs, assured the committee, 'we can be humanitarian and do good science' (Marshall, 1989).

Just what would constitute the good and humanitarian drug research invoked by Fauci that would also satisfy the AIDS activists remains undefined. But, as his critics have indicated, it is clear that it would entail a shift away from the current emphasis on randomized controlled trials. If experimental drugs were made freely available to AIDS patients, it is unlikely that they would submit themselves voluntarily to the lottery of the randomized trial and to the dictates of its designers. The outcome would be, as Ralph Nader's Health Research Group predicted, an 'extraordinary conflict' between researchers and patients (Marshall, 1989), as they contested the control of the drugs and their new criteria of assessment. And, in the absence of any guidelines on matters of drug profitability or liability, it could be argued that the political and economic reality of this rhetorical ideal of a good and humanitarian science might well be less than humanitarian. AZT, the first of the experimental drugs to be made available under the TINDs scheme, has been the source of ongoing bitter disputes among AIDS patients and activists, health insurance companies, Federal officials (who fear they may have to foot a bill estimated at between $1 and $10 billion a year for AZT treatment for impoverished patients), and the manufacturer and distributor, Burroughs Wellcome (currently charging patients about $8,000 a year for a full course of treatment) (Anon, 1989b; Mathiessen, 1989). In an uncontrolled and deregulated market, the real beneficiaries of the struggle for freedom of choice in AIDS therapies are more likely to be the immensely profitable and powerful pharmaceutical corporations, together with a self-selected coterie of researchers and entrepreneurs who have jumped aboard the AIDS bandwaggon, than the patients in whose name the struggle is being waged.

Those campaigners for freedom of choice in cancer therapies who want to draw lessons from the greater impact of their AIDS counterparts should note also that AIDS campaigners have been far less successful in promoting alternative AIDS treatments than in gaining access to the experimental drugs ratified by orthodoxy. As alternative AIDS treatments have burgeoned alongside the 'legitimate' experimental drugs, they have become the target of the antiquackery crusaders. And, ironically, the faster FDA-release route – trail-blazed by AIDS activists and their allies – seems set to become the designated early-release route for the contentious and toxic experimental cancer drugs so stigmatized by alternative critics (Marx, 1989).

This does not mean that consumer opposition or resistance to the judge-ments of professional medicine, or lay challenges to medical authority through alternative approaches, is inevitably rendered ineffectual or coopted to medicine's own ends. The current pressures and possibilities for change in the politics of therapeutic evaluation have never been so widespread, nor the need so urgent. And much of the impetus for change has come from consumer pressure groups, particularly from those associated with alternative medicine.

In the United States, as we saw, it was such pressures that mobilized Congressional support and initiated the Office of Technology Assessment investigation of unorthodox cancer treatments. These same pressures have sustained the continuing dispute and delayed the release of the contentious OTA draft report (see sections 2.6 and 6.5). In Britain, consumer pressure, reflected in the significant proportion of conventional general practice trainees who were already using or who wished to train in alternative methods (Reilly, 1983), forced a reluctant British Medical Asso-ciation (BMA) to carry out a formal evaluation of alternative medicine at the instigation and under the patronage of Prince Charles (British Medical Association, Board of Science and Education, 1986). The publication of this report, which dealt dismissively with alternative medicine as largely untested, ineffective, sometimes harmful, and inconsistent with natural laws, provoked a powerful backlash which included a well-supported Parliamentary motion deploring the report and calling for an enquiry. As a result, and contrary to the BMA claim that all alternative therapies are in principle evaluable by conventional controlled clinical trials and that it was the responsibility of alternative practitioners to mount such trials, the UK Medical Research Council finally moved to support the appointment, together with the Research Council for Complementary Medicine, of a Fellow in Research Methodology for Complementary Medicine at Glasgow University to examine how alternative medicine might best be evaluated (Fulder, 1988).

Rather than expend their energy and efforts on the limited reforms they might achieve via their campaign for the neutral or unprejudiced evaluation of alternative treatments by accredited medical experts, those advocating freedom of choice in cancer treatments might do better to adopt the goal of 'structured coexistence' of conventional and alternative medical systems. This is a situation where, on the basis of strong historical or traditional utilization of or public demand for the services of alternative health practitioners, the parallel existence of two or more separately conceptualized therapy systems is officially or legally recognized and regulated (Unschuld, 1980). This model is in place in some non-western societies, especially in China. But it has also been adopted by certain highly industrialized western countries, notably by West Germany, where there is a long tradition of utilization of alternative therapy systems which are still in demand by a significant proportion of the German population.

The other major factor shaping German *Therapiefreiheit* (the freedom to select a mode of therapy in conformity with the world view of the patient or practitioner) is the well-documented resistance of the extremely powerful German pharmaceutical industry to government regulation or control. Until 1976, the pharmaceutical industry enjoyed nearly total freedom to produce, register and market drugs with only minimal regulation, a freedom which the promoters of alternative therapeutic products also enjoyed under the shelter of the deliberately vague and all-embracing definition of a drug enshrined in the old legislation. The 1976 'Law to Restructure Drug Legislation' was forced upon the legislature by the necessity to conform with European Community guidelines which insisted on proof of efficacy as a precondition for the legal admission of any drug. At the same time, the legislature was also forced to take account of the pluralism of therapeutic world views which the earlier legislation had fostered. The new drug legislation resolved the difficulty by distinguishing between 'admitted' and 'registered' drugs. 'Admitted' drugs must satisfy strict criteria including clinical testing concerning their efficacy and safety; these criteria are not required for 'registered' drugs, such as homeopathic remedies, for which a direct effect cannot be demonstrated by currently available scientific methods.

As well, the legislature, after intense political lobbying by the adherents of alternative therapeutic systems, introduced the institution of 'external expert committees' which have the responsibility of evaluating the data and performing the clinical trials for efficacy and safety and making recommendations for the 'admission' of therapies. Under the terms of the legislation, these committees must be composed of experts from the specific therapy system. In effect, the decision concerning the efficacy of a particular therapy remains entirely in the hands of the adherents of that therapeutic system, and the coexistence of alternative and orthodox systems is legally guaranteed. The legislation goes so far in meeting its political goal of reflecting the existing pluralism in therapeutic systems, as to attribute equality of 'scientific' status and 'scientific knowledge' to those 'experts', whether of alternative or orthodox persuasion, who comprise the external evaluative committees (Roth, 1976; Unschuld, 1980).

The West German system of structured coexistence has resolved the socio-political problem of the evaluation of alternative therapies by ensuring that they are assessed by their own experts within their own conceptual frameworks, and, in the process, has even legislatively redefined 'science' in its terminological upgrading of competing alternative medical doctrines. But, as Unschuld points out, it has not addressed the problem of the proliferation of drugs marketed within the conceptual frameworks of orthodox or alternative systems. Nor has the legislature attempted to assess or to redress the potential undue influence of a powerful pharmaceutical industry on policy making and drug legislation in a free market economy (Unschuld, 1980). Nor, although it has yielded to consumer pressure by legislatively safeguarding the continued coexistence of alternative therapies, has the legislature given consumers any recognized decision-making role in the process. The evaluation of therapies remains firmly under the control of accredited experts, whether conventional or alternative, and subject to the uncontested play of their respective occupational and larger socioeconomic interests.

The proposed model for the structured coexistence of alternative and conventional medicine in the Netherlands promises to be more representative of social values and consumer interests and less open to the undue influences of market forces and occupational self interest. This comprehensive proposal resulted from an intense public campaign for freedom of choice in medicine that led to the setting up of the government-appointed Commission for Alternative Systems of Medicine. The Commission (which consisted of equal numbers defending the position of conventional medicine and of those arguing for alternative medicine and included consumer representation) surveyed and held hearings with all the relevant organizations and examined the available international literature on alternative medicine. It also sponsored a detailed survey of the nature and distribution of use and of the degree of satisfaction with the practices of alternative medicine. The Commission found that the consensus of public opinion was no longer behind the legally-enforced monopoly of orthodox medicine, that the public demand to choose freely alternative healers and methods of treatment was based on personal experience and confidence in finding help and relief for disorders not alleviated by conventional medicine, and that this public demand for and confidence in alternative medicine should be reflected in government policy and Dutch law. In particular, the Commission rejected the conventional evaluative methodology of randomised controlled trials as 'not practicable' in the case of alternative systems of medicine which are so conceptually different from orthodox reductionist medicine. It suggested 'less ambitious' methods which would include the registration of consumption and satisfaction among patients.

Most significantly, the Commission stated its belief that the division between alternative and orthodox medicine is not primarily of a scientific nature, but 'owes its origins and its continued existence to both politico-social and scientific factors', and that this implied that the gap could not be closed 'simply by making scientific recommendations'. On this basis, it argued that the demand that alternative practitioners must demonstrate the effectiveness of their treatments before they could be granted any form of recognition was 'indefensible'. Its recommendations include the institution and implementation of a national information and documentation centre on alternative medicine; government funding of research and tertiary training in alternative forms of treatment; the provision of information on alternative forms of treatment in existing professional medical courses; the adequate training and qualification of alternative practitioners and support and encouragement for the upgrading of their occupational organizations and standards; vigorous opposition to charlatanry and fraud within both conventional and alternative medicine; the inclusion of alternative systems of medicine in health insurance schemes; and statutory provision for the legal recognition and status of appropriately qualified alternative practitioners and their practices (Commission for Alternative Systems of Medicine, 1981; Fulder, 1988).

The Netherlands model is not yet operative and there are many problems to be resolved before it can be fully implemented. But it represents the most comprehensive and democratic attempt to date to come to grips with the political realities of the consumption and assessment of alternative medicine in a western society. From the point of view of this study, its most notable innovations are its explicit recognition of the essentially sociopolitical nature of the division between conventional and alternative medicine and of the limitations of the randomized controlled trial in evaluating alternative treatments, and its proposal to take patterns of patient consumption and satisfaction into account in assessing and recognizing alternative therapies.

The problem with models for structured coexistence is that they do not confront the larger and more pressing social problem of the evaluation of the therapies of the dominant system of orthodox medicine. While the Netherlands model presents the best option so far discussed for the recognition and evaluation of alternative treatment systems, its inherent limitation is that its innovations are restricted to the assessment of alternative medicine. But while they do not of themselves provide a basis for assessing conventional treatments, they point the way towards one. It is, moreover, a way that is supported by this study and the new understanding of medical knowledge that it advocates.

IMPLICATIONS OF THIS STUDY FOR THE EVALUATION AND SOCIAL IMPLEMENTATION OF THERAPIES

We need a perspective on the use and advocacy of alternative systems of medicine in western societies that does not dismiss them as manifestations of irrationality or antiscience, that recognizes these epithets as the rhetorical and marginalizing labels of orthodoxy, and that positively reevaluates alternative medical systems as an attempt by some sections of the public to seek – or even to present – a better approach to health care. At the very least, the current widespread use and advocacy of alternative medicine must be understood as a significant measure of the growing dissatisfaction with the practices and therapies of conventional medicine. But more than this, in their efforts to secure the recognition and legality of alternative treatment systems, their advocates have been forced to confront and to contest their evaluation by the accredited experts of the dominant system of orthodox medicine. These confrontations and disputations between the advocates of such different conceptual treatment systems have laid bare the socioeconomic and political ramifications of the processes of therapeutic assessment of alternative treatments and created the opportunity for their recognition and study. The insights gained from the analysis of rejected alternative knowledge may then be applied to the evaluation of successful conventional treatments. In this book I have tried to show how such a comparison generates a more adequate and realistic understanding of the processes of therapeutic evaluation than the conventional ideal of neutral, objective assessment by impartial experts. In this final section I will discuss briefly some of the more important implications of the new understanding of medicine that I am advocating.

One of its most significant consequences is that we can no longer view the medical expert as a neutral or apolitical arbiter of medical truth. I have argued that an inescapable dimension of medical controversy is the essentially political mobilization of claims and counterclaims – that there are no impartial experts on whom we may call for a neutral or disinterested judgement of the issues. This does not mean that we have to impute self-interested motives of 'bias' or 'conspiracy' to the individuals concerned. Nor should we assume that medical experts will consciously manipulate data to suit their vested interests. While fraud and corruption do occur in medicine as elsewhere, there are also many sincere medical researchers who are motivated by high humanitarian ideals and concerns, just as there are also many caring doctors who want to do the best for their patients. Professionals are also private individuals with diverse personal affiliations and commitments and moral and political views. Their professional and personal diversity notwithstanding, in the larger structural sense, their findings and judgements inevitably will be constrained by the values and interests of the profession or specialty to which they belong. We must expect that they will act in ways consistent with their lengthy training and socialization and to protect their highly valued technical competences and cognitive and social authority. We also must take into account the ways in which wider social, political and economic forces may impinge upon and structure professional judgements of the efficacy or risks of medical therapies and technologies. Again, this does not mean, as their critics have sometimes alleged, that medical experts are the witting tools or the unwitting dupes of the multinational pharmaceutical industry, politicians, corporate capitalism, or whatever. Nor does it mean that they are, as they have on occasion represented themselves, the reluctant captives of media criticism or of increasingly demanding and litigious patients. Rather it is to recognize that they are not immune from any or all of these pressures by virtue of their specialist access to some rigorous scientific testing process that can guarantee the neutrality and objectivity of their judgements.

This revised view of medical knowledge that I am advocating therefore implies the compelling need for a thoroughgoing reappraisal of the expert's role in therapeutic evaluation. The medical expert must be seen as a necessarily 'partisan participant' in a political debate (Albury, 1983), not as an apolitical arbiter of medical truth. In other words, the essentially political role of the expert must be made overt. No longer should medicine be permitted to obscure behind a convenient rhetorical smokescreen of objective assessment, an essential feature of its evaluative processes – namely the structure of sociopolitical institutions and interests that create and perpetuate therapies and technologies.

The logical solution is to shift our evaluative focus from the unrealizable and obscuring idealization of objective assessment, that claims but inevitably fails to exclude all social influences on therapies and technologies, to one that acknowledges and embraces their social and political dimensions. It is important to understand that by this I am not endorsing the praiseworthy but weaker argument of some economists and sociologists: that we may simply add on a social or economic component to the clinical trial; that as well as evaluating therapies and technologies scientifically or objectively, we must also evaluate and take into account their economic and social impacts. This proposal is based on the acceptance of the misleading separation of the scientific from the socio-economic aspects of treatment assessment. I am proposing instead the explicit injection of social values and needs into the evaluative process. This involves the identification and evaluation of the interests and social objectives embodied in competing therapeutic claims as an acknowledged and integral part of the process of therapeutic assessment. The analysis that I have presented in this book suggests some of the ways in which this might be approached.

It follows that the socio-political appraisal of therapies that I advocate is something that can not be left to medical experts. It necessitates the active participation of non-experts, of patients and the public at large, in the processes of treatment assessment and decision-making. To date, under the terms of the standard view of medicine, patients and the public, the major consumers of medicine, have been excluded from the formal evaluative process. In the interests of the medical promotion of its claims to maximal objectivity, the randomized controlled clinical trial has been expressly designed to eliminate the patient's own 'subjective' impressions of treatment effectiveness or choice of available treatments. But if the focus of treatment assessment were to shift from the futile and unrealizable goal of neutral or value-free assessment to the identification and evaluation of the interests and social objectives embodied in the claims made by therapists, then the way is opened for an active and acknowledged evaluative role for the patient and the public. We are all our own experts when it comes to asking and answering the crucial question: do these interests and objectives reflect the kind of medicine we want? To put it another way: do we want our therapies and medical technologies to be evaluated against the values and objectives of a powerful coalition of institutional, economic and professional interests or by a socially broader-based set of evaluative criteria?

There are of course dangers in glib talk of the innovation of socially broader-based sets of indices by which to assess treatments without the concomitant recognition of the need to include institutional changes in the process (Wynne, 1975). Nor am I assuming that the values and social objectives of the different sectors of medical consumers and pressure groups are compatible with one another. On the contrary, on the basis of this study and others, I can predict with confidence that medical politics will continue to be the subject of criss-crossing and contradictory pressures exerted by different groups with their own disparate interests and agendas (Willis, 1983; Turner, 1987). But within the new conception of therapeutic evaluation I am envisaging there will be no illusion that such conflicts of interest can be resolved in the non-political arena of the clinical trial. If, as I have tried to show, therapeutic evaluation is a political process which systematically favours the interests of a medical elite and of other powerful groups in society, then it follows that its democratic reform requires the maximum of political participation by all members of society and the subordination of the technical expertise of medical experts to the democratic political process. Until now, the political argument from medical expertise has been: here is objective reality and you must adapt your values and interests to it. The situation I am advocating is: here are our values and interests and medicine must adapt its assessments and practices to them (Albury, 1983; Larson, 1984). In other words, what I am proposing is a radical reversal of the current ground rules; a reversal of rules that would empower consumers in their confrontations with medical authority and medical judgements. If medicine is unable to retreat to its privileged position of impartial, objective adjudication of treatments, then a more equitable representation of different social interests in the evaluation and choice of available treatments becomes a real political possibility.

This is where I think we might apply some of the insights to be gained from the previously discussed Netherlands model. Dutch policy makers, in recognizing the sociopolitical dimensions of the division between orthodox and alternative medicine, have recommended less ambitious methods for the assessment of alternative treatments than those conventionally used. We also might consider including measures of consumer satisfaction in the evaluation of conventional treatments. This might be done at both the institutional level – as with the Netherlands proposal for the implementation of a national information and documentation centre on alternative medicine – and at the level of individual experience within the clinical trial.

From the comparative and historical viewpoint of this study, it is clear that the randomized controlled clinical trial is an inappropriate and increasingly redundant method of treatment assessment. In the first place, it cannot deliver what it promises. Its pretensions to objective and neutral assessment have been shown to be incapable of realization. Secondly, whatever limited effectiveness it may have had as an evaluative tool is increasingly compromised by patient and consumer resistance to its principle of randomization and by professional resistance to the implementation of those of its findings that conflict with established professional practices. Thirdly, its methodological exclusion, in the name of maximal objectivity, of any but quantifiable factors from the evaluative process is inconsistent with the growing emphasis on quality of life in treatment assessment. In the last analysis, quality of life can only be assessed by the patient, by the consumers of medical treatment; but the randomized controlled trial is specifically designed to exclude their subjective input. It is this explicit exclusion of the patient's perceptions of treatment effectiveness or harm that renders the randomized controlled trial such an obsolete evaluative tool in the contemporary climate of growing public disillusionment with medicine and its pretensions to neutral assessment, and consumer demand for a greater and better informed evaluative role. Finally, the goal of neutral assessment is totally out of place in the revised and more realistic system of therapeutic evaluation supported by this study, where not only the subjective perceptions of the consumer, but also wider socio-economic and political criteria, are recognized as legitimate and integral to the processes of assessment and decision-making.

Rather than continue with the heavy economic and social investment in ever more tightly organized and rigorously controlled clinical trials in pursuit of the ever elusive goal of certain medical knowledge of disease and its treatment, we would do better to learn to live with the reality of uncertainty entailed in the new understanding of medical knowledge presented in this study. This does not mean that we must abandon all attempts at treatment evaluation. On the contrary, a responsible health care system must try to ensure that available treatments do not harm patients and that they satisfy socially-acceptable standards of treatment effectiveness. The system I am proposing requires, among other reforms, the redesigning of the clinical trial specifically to include the patient's perceptions of treatment effects in the processes of appraisal and decision-making. We might borrow again from some of the suggestions that have been made for the evaluation of alternative medicine, such as the 'co-operative enquiry' in which the investigator and subject form a team to explore the treatment's effects (Fulder, 1988). Or, some of the currently available conventional methods, such as non-randomized trials and computerized data bases, might be broadened to include the subjects' own appraisals of treatment effects as well as broader-based social criteria. These proposals for the abandonment of the unattainable goal of neutral assessment and the adoption of more flexible, socially-based methods of assessment, would also do away with many of the previously discussed ethical and other dilemmas surrounding the randomized controlled trial (1.4).

As for those individuals faced with the necessity of choosing a treatment, the radical reversal of the current ground rules that I am proposing would have the effect of enhancing their control over the choice of available treatments and of broadening their options. It would mean that they would be better able to resist the pressures to attempt or continue with highly toxic, invasive, or expensive therapies and to opt for treatments more appropriate to their own values and concerns. Unlike the hypothetical judge conjured up by Pauling's attorney, they *could* presume to decide between Linus Pauling and the Mayo Clinic. When it comes to the making of value judgements the consumer is at least as well equipped to make such judgements as a Nobel Laureate or the doctors from the world's leading medical clinic. The understanding of medical knowledge that I have presented in this book makes it clear that different forms of knowledge shaped by and for different social objectives are possible and viable, and that the demand for therapies more appropriate to the consumer's social interests is entirely defensible.

The proposals I have outlined require that such different forms of treatments must be available to the consumer, and this again highlights the importance of alternative therapeutic systems in creating and promoting treatment options. It must not be taken for granted, however, that alternative systems of medicine are necessarily more representative of broader social interests than orthodox medicine. Holistic medicine, for instance, which has often been presented as a progressive movement generated from cultures of protest, does not offer a clearcut and unproblematic alternative to the conventional medical system. 'Quackery' and 'charlatanry' might best be understood as the marginalizing labels of orthodoxy, but fraud and deception undoubtedly do occur in alternative medicine. Nor are alternative practitioners immune from occupational self-interest, nor from attachment to the interests of other powerful sectors of society. Alternative treatments must not be exempt from the same critical scrutiny of their social objectives and relevant interests that I have proposed for the treatments of orthodox medicine.

In the meantime, the treatment options provided by both alternative and conventional medicine may be deployed in the struggle to achieve a medicine that is more representative of all affected interests. For neither should it be assumed that all conventional treatments must be abandoned in this political process of struggle and compromise. There are, no doubt, many orthodox therapies and technologies that might withstand critical social appraisal or that might be adapted to it. William Arney, for instance, has argued that, despite a veneer of belligerence, women and obstetricians have evolved more flexible childbirth technologies and practices through a conjunction of interests in changing professional and social contexts (Arney, 1982). And, in the light of my previous analysis, we may expect that some sectors of the medical profession would be prepared to concede some of their autonomy with respect to the socio-political evaluation of their work, if they were to be convinced that it was in their interests to do so (Bartels, 1983). I have indicated some of the factors that might convince them that it would be beneficial rather than harmful to cooperate with the demand for democratic participation in treatment assessment.

Within the specificities of cancer treatment and research, the indications are that, for a complexity of medical, social and economic reasons, and as Arney found in his analysis of child-birth technology, the interests of cancer patients, alternative activists, government regulators, doctors and researchers are converging. In a situation where many prominent oncologists and biostatisticians have conceded the lack of effective treatments for many cancers, the toxicity and risks of conventional treatment, and the uncertainty of long-term survival even after apparently successful treatment; where the distinction between conventional and unconventional cancer treatment is becoming progressively blurred; where both doctors and alternative activists have declared their commitment to more humane and caring treatment and research; where the patient's experience of quality of life is becoming a more prominent issue in treatment assessment; where certain leading experts are engaged in their own attempts at evaluative reform within cancer medicine and research. . . .there is more potential for fundamental agreement between activists and professionals on cancer treatment and its evaluation than either side as yet is willing to recognize.

Given the current pressures for change in evaluative criteria and procedures, we may expect the issue of therapeutic evaluation to become increasingly politicized. As these criss-crossing pressures are brought to bear upon the internal politics of medicine, they will create opportunities for intervention and reform. It remains to be seen whether these opportunities will be recognized and acted upon. As I have tried to show, medicine is deeply embedded in the culture and social structure of human societies, and any proposals for the social reform of evaluative criteria and assessment procedures will require institutional, legislative, and other social changes and be influenced by the existing pattern of values and institutions within a given society. The prediction of social change is a risky business. But I am convinced that effective strategies for coping with the challenge of evaluative reform are more likely to emerge from the more realistic understanding of the politics of therapeutic evaluation presented in this study, than from the sterile pursuit of the obscuring and unattainable ideal of neutral, objective treatment assessment.

Epilogue

On 5 September, 1989, Linus Pauling held a seminar at the Mayo Clinic at the invitation of the Biochemistry and Molecular Biology Graduate Students Association. Simultaneously, the Linus Pauling Institute issued a press release: '"Mayo Vitamin C Study was Flawed," Linus Pauling tells Mayo Clinic Grads.' On the same day, a paper by Pauling and his research associate, Dr Zelek Herman, was published in the *Proceedings of the National Academy of Sciences*. This paper contained a biostatistical analysis of the second Mayo Clinic trial, purporting to show that the trial had no validity (Pauling and Herman, 1989).

Pauling's Mayo Clinic seminar and the subsequent televised news conference he gave in Rochester, were the culmination of a carefully planned and well-coordinated renewal of their campaign by Pauling and the vitamin C 'believers'. The groundwork for this media event had been strategically laid by Pauling some months previously. He had then published an earlier paper in the *PNAS* which contained an account of a new method he had formulated for the biostatistical analysis of mortality data for groups of cancer patients (Pauling, 1989). Following this, Pauling and Herman applied the new method to the formulation of three criteria by means of which, they claimed, the validity of a clinical study of the mortality of a group of cancer patients may be tested. They analysed more than 200 published reports of cancer clinical trials, and 'essentially all' of these passed the test, satisfying the three criteria. The Mayo Clinic trial, however, violated all three criteria.

According to Pauling and Herman, this means that the conclusion reached in that study – that vitamin C had no more value than placebo in extending the survival of patients with advanced colorectal cancer – 'is not justified'. Further, they claim, their analysis supports their conclusion that the life expectancy of patients in the trial was decreased by withdrawal of vitamin C and the administration of cytotoxic chemotherapy (Pauling and Herman, 1989).

Pauling's seminar and his meeting with a group of faculty at the Mayo Clinic was instigated by Robert Horton, a graduate student in molecular biology. In 1985 Horton had submitted a letter to the *New England Journal of Medicine*, commenting on the relevance of the rebound effect to the results obtained in the second Mayo Clinic trial. Horton's letter was rejected on the ground that his point of view was 'adequately represented' among the other letters received on this subject and 'already accepted for publication' (Salzman to Horton, 22 April 1985). As Horton informed the media at

237

Pauling's press conference, the *New England Journal of Medicine* had never published any of the critical letters or papers submitted: 'I thought it would be a good thing if Dr Pauling could come here and speak and improve communication' (McAuliffe, 1989).

According to the same newspaper report, Mayo Clinic researchers 'reserved judgment' on Pauling's latest paper until they had time to study it. Dr John S. Kovach, the current Chairman of the Oncology Department at Mayo and director of the Clinic's Comprehensive Cancer Center, was quoted as saying:

> We appreciate Dr Pauling's emphasis on the importance of effective dialogue among various scientific disciplines regarding the nature and management of the multitude of diseases which comprise human cancer. The significance of Dr Pauling's approach to the biostatistical analysis of mortality data for cancer patients . . . remains to be assessed by the scientific community. (McAuliffe, 1989)

Pursuing his case on yet another front, the indomitable Pauling has also managed to reopen negotiations with the new head of the NCI, Dr Samuel Broder. His interview with Broder, grudgingly scheduled for half an hour on 5 April 1989, was extended to two and a half hours, after Broder's initial antagonism to Pauling's shock opener of 'criminal' neglect by the NCI of vitamin C and cancer research was overcome. According to Pauling's account and that of the associate who accompanied him, Broder gave a careful hearing to Pauling's critique of the two Mayo Clinic trials and to the theoretical arguments and the cases of complete remission claimed by Pauling for high-dose ascorbate treatment. Broder's own view was the standard NCI one: that vitamin C might have value as an adjuvant therapy in cancer prevention but not its treatment. Still, as a result of Pauling's representations, he invited Pauling to talk to the Scientific Board of the NCI Division of Cancer Prevention and Control, with a view to instituting a possible new NCI trial of high dose vitamin C according to a protocol involving Pauling and Cameron. At the same time, Broder cautioned that if this further trial were undertaken by the NCI and showed no positive result, Pauling should accept this and cease his public criticism of the NCI's role in vitamin C and cancer research.

In a cordial follow-up letter, Broder stressed the general consensus among clinicians and scientists that vitamin C had been adequately tested and failed to yield a positive result. While he assured Pauling that he fully understood Pauling's point of view and his explanation for the negative results of the Mayo Clinic trials, Broder thought that this general medical perception of the lack of an objective database for vitamin C was not conducive to further trials by the groups associated with the standard clinical trials mechanism of the NCI. It was because of this and Pauling's objections to certain of these groups that Broder had suggested that the Division of Cancer Prevention and Control should serve as the administrative contact point for vitamin C issues. It was up to Pauling to make an appropriate submission which would be fairly heard in an open forum and submitted to fair review by the usual peer review process. The ball, Broder concluded, was in Pauling's court, and he wished him every success (Broder to Pauling, 24 April 1989).

After further negotiations, Ewan Cameron returned to Vale of Leven Hospital to collect and follow up the files of the 'best cases' for a report to the NCI's Division of Cancer Prevention and Control. This report was submitted in December 1989. In January 1990, the National Institutes of Health announced that it would host a three-day international symposium on Vitamin C and Cancer to be held in the National Library of Medicine, Washington, with Linus Pauling as a featured speaker.

The vitamin C and cancer controversy is clearly not over. It continues with its familiar mix of medicine and politics.

In the meantime, Dr Charles Moertel reportedly has been at the centre of another controversy among top cancer researchers over a new drug therapy for colon cancer. Two clinical trials carried out under Moertel's direction have indicated that the new drug, levamisole, in combination with 5-fluorouracil, can delay or prevent the recurrence of colon cancer in certain patients who have had their original tumours surgically removed. Moertel's dispute with other cancer researchers and bureaucrats centred on what constitutes a positive result in a cancer clinical trial, and when experimental therapies should be made available to patients with a life-threatening disease. Moertel maintained that the levamisole-5-fluorouracil results were not yet firm enough to warrant clinical application. 'The survival advantage is what counts', Moertel was quoted as saying. 'Response rates don't mean a hoot'. He argued that, although the results of the first colon cancer study were encouraging, the patients in the second more extensive test had not been followed long enough to determine whether the drugs have any significant impact on their five-year survival rates. According to Moertel, levamisole, which was originally licensed as a drug for the treatment of worms in farm animals, has had a notoriously chequered career in the fifteen years of its investigation as an anti-cancer drug: 'One investigator would do a study and find miraculous things. Another would do a more careful study and find nothing.' Moertel also claimed that the levamisole-5-fluorouracil therapy was too toxic to administer without proof of efficacy. One patient had already died of its side effects (Marx, 1989; Shereff, 1989).

Moertel's claims were 'vehemently' disputed by Vincent DeVita, ex-NCI director: 'You could save 12,000 lives per year with this therapy. Why wait?' DeVita alleged that Moertel was reluctant to announce the results of the levamisole-5-fluorouracil studies because he did not want to jeopardize the recruitment of patients to his new placebo-controlled trial of yet another drug combination, leucovorin and 5-fluorouracil. Moertel took what was described in the *Science* report of the conflict as 'strong umbrage' at DeVita's suggestion. He claimed that the leucovorin combination may hold even greater promise than the levamisole one for colon cancer patients: 'We're trying to defend that study because we feel it is in the best interest of cancer patients' (Marx, 1989).

In October 1989, three months after the report of this dispute was published, the FDA announced the release of levamisole to be used in combination with the approved agent 5-fluorouracil as a treatment for colorectal cancer under the new TINDs guidelines. The FDA had acted on the recommendation of the NCI, which reported that preliminary data from the disputed trial had shown that the 5 FU-levamisole combination delayed or halted tumour recurrence, although the trend for improved survival was 'only suggestive'. The treatment will be used for an estimated 25,000 patients a year (Horwitz, 1989a).

I leave it to readers to carry out their own analysis of these new developments.

Bibliography

Aakster, C.W. (1986). Concepts in Alternative Medicine. *Social Science and Medicine*, 22, 265–73.

ACS (1976). *Unproven Methods of Cancer Management – 1976*, American Cancer Society, New York.

ACS (1985a). *Cancer Facts and Figures*, American Cancer Society, New York.

ACS (1985b). *Nutrition, Common Sense, and Cancer*, American Cancer Society, New York.

ACS (1987). *Unproven Methods of Cancer Management*, Active Statements, 1987, American Cancer Society, New York.

Adams, S. (1984). *Roche versus Adams*, Jonathan Cape, London.

Albury, R. (1983). *The Politics of Objectivity*, Deakin University Press, Geelong, Victoria.

Alcantara, E.N. and Speckmann, E.W. (1977). Diet, Nutrition and Cancer. *American Journal of Clinical Nutrition*, 30, 662.

Altman, L.K. (1988). Medical Guardians: Does New England Journal Exercise Undue Power on Information Flow? *New York Times* (28 January), 1, 13.

American Society of Clinical Oncology Subcommittee on Unorthodox Therapies (1983). Ineffective Cancer Therapy: A Guide for the Layperson. *Journal of Clinical Oncology*, 1, 154–63.

Anderson, I. (1985). Pauling Claims Fraud in Vitamin Study. *New Scientist*, 105 (24 January), 22.

Anderson, T.W. (1977). New Horizons for Vitamin C. *Nutrition Today*, 12, 6–13.

Anonymous (1966). Linus Pauling Takes the Stand. *National Review*, 17 May, 459–66.

Anonymous (1975a). Scientists and their Images. *New Scientist*, 67, 471–5.

Anonymous (1975b). Chemical Profile: Ascorbic Acid, *Chemical Marketing Reporter*, 29 December, 9.

Anonymous (1979a). The Vitamin Giant that would Brook no Competitor. *The Economist*, 270, 58–9.

Anonymous (1979b). No Vitamin-C Benefit Found in Cancer Trial. *Medical World News*, 25 June, 19.

Anonymous (1980a). Interferon Research. *Cancer Nursing*, 3, 190.

Anonymous (1980b). Interferon Sales Could Reach $3 Billion by End of Decade. *European Chemical News*, April 14, 18.

Anonymous (1980c). The Big IF in Cancer. *Time* Magazine, 31 March, 40–6.

Anonymous (1982). Deaths Halt Interferon Trials in France. *Science*, 218, 772.

Anonymous (1983a). Pauling Institute: Lawsuit Settled Out of Court. *Nature*, 303, 103.

Anonymous (1983b). Vitamin C Goes Down for the Count in Advanced-Cancer Controlled Trial. *Medical World News*, 22 August, 69.

Anonymous (1984). Chemical Profile: Ascorbic Acid. *Chemical Marketing Reporter*, 2 Jan., 62.

Anonymous (1985a). Pauling May Sue over Vitamin C Report. *New Scientist*, 105, 8.

Anonymous (1985b). Ascorbic Acid Does Not Cure Cancer. *Nutrition Reviews*, 43, 146–7.

Anonymous (1989a). Insurers Target Chemotherapy Payments. *Wall Street Journal*, 11 May, 14.

Anonymous (1989b). Burroughs Agrees to Cut AZT Price. *The Nation's Health*, Oct.–Nov., 5.

APA Task Force Report on Vitamin Therapy in Psychiatry (1973). *Megavitamin Therapy and Orthomolecular Therapy in Psychiatry*, American Psychiatric Association, Washington D.C.

Arney, W.R. (1982). *Power and the Profession of Obstetrics*, University of Chicago Press, Chicago and London.

Associated Press. (1985). Half of All Americans Would Risk Unorthodox Cures, Poll Indicates. *The Tribune*, San Diego, 11 Nov., A–4.

Bailar, J.C. and Smith, E. (1986). Progress Against Cancer? *New England Journal of Medicine*, 314, 1226–32.

Barnes, B. (1977). *Interests and the Growth of Knowledge*, Routledge & Kegan Paul, London and Boston, MA.

Barnes, B. (1985). *About Science*, Basil Blackwell, Oxford and New York.

Barnes, B. and Edge, D. (eds) (1982). *Science in Context: Readings in the Sociology of Science*, The Open University Press, Milton Keynes, Bucks, MIT Press, Cambridge, MA.

Barnes, D.M. (1987). Biologics Gain Influence in Expanding NCI Program. *Science*, 237, 848–50.

Barrett, S. and Knight, G. (1976). *The Health Robbers: How to Protect Your Money and Your Life*, George F. Stickley Co., Philadelphia.

Bartels, D. (1983). Public Participation in Scientific Decision Making. In R. Albury, *The Politics of Objectivity*, Deakin University Press, Geelong, Victoria.

Basu, T.K. and Schorah, C.J. (1982). *Vitamin C in Health and Disease*, Croom Helm, London.

Benade, L., Howard, T. and Burk, D. (1969). Synergistic Killing of Ehrlich Ascites Carcinoma Cells by Ascorbate and 3-Amino-1, 2, 4-Triazole. *Oncology*, 23, 33–43.

Berliner, H.S. and Salmon, J.W. (1979a). The Holistic Health Movement and Scientific Medicine: The Naked and the Dead. *Socialist Review*, 43, 31–52.

Berliner, H.S. and Salmon. J.W. (1979b). To the Editor. *New England Journal of Medicine*, 300, 1222.

Berliner, H.S. and Salmon, J.W. (1980). The Holistic Alternative to Scientific Medicine: History and Analysis. *International Journal of Health Services*, 10, 133–47.

Bishop, J.E. (1985). Vitamin C Therapy for Cancer Patients is Challenged Again: Second Study at Mayo Clinic Fails to Confirm Benefit Claimed by Linus Pauling. *Wall Street Journal*, 17 Jan., 16.

Bjelke, E. (1974), Epidemiological Studies of Cancer of the Stomach, Colon and Rectum, with Special Emphasis on the Role of Diet. *Scandinavian*

Journal of Gastroenterology, 9 (Suppl.31), 1–235.

Bloor, D. (1976). *Knowledge and Social Imagery*, Routledge and Kegan Paul, London.

Boly, W. (1989). Cancer, Inc., *Hippocrates Magazine*, January/February.

Braithwaite, J. (1984). *Corporate Crime in the Pharmaceutical Industry*, Routledge and Kegan Paul, London, Boston, Melbourne and Henley.

Brandt, A. M. (1985). *No Magic Bullet: A History of Venereal Disease in the United States since 1880*, Oxford University Press, Oxford and New York.

British Medical Association, Board of Science and Education (1986). *Alternative Therapy*, Report of the Board of Science and Education, British Medical Association, London.

Broad, W.J. (1979). NIH Deals Gingerly with Diet–Disease Link. *Science*, 204 (15 June), 1175–8.

Budiansky, S. (1983). Pauling Backs Wonder Cures. *Nature*, 303, 275.

Burns, J.J., Rivers, J.M., and Machlin, L.J. (1987). *Third Conference on Vitamin C (Annals of the New York Academy of Sciences*, 498), The New York Academy of Sciences, New York, New York.

Bury, M.R. (1986). Social Constructionism and the Development of Medical Sociology. *Sociology of Health and Illness*, 8, 137–69.

Bush, H. (1984). CURE. Despite claims to the contrary, treatment today offers little more hope than it did a generation ago. *Science 84 Magazine* (September), 34–5.

Buyse, M.E., Staquet, M.J. and Sylvester, R.J. (eds) (1984). *Cancer Clinical Trials: Methods and Practice*, Oxford University Press, Oxford, New York and Toronto.

Buyse, M., Zeleniuch-Jacquotte, A., and Chalmers, T.C. (1988). Adjuvant Therapy of Colorectal Cancer: Why We Still Don't Know. *Journal of the American Medical Association*, 259, 3571–8.

Byrski, L. (1989). *Facing Cancer: Searching For Solutions*, Collins Dove, Melbourne.

Cairns, J. (1978). *Cancer: Science and Society*, W.H. Freeman and Co., San Francisco.

Cairns, J. (1985m). The Treatment of Diseases and the War against Cancer. *Scientific American*, 253 (November), 31–9.

Cameron, E. (1966). *Hyaluronidase and Cancer*, Pergamon Press, New York.

Cameron, E. (1972). *Cancer – the Cellular Rebellion* (unpublished paper, written and communicated to Pauling, March, 1972), 1–4.

Cameron, E. (1980). To the Editor. *New England Journal of Medicine*, 302 (31 January), 299.

Cameron, E. (1982). Vitamin C and Cancer: An Overview. In Hanck, A. (ed.), *Vitamin C: New Clinical Applications in Immunology*, Lipid Metabolism and Cancer, 115–27

Cameron, E. (1985). Statement Prepared by Dr Ewan Cameron for Hearing of U.S. House of Representatives, House Subcommittee on Science and Technology. Originally scheduled for 25 March 1985, but subsequently cancelled 12 Oct. 1985.

Cameron, E. and Baird, G. (1973). Ascorbic Acid and Dependence on Opiates in Patients with Advanced Disseminated Cancer. *International Research Communications Systems*, Letter to the Editor, August.

Cameron, E. and Campbell, A. (1974). The Orthomolecular Treatment of Cancer: II. Clinical Trial of High-Dose Ascorbic Acid Supplements in Advanced Human Cancer. *Chemico-Biological Interactions*, 9, 285–315.

Cameron, E., Campbell, A. and Jack, T. (1975). The Orthomolecular Treatment of Cancer: III. Reticulum Cell Sarcoma: Double Complete Regression Induced by High-Dose Ascorbic Acid Theraphy. *Chemico-Biological Interactions*, 11, 387–93.

Cameron, E., Moffat, L., Campbell, A. and Marcuson, R. (1984). Supplemental Ascorbate in Incurable Cancer. Unpublished manuscript, submitted to *New England Journal of Medicine*, Dec. 1984.

Cameron, E. and Pauling, L. (1973). Ascorbic Acid and the Glycosaminoglycans: An Orthomolecular Approach to Cancer and Other Diseases. *Oncology*, 27, 181–92.

Cameron, E. and Pauling, L. (1974). The Orthomolecular Treatment of Cancer: 1. The Role of Ascorbic Acid in Host Resistance. *Chemico-Biological Interactions*, 9, 273–83.

Cameron, E. and Pauling, L. (1976), Supplemental Ascorbate in the Supportive Treatment of Cancer: Prolongation of Survival Times in Terminal Human Cancer. *Proceedings of the National Academy of Sciences*, 73, 3685–9.

Cameron, E. and Pauling, L. (1978a). Ascorbic Acid as a Therapeutic Agent in Cancer. *Journal of the International Academy of Preventative Medicine*, 5, 8–29.

Cameron, E. and Pauling, L. (1978b). Supplemental Ascorbate in the Supportive Treatment of Cancer: Reevaluation of Prolongation of Survival Times in Terminal Human Cancer. *Proceedings of the National Academy of Sciences*, 75, 4538–42.

Cameron, E. and Pauling, L. (1978c). Experimental Studies Designed to Evaluate the Management of Patients with Incurable Cancer. *Proceedings of the National Academy of Science*, 75, 6252.

Cameron, E. and Pauling, L. (1979a). Ascorbate and Cancer. *Proceedings of the American Philosophical Society*, 123, 117–23.

Cameron, E. and Pauling, L. (1979b). *Cancer and Vitamin C*, The Linus Pauling Institute of Science and Medicine, Menlo Park, CA.

Cameron, E., Pauling, L. and Leibovitz, B. (1979). Ascorbic Acid and Cancer: A Review. *Cancer Research*, 39, 663–81.

Cameron, E. and Rotman, D. (1972). Ascorbic Acid, Cell Proliferation, and Cancer. *Lancet*, 1, 542.

Carpenter, K.J. (1986). *The History of Scurvy and Vitamin C*, Cambridge University Press, Cambridge.

Carroll, J. (1979). The Perils of Pauling. *New West* (8 October), 39–54.

Carter, S.K. (1984). In Buyse, M.E., Staquet, M.J. and Sylvester, R.J. (eds), *Cancer Clinical Trials: Methods and Practice*, Oxford University Press, Oxford, 223–38.

Cassileth, B.R., Lusk, E.J., Strouse, B.A., Bodenheimer, B.J. (1984). Contemporary Unorthodox Treatments in Cancer Medicine: A Study of Patients, Treatments, and Practitioners. *Annals of Internal Medicine*, 101, 105–12.

Cassileth, B. and Brown, H. (1988). Unorthodox Cancer Medicine. *Ca – A Cancer Journal for Clinicians*, 38, 176–86.

Chalmers, T.C. (1974). The Impact of Controlled Trials on the Practice of Medicine. *Mt. Sinai Journal of Medicine*, 41, 753–8.

Chalmers, T.C. (1981). The Clinical Trial. *Milbank Memorial Fund Quarterly / Health and Society*, 59, 324–39.

Chase, M. (1986). Latest Findings on Cancer Drug Fall Short of Dazzling First Results. *The Wall Street Journal (12 November)*, 37.

Cheraskin, E., Ringsdorf, W.M. and Sigley, E.L. (1983). *The Vitamin C Connection*, Harper & Row, New York.

Chowka, P.B. (1978). The Cancer Charity Ripoff. WARNING: The American Cancer Society May be Hazardous to Your Health, *East–West Journal* (July), 23–9.

Chowka, P.B. (1988). Cancer 1988: Is a Healing Peace in the Government's War on Cancer Finally at Hand? Adapted from an article that appeared in *East West* (December), 1987, distributed by Project CURE, Centre for Alternative Cancer Research, Washington, D.C.

Cochrane, A.L. (1972). *Effectiveness and Efficiency: Random Reflections on the Health Services*, Nuffield Provincial Hospitals Trust/Oxford University Press, London.

Cohen, J.M. (1979). Ethical Questions in Chemotherapy of Patients with Gastrointestinal Cancer. *New England Journal of Medicine*, 300, 436.

Collier, P. (1978). The Old Man and the C. *New West* (24 April), 1–4.

Collins, H.M. (1975). The Seven Sexes: A Study of the Sociology of a Phenomenon, or the Replication of Experiments in Physics. *Sociology*, 9, 205–24.

Collins, H.M. (1981). Knowledge and Controversy: Studies of Modern Natural Science. *Social Studies of Science*, 11, 3–158.

Collins, H.M. (1982). *Sociology of Scientific Knowledge: A Source Book*, Bath University Press, Bath.

Collins, H.M. (1983). An Empirical Relativist Programme in the Sociology of Scientific Knowledge. In Knorr-Cetina, K.D. and Mulkay, M. (eds), *Science Observed: Perspectives in the Social Study of Science*, Sage, London, 85–113.

Collins, H.M. (1985). *Changing Order*, Sage, London.

Collins, H.M. and Pinch, T.J. (1979), The Construction of the Paranormal: Nothing Unscientific is Happening. In Wallis, R. (ed.), *On the Margins of Science: The Social Construction of Rejected Knowledge* (University of Keele, Sociological Review Monograph No. 27, Keele, Staffs.), 237–70.

Collins, H.M. and Pinch, T. (1982). *Frames of Meaning: The Social Construction of Extraordinary Science*, Routledge & Kegan Paul, London

Collins, H.M. and Shapin, S. (1989). Experiment, Science Teaching, and the New History and Sociology of Science. In Shortland, M. and Warwick, A. (eds), *Teaching the History of Science*, The British Society for the History of Science, Basil Blackwell, 67–79.

Commission for Alternative Systems of Medicine (1981). *Alternative Medicine in the Netherlands. Summary of the Report of the Commission for Alternative Systems of Medicine*. In *Alternative Therapy*, Report of the Board of Science and Education, British Medical Association, London, 1986, 113–58. The original report of the Commission (4640 pp. in Dutch) is available from: Staatsuitgeverij, C. Plantijnstraat 2, Is Gravenhage, The Netherlands.

Committee on Diet, Nutrition, and Cancer, Assembly of Life Sciences, (1982). National Research Council, *Diet, Nutrition and Cancer*, National Academy Press, Washington, DC.

Commitee on Interstate and Foreign Commerce, House of Representatives, (1974). *Hearings before the Subcommittee on Public Health and Environment*, 93rd Congress. To Amend the Federal food, Drug and Cosmetic Act to include a Definition of Food Supplements and for other Purposes, 29–31 October 1973, US GPO, Washington, DC. Statement of Linus Pauling, Professor of Chemistry, Stanford University, Part 2, 833–6.

Comroe, J.H. (1978). Experimental Studies Designed to Evaluate the Management of Patients with Incurable Cancer. *Proceedings of the National Academy of Sciences*, 75, 4543.

Cousins, N. (1977). To the Editor. *New England Journal of Medicine*, 296, 763.

Coward, R. (1989). *The Whole Truth: The Myth of Alternative Health*, Faber & Faber, London and Boston.

Crawford, R. (1980). Healthism and the Medicalization of Everyday Life. *International Journal of Health Services*, 10, 365–88.

Crawford, R. (1984). A Cultural Account of 'Health': Control, Release, and the Social Body. In McKinlay, J.B. (ed.), *Issues in the Political Economy of Health Care*, Tavistock Publications, New York and London, 60–103.

Creagan, E.T. and Moertel, C.G. (1979). Vitamin C Therapy of Advanced Cancer. *New England Journal of Medicine*, 301, 1399.

Creagan, E.T., Moertel, C.G., O'Fallon, J.R., Schutt, A.J., O'Connell, M.J., Rubin, J. and Frytak, S. (1979). Failure of High-dose Vitamin C (Ascorbic Acid) Therapy to Benefit Patients with Advanced Cancer. *New England Journal of Medicine*, 301, 687–90.

Creagan, E.T. and Moertel, C.G. (1980). To the Editor, *New England Journal of Medicine*, 302, 299–300.

Culbert, M.J. (1983). *What the Medical Profession Won't Tell You That Could Save Your Life*, Donning, Norfolk Beach, Virginia.

Cullinan, S.A., Moertel, C.G., Fleming, T.R., Rubin, J.R., Krook, J.E., Everson, L.K., Windschitl, H.E., Twito, D.I., Marschke, R.F., Foley, J.F., Pfeifle, D.M., Barlow, J.F., for the North Central Cancer Treatment Group (1985). A Comparison of Three Chemotherapeutic Regimens in the Treatment of Advanced Pancreatic and Gastric Carcinoma. *Journal of the American Medical Association*, 253, 2061–7.

Culliton, B.J. (1972). Academy Turns Down a Pauling Paper. *Science*, 177, 409.

Culliton, B.J. and Waterfall, W.K. (1979). War on Cancer – Interferon. *British Medical Journal*, 279, 195–6.

Currie, G.A. (1972). Eighty Years of Immunotherapy: A Review of Immunological Methods Used for the Treatment of Human Cancer. *British Journal of Cancer*, 26, 141–53.

Dale, D. (1987). Vitamins have their ups and downs as the experts brawl. *The Sydney Morning Herald* (10 February), 13.

Daly, P. (1985). *The Biotechnology Business, A Strategic Analysis*, Francis Pinter (Publishers) Ltd., London, Rowman and Allanheld Publishers, Totowa NJ.

DeCosse, J.J. (1984). Are We Doing Better With Large Bowel Cancer? *New*

England Journal of Medicine, 310, 782–3.

DeCosse, J.J., Adams, M.B., Kuzma, J.F., LoGerfo, P., and Gordon, R.E. (1975). Effect of Ascorbic Acid on Rectal Polyps of Patients with Familial Polyposis. *Surgery*, 78, 608–12.

Deutsch, R.M. (1977). *The New Nuts Among the Berries*, Bull, Palo Alto, CA.

DeVita, V.T. and Roper, M. (1987). The Emergence of Biologicals as Cancer Treatment: The Good News and The Bad. *Hospital Practice*, 22, 15–16.

Diesendorf, M. (ed.). (1976). *The Magic Bullet; Social Implications and Limitations of Modern Medicine; An Environmental Approach*, Society for Social Responsibility in Science, Canberra.

Dixon, B. (1978). *Beyond the Magic Bullet*, George Allen and Unwin, Boston and Sydney.

Doll, R. and Peto, R. (1981). *The Causes of Cancer*, Oxford University Press, Oxford.

Doyal, L. and Doyal, L. (1984). Western Scientific Medicine: A Philosophical and Political Prognosis. In Birke, L. and Silvertown, J. (eds), *More Than the Parts: Biology and Politics*, Pluto Press, London and Sydney, 82–109.

Doyal, L. with Pennell, I. (1979). *The Political Economy of Health*, Pluto Press, London.

Doyle, R.P. (1983). *The Medical Wars*, William Morrow and Co., New York.

Dunham, W. B., Zuckerkandl, E., Reynolds, R., Willoughby, R., Marcuson, R., Barth, R., and Pauling, L. (1982). Effects of Intake of L-ascorbic Acid on the Incidence of Dermal Neoplasms Induced in Mice by Ultraviolet Light. *Proceedings of the National Academy of Sciences*, 79, 7532–6.

Edelhart, M. and Lindenmann, J. (1981), *Interferon: The New Hope for Cancer*, Ballantine Books, New York.

Edsall, J.T. (1972). Linus Pauling and Vitamin C. *Science*, 178, 696.

Ellison, N.M., Byar, D.P. and Newell, G.R. (1978). Special Report on Laetrile: The NCI Laetrile Review, *New England Journal of Medicine*, 299, 494–552..

Engel, G.L. (1977). The Need for a New Medical Model: A Challenge for Biomedicine. *Science*, 196, 129–35.

Engelhardt, T. and Caplan, A.L. (eds) (1987). *Scientific Controversies; Case Studies in the Resolution and Closure of Disputes in Science and Technology*, Cambridge University Press, Cambridge.

Epstein, S.S. (1979). *The Politics of Cancer*, revised edn, Anchor Books, New York.

Faucault, M. (1973). *The Birth of the Clinic*, Tavistock, London.

Faulder, C. (1985). *Whose Body Is It? The Troubling Issue of Informed Consent*, Virago, London.

Fee, E. and Fox, D.M. (eds) (1988). *AIDS: The Burdens of History*, University of California Press, Berkeley, Los Angeles, London.

Feinstein, A.R. (1972). The Need for Humanised Science in Evaluating Medication. *Lancet*, 2, 421–3.

Feinstein, A.R. (1977). *Clinical Biostatistics*, C.V. Mosby, St. Louis, MO.

Feinstein, A.R. (1985). *Clinical Epidemiology: The Architecture of Clinical Research*, W. B. Saunders and Co., Philadelphia, London, Toronto

Figlio, K. (1977). The Historiography of Scientific Medicine: An Invitation to the Human Sciences. *Comparative Studies in Science and History*, 19, 262–86.

Fink, J.M. (1988). *Third Opinion: An International Directory to Alternative Therapy Centers for the Treatment and Prevention of Cancer*, Avery Publishing Group, New York.

Finney, D.J. (1982). The Questioning Statistician. *Statistics in Medicine*, 1, 5–13.

Fitzgerald, J.C. (1979). Ethical Questions in Chemotherapy of Patients with Gastrointestinal Cancer. *New England Journal of Medicine*, 300 (22 February), 436–7.

Fried, J. (1984). *Vitamin Politics*, Prometheus Books, Buffalo, NY.

Freidson, E. (1970). *Profession of Medicine: A Study of the Sociology of Applied Knowledge*, Harper & Row, New York and London.

Freidson, E. (1986). *Professional Powers: A Study of the Institutionalization of Formal Knowledge*, The University of Chicago Press, Chicago and London.

Fulder, S. (1989). *The Handbook of Complementary Medicine*, 2nd. ed., Coronet Books, London.

Garb, S. (1968). *Cure for Cancer: A National Goal*, Springer, New York.

Garfield, E. (1989). In Tribute to Linus Pauling: A Citation Laureate, The *Scientist*, 3, 10.

Gastrointestinal Tumor Study Group (1984). Adjuvant Therapy of Colon Cancer – Results of a Prospectively Randomized Trial. *New England Journal of Medicine*, 310, 737–43.

Geehan, E. and Freireich, E.J. (1974). Non-randomized Controls in Cancer Clinical Trials. *New England Journal of Medicine*, 290, 198–203.

Gieryn, T.F. (1983). Making the Demarcation of Science a Sociological Problem. In Laudan, R. (ed.), *Working Papers in Science and Technology*, 2, Center for the Study of Science in Society, Virginia Polytechnic Institute, Blacksburg, VA, 60–86.

Glymour, C. and Stalker, D. (1983). Engineers, Cranks, Physicians and Magicians. *New England Journal of Medicine*, 308, 960–3.

Goldenring, J. (1979). To the Editor. *New England Journal of Medicine*, 300, 1221.

Goodell, R. (1987). The Role of the Mass Media in Scientific Controversy. In Engelhardt, H. T. and Caplan, A. L. (eds), *Scientific Controversies: Case Studies in the Resolution and Closure of Disputes in Science and Technology*, Cambridge University Press, Cambridge, 585–97.

Goodfield, J. (1975). *The Siege of Cancer*, Random House, New York.

Grabowski, H.G. (1976). *Drug Regulation and Innovation*, American Enterprise Institute for Public Policy Research, Washington D.C.

Grant, J. (1979). Of Mice and Men: The Linus Pauling Institute is Plunged into Controversy. *Barron's*, 59, 4–5.

Grauerholz, J. (1984). The Nobel Fakery of Linus Pauling, interview with Dr Arthur Robinson, *EIR: Executive Intelligence Review*, 14, 10–13.

Greenberg, D.S. (1974). The 'War' on Cancer: Official Figures and Harsh Facts. *Science and Government Report*, 4, 1–3.

Greenberg, D.S. (1975). 'Progress' in Cancer Research – Don't Say It Isn't So. *New England Journal of Medicine*, 292, 707–8.

Greenberg, D.S. (1977). The Unhappy Lessons of Cancer Politics. *The Washington Post* (17 November), A19.

Greenberg, D.S. (1981). Cancer Offensive. *New Scientist*, 90, 105–6.

Greenberg, D.S. (1981). Congress versus Cancer. *Nature*, 294, 1–2.

Greenwald, P. (1986). Nutrition and Cancer. *Cancer Facts*, Office of Cancer Communications, National Cancer Institute, Bethesda, MD.

Gupp, T. and Neumann, J. (1981). Cancer Cures Often a Curse. *Washington Post*, (18 October) A–14. Section 2, 1.

Guttmacher, S. (1979). Whole in Body, Mind and Spirit: Holistic Health and the Limits of Medicine. *The Hastings Centre Report*, 9, 15–20.

Hanlon, J. (1976). Is Vitamin C an Effective Cancer Treatment? *New Scientist*, 71, 30–31.

Harper, A.E. (1977). Nutritional Regulations and Legislation – Past Developments, Future Implications. *Journal of American Dietetic Association*, 71, 601–9.

Herberman, R.B. (1985). Design of Clinical Trials With Biological Response Modifiers. *Cancer Treatment Reports*, 69, 1161–4.

Herbert, V. (1978). Facts and Fictions about Megavitamin Therapy. *Resident and Staff Physician* (December), 43–50.

Herbert, V. (1980a). The Vitamin Craze. *Archives of Internal Medicine*, 140, 173–6.

Herbert, V. (1980b). *Nutrition Cultism: Facts and Fictions*, George F. Stickley Co., Philadelphia.

Herbert, V. (1986). Unproven (Questionable) Dietary and Nutritional Methods in Cancer Prevention and Treatment. *Cancer*, 58, 1930–41.

Herbert, V. and Barrett, S. (1981). *Vitamins and Health Foods: The Great American Hustle*, George F. Stickley Co., Philadelphia.

Hoffer, A. (1980). Megavitamins. *Biological Psychiatry*, 15, 821–2.

Hoffer, M.D. and Osmond, H. (1960). Double Blind Clinical Trials. *Journal of Neuropsychiatry*, 2, 221–7.

Hoffer, M.D. and Walker, M. (1978). *Orthomolecular Nutrition: New Lifestyle for Super Good Health*, Keats Publishing, New Canaan, Conn.

Holland, J.C. (1982). Why Patients Seek Unproven Cancer Remedies: A Psychological Perspective. Reprinted from *Ca – A Cancer Journal for Clinicians*, by The American Cancer Society, Professional Education Publications.

Horwitz, N. (1985). Linus Pauling Counters Attack on Vitamin C Theory. *Nutrition Health Review* (Spring), 9.

Horwitz, N. (1989a). Colorectal Cancer Rx Gets Quick Approval From FDA. *Medical Tribune*, 26 Oct., 8, 9, 14.

Horwitz, N. (1989b). 'Family Physicians Have Cause to Be Concerned'. *Medical Tribune*, 9 Dec., 9.

Houston, R.G. (1987). *Repression and Reform in the Evaluation of Alternative Cancer Therapies*, Project Cure, Washington, D.C.

Huemer, R.P. (ed.) (1986). *The Roots of Molecular Medicine: A Tribute to Linus Pauling*, W. H. Freeman, New York.

Hussain, F. (1977). The Linus Pauling Institute: An Investigation. *New Scientist*, 75, 216–20.

Illich, I. (1977). *Limits to Medicine*, Penguin, Harmondsworth, Middlesex.

Inglis, B. (1983). *The Diseases of Civilization: Why We Need a New Approach to Medical Treatment*, Granada, London, Toronto, Sydney and New York.

Jackson, T. (1985). Drug Giants Bury Hatchet: Accord Clears Way for Interferon Production. *Financial Review* (21 May), 25.

Jacobs, P. (1980). Pauling Foes to Redo Tests on Vitamin C. *Los Angeles Times*, 2 April.

Jamous, H. and Peloille, B. (1970). The French University–Hospital System. In Jackson, J. A. (ed.), *Professions and Professionalization*, Cambridge University Press, Cambridge, 111–52.

Jarvis, W. (1986). Helping Your Patients Deal with Questionable Cancer Treatments. Reprinted from *Ca – A Cancer Journal for Clinicians*, by The American Cancer Society, Professional Education Publications.

Johnson, T.J. (1972). *Professions and Power*, Macmillan, London.

Jukes, T.H. (1975). Megavitamin Therapy. *Journal of the American Medical Association*, 233, 550–1.

Jukes, T.H. (1986). From Pauling, Too Much of a Good Thing. *Washington Post*, Health Magazine (30 April).

Kennedy, I. (1981). *The Unmasking of Medicine*, Allen and Unwin, London.

Kenney, M. (1986). *Biotechnology: the University–Industrial Complex*, Yale University Press, New Haven and London.

Knorr-Cetina, K.D. (1979). Tinkering Towards Success: Prelude to a Theory of Scientific Practice. *Theory and Society*, 8, 347–76.

Knorr-Cetina, K.D. (1981). *The Manufacture of Knowledge: An Essay on the Constructivist and Contextual Nature* of Science, Pergamon Press, Oxford.

Kopelman, L. (1986). Consent and Randomized Clinical Trials: Are There Moral or Design Problems? *The Journal of Medicine and Philosophy*, 11, 317–45.

Koplan, J.P., Annest J.L., Layde P.M. and Rubin G.L. (1986). Nutrient Intake and Supplementation in the United States. *American Journal of Public Health*, 76, 287–9.

Krown, S. (1986). Interferons and Interferon Inducers in Cancer Treatment. *Seminars in Oncology*, 13, 207–17.

Kuhn, T.S. (1962). *The Structure of Scientific Revolutions*, Chicago University Press, Chicago. 2nd. enlarged edition, 1970.

Kushner, R. (1984). Is Aggressive Adjuvant Chemotherapy the Halsted Radical of the 80s? *Ca – A Cancer Journal for Clinicians*, 34, 345–51.

Ladas, H.S. (1988). The War on Cancer: Reactions to Innovative Treatments. *Holistic Medicine*, 3, 99–108.

Lansky, S.B., Black, J.L., and Cairns, N.U. (1983) Childhood Cancer; Medical Costs. *Cancer*, 52, 762–6.

Larson, M.S. (1979). Professionalism: Rise and Fall. *International Journal of Health Sciences*, 9, 607–27.

Larson, M.S. (1984). The Production of Expertise and the Constitution of Expert Power. In Haskell, T. L. (ed.), *The Authority of Experts: Studies in History and Theory*, Indiana University Press, Bloomington, IN., 28–79.

Latour, B. (1987). *Science in Action: How to Follow Scientists and Engineers Through Society*, Open University Press, Milton Keynes.

Latour, B. and Woolgar, S. (1979). *Laboratory Life: The Social Construction of Scientific Facts*, Sage Publications, Beverly Hills and London.

Laurence, I. (1983). *Some Historical Aspects of the Commercial Developments of Interferon*. Unpublished MSc Thesis, University of Manchester.

Leary, W.E. (1989). Outspoken and Impatient Scientist Takes Charge of War on Cancer. *New York Times* (7 February), Y19.

Le Shan, L. (1984). *Holistic Health: How to Understand and Use the Revolution in Medicine*, Turnstone Press, Wellingborough, Northants.

Lesser, M. (1980). *Nutrition and Vitamin Therapy*, Bantam Books, Toronto, New York, London, Sydney.

Levin, B. and O'Connell, M.J. (1988). Colorectal Cancer Chemotherapy: Meta-analysis or Large-Scale Trials? *Journal of the American Medical Association*, 259, 3611.

Levine, M. (1986). New Concepts in the Biology and Biochemistry of Ascorbic Acid. *New England Journal of Medicine*, 314, 892–902.

Lewin, S. (1976). *Vitamin C: Its Molecular Biology and Medical Potential*, Academic Press, London and New York.

Lewis, B.J. (1976). Report to Associate Director for Program Planning and Evaluation of the Department of Health, Education and Welfare, 8 Dec. National Cancer Institute.

Linus Pauling Institute of Science and Medicine (1985a). Transcript of Staff Seminar. 17 Jan.

Linus Pauling Institute of Science and Medicine (1985b). Press Release. 26 Jan.

Linus Pauling Institute of Science and Medicine (1985c). Transcript of Consultation with Attorney. 5 March.

Long, R.Y. (1983). *Crackdown on Cancer With Good Nutrition*, Nutrition Education Association, Houston, Texas.

Lortat-Jacob, J.L., Mathe, G., and Servier, J. (1978). International Meeting on Comparative Therapeutic Trials. *Biomedicine* (Special Issue), 28, 2–63.

Mae, E. with Loeffler, C. (1975). *How I Conquered Cancer Naturally*, Harvest House Publishers, Irvine, CA.

Mannisto, M. (1988). Proposed Payment Changes Raise Quality, Innovation and Medical Judgement Issues. *The Journal of Cancer Program Management*, 3, 9–15.

Markle, G.E. and Petersen, J.C. (1987). Resolution of the Laetrile Controversy: Past Attempts and Future Prospects. In Engelhardt, H. T. and Caplan, A. L. (eds), *Scientific Controversies: Case Studies in the Resolution and Closure of Disputes in Science and Technology*, Cambridge University Press, Cambridge, 315–32.

Markman, M. (1985). Medical Complications of 'Alternative' Cancer Therapy. *New England Journal of Medicine*, 312, 1640.

Marshall, C.W. (1983). *Vitamins and Minerals: Help or Harm?* George F. Stickley, Philadelphia, PA.

Marshall, E. (1985). The Academy Kills a Nutrition Report. *Science*, 230, 420–1.

Marshall, E. (1989). Quick Release of AIDS Drugs. *Science*, 245, 345–7.

Martin, B. (1988). Analyzing the Fluoridation Controversy: Resources and Structures. *Social Studies of Science*, 18, 331–63.

Marx, J.L. (1989). Drug Availability Is an Issue for Cancer Patients Too. *Science*, 245, 346–7.

Mathiessen, C. (1989). Uninsurance. *Hippocrates*, Nov/Dec., 36–46.

Mayo Clinic (1985). The Mayo Clinic Responds. *Science 85*, July, August, 15.

McAuliffe, B. (1989). Study Supports Vitamin C Therapy, Pauling Says. *Star Tribune*, Minneapolis, 6 Sept., A7.

McCormick, W.J. (1959). Cancer: A Collagen Disease, Secondary to a Nutritional Deficiency? *Archives of Pediatrics*, 76, 166–71.

McCracken, K. (1979). Mayo Study: Pauling Wrong on Vitamin C for Cancer. *Post–Bulletin*, Rochester, 12 Sept., 22.

McGovern, G. (1980). Foreword. In Lesser, M., *Nutrition and Vitamin Therapy*, Bantam Books, Toronto, New York, London, Sydney.

McKeown, T. (1979). *The Role of Medicine*, Blackwell, Oxford.

McKinlay, J.B. (1981). From 'Promising Report' to 'Standard Procedure': Seven Stages in the Career of a Medical Innovation. *Milbank Memorial Fund Quarterly*, 59, 374–411.

McMichael, A.J. (1981). Orthomolecular Medicine and Megavitamin Therapy. *Medical Journal of Australia*, 1, 6–8.

Melville, A. and Johnson, C. (1983). *Cured to Death: The Effects of Prescription Drugs*, New English Library, London.

Moertel, C.G., Schutt, A.J., Hahn, R.G. and Reitmeier, R.J. (1974). Effects of Patient Selection on Results of Phase II Chemotherapy Trials in Gastrointestinal Cancer. *Cancer Chemotherapy Reports*, 58, 257–9.

Moertel, C.G. (1976). Fluorouracil as an Adjuvant to Colorectal Cancer Surgery: The Breakthrough That Never Was. *Journal of the American Medical Association*, 236, 1935–6.

Moertel, C.G. (1978a). A Trial of Laetrile Now. *New England Journal of Medicine*, 298, 218–19.

Moertel, C.G. (1978b). Current Concepts in Cancer: Chemotherapy of Gastrointestinal Cancer. *New England Journal of Medicine*, 299, 1049–52.

Moertel, C.G. (1979). Ethical Questions in Chemotherapy of Patients with Gastrointestinal Cancer *New England Journal of Medicine*, 300, 436–7.

Moertel, C.G. (1986a). A Proposition: Megadoses of Vitamin C are Valuable in the Treatment of Cancer. Negative. *Nutrition Reviews*, 43, 30–2.

Moertel, C.G. (1986b). On Lymphokines, Cytokines, and Breakthroughs. *Journal of the American Medical Association*, 256, 3141.

Moertel, C.G. (1989). Interview on 'Health Report', ABC Radio National, 7 August.

Moertel, C.G. and Creagan, E.T. (1980). To the Editor, *New England Journal of Medicine*, 302, 694–5.

Moertel, C.G., Fleming, T.R., Creagan, E.T., Rubin, J., O'Connell, M.J., and Ames, M.M. (1985). High-Dose Vitamin C Versus Placebo in the Treatment of Patients with Advanced Cancer who have had no prior Chemotherapy. *New England Journal of Medicine*, 312, 137–41.

Moertel, C.G., Fleming, T.R., Rubin, J., Kvols, L.K., Sarna, G., Koch, R., Currie, V.E., Young, C.M., Jones, S.E., and Davignon, J.P. (1982). A Clinical Trial of Amygdalin (Laetrile) in the Treatment of Human Cancer. *New England Journal of Medicine*, 306, 201–6.

Moertel, C.G. and Hanley, J.A. (1976). The Effect of Measuring Error on the Results of Therapeutic Trials in Advanced Cancer. *Cancer*, 38, 388–94.

Moll, L. (1987). Medical Care: Where's the Choice? Distributed by Project CURE, Centre for Alternative Cancer Research, Washington, D.C.

Monaco, G.P. and Gottleib, M.G. (1987). Treatment INDs: Research for Hire? *Journal of the American Medical Association*, 258, 3296–7.

Morishige, F. and Murata, A. (1979). Prolongation of Survival Times in Terminal Human Cancer by Administration of Supplemental Ascorbate. *Journal of the International Academy of Preventive Medicine*, 5, 47–52.

Mortenson, L.E. (1988). Audit Indicates Half of Current Chemotherapy Uses Lack FDA Approval. *Journal of Cancer Program Management*, 3, 21–5.

Moss, R.W. (1980). *The Cancer Syndrome*, Grove Press, New York.

Mulkay, M. (1979). *Science and the Sociology of Knowledge*, Allen & Unwin, London.

Mulkay, M. and Gilbert, G.N. (1982). What is the Ultimate Question? Some Remarks in the Defence of the Analysis of Scientific Discourse. *Social Studies of Science*, 12, 309–19.

Mulkay, M., Potter, J. and Yearley, S. (1983). Why an Analysis of Scientific Discourse is Needed. In Knorr-Cetina, K.D. and Mulkay, M. (eds), *Science Observed*, Sage, London, 171–203.

NCI (1981). Statement on Laetrile. Press release, 30 April 1981.

NCI (1984). Cancer Chemotherapy. *Fact Sheet*, National Cancer Institute/Office of Cancer Communications.

NCI (1985a). *NCI Fact Book. National Cancer Program 1985*, US Department of Health and Human Services, Public Health Service, National Institutes of Health, Washington, DC.

NCI (1985b). *Chemotherapy & You: A Guide to Self-Help During Treatment*, U.S. Department of Health and Human Services, Public Health Service, National Institutes of Health. NIH Publication No.85–1136.

NCI (1986). PDQ: The National Cancer Institute's New Computerized Database for Physicians. National Cancer Institute, Scientific Information Branch, Bethesda, MA.

NCI (1988). National Cancer Institute Statement: Vitamin C. The Cancer Information Service, Office of Cancer Communciations, Memorial Sloan–Kettering Cancer Centre, New York, 7 March.

Nethersell, A. and Sikora, K. (1985). Interferons and Malignant Disease. In Taylor-Papadimitriou, J. (ed.), *Interferons: their Impact in Biology and Medicine*, Oxford University Press, Oxford, 127–45.

Nelkin, D. (ed.) (1979). *Controversy: Politics of Technical Decisions*, Sage, Beverly Hills.

Newbold, H.L. (1979). *Vitamin C Against Cancer*, Stein & Day, New York.

Newmark, P. (1981). Interferon: Decline and Stall. *Nature*, 291, 106.

Nicolson, M. and McLaughlin, C. (1987). Social Constructionism and Medical Sociology: A Reply to M.R. Bury. *Sociology of Health and Illness*, 9, 107–26.

Nightingale, S.L. (1979). To the Editor. *New England Journal of Medicine*, 300, 1222.

O'Connell, M.J., Moertel, C.G., Rubin, J., Hahn, R.G., Kvols, L.K., Schutt, A.J. (1984). Clinical Trial of Sequential N-Phosphonacetyl -l-Aspartate, Thymidine, and 5-Fluorouracil in Advanced Colorectal Carcinoma. *Journal of Clinical Oncology*, 2, 1133–8.

Oldham, R.K. (1982). Biological Response Modifiers Program. *Journal of Biological Response Modifiers*, 1, 81–100.

Page, H.S. and Asire, A.J. (1985). National Cancer Institute. *Cancer Rates and Risks*, 3rd edn, US Department of Health and Human Services, Public Health Service, National Institutes of Health, NIH Publication No. 85691, Washington, DC.

Panem, S. (1984). *The Interferon Crusade*, The Brookings Institution, Washington, DC.

Paradowski, R.J. (1986). In Pauling, L., *How to Live Longer and Feel Better*, W.H. Freeman and Co., New York, 307–12.

Patel, M.S. (1987a). Evaluation of Holistic Medicine. *Social Science and Medicine*, 24, 169–75.

Patel, M.S. (1987b). Problems in the Evaluation of Alternative Medicine. *Social Science and Medicine*, 25, 669–78.

Patterson, J.T. (1987). *The Dread Disease: Cancer and Modern American Culture*, Harvard University Press, Cambridge (Mass.).

Pauling, L. (1968). Orthomolecular Psychiatry. *Science*, 160, 265–71.

Pauling, L. (1970a). *Vitamin C and the Common Cold*, W. H. Freeman, San Francisco, CA.

Pauling, L. (1970b). Evolution and the Need for Ascorbic Acid. *Proceedings of the National Academy of Science*, 67, 1643–8.

Pauling. L. (1972). Vitamin C. *Science*, 177, 1152.

Pauling, L. (1976). *Vitamin C, the Common Cold and the Flu*, W. H. Freeman & Co., 2nd edn, San Francisco, CA.

Pauling, L. (1978). William Fulton Cathcart, III, M.D.: On Orthomolecular Physicians. *The Linus Pauling Institute of Science and Medicine, Newsletter*, 1, 1.

Pauling, L. (1979). The Mayo Clinic Trial of Vitamin C and Cancer. *The Linus Pauling Institute of Science and Medicine, Newsletter*, 1 (7), 3.

Pauling, L. (1980). Vitamin C Therapy of Advanced Cancer. *New England Journal of Medicine*, 302, 694.

Pauling, L. (1982). Laetrile. *New England Journal of Medicine*, 306, 118–19.

Pauling, L. (1983). The Laetrile Controversy. *The Linus Pauling Institute of Science and Medicine, Newsletter*, 2 (3), 2.

Pauling, L. (1986). *How to Live Longer and Feel Better*, W.H. Freeman & Co., New York.

Pauling, L. (1989). Biostatistical Analysis of Mortality Data for Cohorts of Cancer Patients. *Proceedings of the National Academy of Sciences*, 86, 3466–8.

Pauling, L. and Herman, Z.S. (1985). An Analysis of a Randomized Double-Blind Study of the Effects of Giving Vitamin C to Patients with Advanced Colorectal Cancer and then Stopping the Vitamin C and Administering Chemotherapy. Unpublished manuscript, submitted to *New England Journal of Medicine*, 17 April 1985, rejected 4 Sept. 1987.

Pauling, L. and Herman, Z.S. (1989). Criteria for the Validity of Clinical Trials of Treatments of Cohorts of Cancer Patients Based on the Hardin Jones Principle. *Proceedings of the National Academy of Sciences*, 86, 6835–7.

Pauling, L., Itano, H.A., Singer, S.J. and Wells, I.C. (1949). Sickle Cell Anemia, A Molecular Disease. *Science*, 110, 543–8.

Pauling, L., Nixon, J.C., Stitt, F., Marcuson, R., Dunham, W.B., Barth, R.,

Bensch. K., Herman, Z.S., Blaisdell, E., Tsao, C., Prender, M., Andrews, V., Willoughby, R., Zuckerkandl, E. (1985). Effect of Dietary Ascorbic Acid on the Incidence of Spontaneous Mammary Tumors in RIII Mice, *Proceedings of the National Academy of Sciences*, 82, 5185–9.

Pauling, L., Willoughby, R., Reynolds, R., Blaisdell, B. E. and Lawson, S. (1982). Incidence of Squamous Cell Carcinoma in Hairless Mice Irradiated with Ultraviolet Light in Relation to Intake of Ascorbic Acid (Vitamin C) and of D, L-a-Tocopheryl Acetate (Vitamin E). In Hanck, A. (ed.), *Vitamin C: New Clinical Applications in Immunology, Lipid Metabolism and Cancer*, Hans Buber Publishers, Bern, Stuttgart & Vienna, 53–82.

PDR (1989). *Physicians' Desk Reference*, Medical Economics Company, Dradell NJ.

Petersen, J.C. and Markle, G.E. (1979a). Politics and Science in the Laetrile Controversy. *Social Studies of Science*, 9, 139–66.

Petersen, J.C. and Markle, G.E. (1979b). The Laetrile Controversy. In Nelkin, D. (ed.), *Controversy: Politics of Technical Decisions*, Sage, Beverly Hills, CA., 159–78.

Petersen, J.C. and Markle, G.E. (1981). Expansion of Conflict in Cancer Controversies. In Kriesberg, L. (ed.), *Research in Social Movements, Conflict and Change*, 4, JAI Press, Greenwich, CT, 143–54.

Pickering, A. R. (1984). *Constructing Quarks: A Sociological History of Particle Physics*, Edinburgh University Press, Edinburgh.

Pinch, T. (1986). *Confronting Nature: The Sociology of Solar-Neutrino Detection*, Reidel, Dordrecht.

Powledge, T.M. (1988). NEJM's Arnold Relman. *The Scientist*, 2, 12–13.

Project Cure (1985). Mailout Leaflet.

Raven, R. W. (1990). *The Theory and Practice of Oncology: Historical Evolution and Present Principles*, Parthenon Publishing Group, Cornforth and Park Ridge (NJ).

Reilly, D.T. (1983). Young Doctors' Views on Alternative Medicine. *British Medical Journal*, 287, 337–9.

Relman, A.S. (1979a). Holistic Medicine. Editorial. *New England Journal of Medicine*, 300, 312–13.

Relman, A.S. (1979b). Note. *New England Journal of Medicine*, 300, 1222.

Relman, A.S. (1980). The New Medical–Industrial Complex. Editorial. *New England Journal of Medicine*, 303, 963–70.

Relman, A.S. (1982a). Closing the Books on Laetrile. Editorial. *New England Journal of Medicine*, 306 (28 January), 236.

Relman, A.S. (1982b). An Institute for Health Care Evaluation. Editorial. *New England Journal of Medicine*, 306, 669–70.

Relman, A.S. (1983). Technology Assessment by Physicians. In Gay, J.R. and Sax Jacobs, B.J. (eds), *The Technology Explosion in Medical Science: Implications for the Health Care Industry and the Public (1981-2001)*, SP Medical and Scientific Books, New York and London, 101–9.

Relman, A.S. (1988). Assessment and Accountability: The Third Revolution in Medical Care. *New England Journal of Medicine*, 319, 1220–1.

Relman, A.S. (1989). Universal Health Insurance: Its Time Has Come. Editorial. *New England Journal of Medicine*, 320, 117–18.

Rettig, A. (1977). *Cancer Crusade: The Story of the National Cancer Act of 1971*, Princeton University Press, Princeton, NJ.

Rice, D.P. and Hodgson, T.A. (1981). *Social and Economic Implications of Cancer in the United States*, NCHS Publ. No.81–1404, U.S. Department of Health and Human Services.

Rich, S. (1986). The Cost in Dollars. *Washington Post*, 'Cancer' Supplement, 30 Sept.

Richards, E. (1983). Darwin and the Descent of Woman. In Oldroyd, D. and Langham, I. (eds), *The Wider Domain of Evolutionary Thought*, Reidel, Dordrecht, 57–111.

Richards, E. (1986). Vitamin C Suffers a Dose of Politics. *New Scientist*, 109, 46–9.

Richards, E. (1987). A Question of Property Rights: Richard Owen's Evolutionism Reassessed. *British Journal for the History of Science*, 20, 129–72.

Richards, E. (1988). The Politics of Therapeutic Evaluation: The Vitamin C and Cancer Controversy. *Social Studies of Science*, 18, 653–701.

Richards, E. (1989a). The 'Moral Anatomy' of Robert Knox: The Interplay Between Biological and Social Thought in Victorian Scientific Naturalism. *Journal of the History of Biology*, 22, 373–436.

Richards, E. (1989b). Huxley and Woman's Place in Science: The 'Woman Question' and the Control of Victorian Anthropology. In Moore, J. (ed.), *History, Humanity and Evolution*, Cambridge University Press, Cambridge, 253–84.

Richards, E. and Schuster, J.S. (1989). The Feminine Method as Myth and Accounting Resource: A Challenge to Gender Studies and the Social Studies of Science. *Social Studies of Science*, 19, 697–720.

Richards, V. (1978). *The Wayward Cell: Cancer, its Origins, Nature, and Treatment*, University of California Press, Berkeley, Los Angeles and London.

Robinson, A.B. (1979). Diet and Cancer. *Barron's*, 59 (3 September), 7, 19.

Rosch, P.J. and Kearney, H.M. (1985). Holistic Medicine and Technology: A Modern Dialectic. *Social Science and Medicine*, 21, 1405–9.

Roth, J.A. (1976). *Health Purifiers and Their Enemies*, Croom Helm, London.

Rudwick, M.J.S. (1985). *The Great Devonian Controversy*, Chicago University Press, Chicago.

Sadler, J. (1978). Ideologies of 'Art' and 'Science' in Medicine. In Krohn, R. and Weingart, P. (eds), *The Dynamics of Science and Technology (Sociology of the Sciences*, 2, 177–215), Reidel, Dordrecht.

Salmon, J.W. (ed.) (1984). *Alternative Medicines: Popular and Policy Perspectives*, Tavistock, New York and London.

Scarr, L. (1978). Deaths Delay Vitamin C Cancer Test Results. *San Diego Union*, 7 Sept.

Schaffner, K. F. (1986). Ethical Problems in Clinical Trials. *The Journal of Medicine and Philosophy*, 11, 297–315.

Schlegel, J.U. (1975). Proposed Uses of Ascorbic Acid in Prevention of Bladder Control. *Annals of New York Academy of Science*, 258, 432–7.

Schuster, J. (1984). Methodologies as Mythic Structures: A Preface to the Future Historiography of Method. *Metascience*, 1, 15–36.

Schuster, J. and Yeo, R. (eds) (1986). *The Politics and Rhetoric of Scientific Method*, Reidel, Dordrecht.

Scott, P., Richards, E., and Martin, B. (1990). Captives of Controversy: The Myth of the Neutral Social Researcher in Controversy Analysis. *Science, Technology, and Human Values,* in press.

Senecker, H. (1977). Vitamin C Giant. *Drug and Cosmetic Industry,* 121 (August), 40–3.

Senecker, H. (1979). Body Building at Hoffmann–La Roche. *Forbes,* 5 February, 92–4.

Serafini, A. (1989). *Linus Pauling: A Man and His Science,* Paragon House, New York.

Shapin, S. (1982). History of Science and its Sociological Reconstructions. *History of Science,* 20, 157–211.

Shapo, M.S. (1979). *A Nation of Guinea Pigs,* The Free Press, New York.

Shereff, R. (1989). Levamisole-5-FU Mix Just One of Many. *Medical Tribune,* 26 Oct., 9.

Shurkin, J.W. (1979). Vitamin C vs. Cancer: A New Look. *Philadelphia Inquirer,* 15 Feb., 17–A.

Siegel, B.V. (1975). Enhancement of Interferon Production by Poly(rl) poly(rC) in Mouse Cell Cultures by Ascorbic Acid. *Nature,* 254, 531–2.

Siegelbaum, M. (1979). To the Editor. *New England Journal of Medicine,* 300, 1221.

Silverman, M. and Lee, P.R. (1974). *Pills, Profits and Politics,* University of California Press, Berkeley.

Silverman, W.A. (1985). *Human Experimentation: A Guided Step into the Unknown,* Oxford University Press, Oxford.

Sikora, K. (1986). Interferon and Malignant Disease. *The British Journal of Clinical Practice,* 40, 406–10.

Smith, D. (1986). Overhyped Interferon Makes a Comeback. *National Times* (7 March), 22.

Smith, T. (1983). Alternative Medicine. Editorial. *British Medical Journal,* 287, 307.

Smyth, J.F., Balkwill, F.R., Cavalli, F., Kimchi, A., Mattson, K., Niederle, N.E., Spiegel, R. J. (1987). Interferons in Oncology: Current Status and Future Directions. *European Journal of Cancer Clinical Oncology,* 23, 887–9.

Sobel, D.S. (ed.) (1979). *Ways of Health,* Harcourt Brace Jovanovich, New York and London.

Sontag, S. (1983). *Illness as Metaphor,* Penguin Books, Harmondsworth, Middx.

Starr, P. (1982). *The Social Transformation of American Medicine,* Basic Books, Inc., New York.

Steward, F. and Wibberley, A.G. (1981). Drug Innovation: What's Slowing It Down? *Nature,* 284, 118–20.

Stockwell, S. (1985). Vitamin C Shown Ineffective Against Cancer: Pauling Disputes Results, Moertel Defends. *Oncology Times,* 7, 1, 22.

Stone, I. (1972). *The Healing Factor: 'Vitamin C' Against Disease,* Grosset & Dunlap, New York.

Stone, I. (1980). The Possible Role of Mega-ascorbate in the Endogenous Synthesis of Interferon. *Medical Hypothesis,* 6, 309–14.

Strander, H. (1977). Anti-Tumour Effects of Interferon and its Possible Use as an Anti-Neoplastic Agent in Man. *Texas Reports on Biology and Medicine,*

35, 429–35.

Strander, H. (1982). Interferon in Cancer: Faith, Hope, and Reality. *American Journal of Clinical Oncology*, 5, 297–301.

Strickland, S.P. (1972). *Politics, Science and Dread Disease*, Harvard University Press, Cambridge, MA.

Studer, K.E. and Chubin, D.E. (1980). *The Cancer Mission: Social Contexts of Biomedical Research*, Sage, Beverly Hills, CA.

Sun, M. (1981a). Interferon: No Magic Bullet Against Cancer. *Science*, 212, 142.

Sun, M. (1981b). Laetrile Brush Fire is Out, Scientists Hope. *Science*, 212, 758–9.

Sun, M. (1981c). At Long Last, Linus Pauling Lands NCI Grant. *Science*, 212, 1126.

Sun, M. (1981d). Cancer Institute's Drug Program Reproved. *Science*, 214, 887–9.

Sylvester, R. (1984). Planning Cancer Clinical Trials. In Buyse, M.E., Staquet, M.J. and Sylvester, R.J. (eds), *Cancer Clinical Trials: Methods and Practice*, Oxford University Press, Oxford, New York and Toronto, 47–63.

Tatkon, M.D. (1968). *The Great Vitamin Hoax*, Macmillan, New York.

Teitelman, R. (1989). The Case of Alpha Interferon: Slow and Steady Wins the Race. *Oncology Times*, 11, 3, 21.

Temin. P. (1980). *Taking Your Medicine: Drug Regulation in the United States*, Harvard University Press, Cambridge (Mass.).

Treaster, J.B. (1980). Orthodox Researchers Quit an 'Alternative' Cancer Parley. *New York Times* (13 October).

Truswell, A.S. (1986). Ascorbic Acid. *New England Journal of Medicine*, 315, 709–10.

Tschetter, L., Creagan, E.T., O'Fallon, J.R., Schutt, A.J., Krook, J.E., Windschitl, H.E., *et al.* (1983). A Community-Based Study of Vitamin C (Ascorbic Acid) Therapy in Patients with Advanced Cancer. *Proceedings of the American Society of Clinical Oncology*, 2, 92.

Turner, B.S. (1987). *Medical Power and Social Knowledge*, Sage, London and Beverly Hills.

United States General Accounting Office (1987). *Cancer Patient Survival: What Progress Has Been Made? Report to the Chairman*, Subcommittee on Intergovernmental Relations and Human Resources, Committee on Government Operations, House of Representatives, General Accounting Office, Washington, D.C. GAO/PEMD–87–13.

Unschuld, P.U. (1980). The Issue of Structured Coexistence of Scientific and Alternative Medical Systems: A Comparison of East and West German Legislation. *Social Science and Medicine*, 148, 15–24.

Van Dam, F.S.A.M., Linssen, C.A.G., and Couzjin, A.L. (1984). Evaluating 'Quality of Life' in Cancer Clinical Trials. In Buyse, M.E., Staquet, M.J. and Sylvester, R.J. (eds), *Cancer Clinical Trials: Methods and Practice*, Oxford University Press, Oxford, New York and Toronto, 26–43.

Wallis, R. (1985). Science and Pseudo-Science. *Social Science Information*, 24, 585–601.

Williams, R. and Kalita, D. (eds) (1977). *A Physician's Handbook on Orthomolecular Medicine*, Pergamon Press, Elmsford, NY.

Willis, E. (1983). *Medical Dominance*, George Allen & Unwin, Sydney, London and Boston, MA.

Wittes, R.E. (1985). Vitamin C and Cancer. *New England Journal of Medicine*, 312, 178–9.

Woodcock, J. (1981). Medicines – The Interested Parties. In Blum, R., Herxheimer, A., Stenzl, C. and Woodcock, J. (eds), *Pharmaceuticals and Health Policy: International Perspectives on Provision and Control of Medicines*, Croom Helm, London, 27–35.

Wright, P. and Treacher, A. (eds) (1982). *The Problem of Medical Knowledge: Examining the Social Construction of Medicine*, Edinburgh University Press, Edinburgh.

Wyke, A. (1987). Molecules and Markets: A Survey of Pharmaceuticals. *The Economist*, 302 (7–13 February, Supplement), 1–17.

Wynne, B. (1975). The Rhetoric of Consensus Politics: A Critical View of Technology Assessment. *Research Policy*, 4, 108–58.

Yetiv, J.Z. (1986). *Popular Nutritional Practices: A Scientific Appraisal*, Popular Medicine Press, Toledo, Ohio.

Yonemoto, R.H., Chretien, P.B., and Fehniger, T.F. (1976). Enhanced Lymphocyte Blastogenesis by Oral Ascorbic Acid. *Proceedings of the American Association for Cancer Research*, 17, 288.

Young, F.E., Norris, J.A., Levitt, J.A. and Nightingale, S.L. (1988). The FDA's New Procedures for the Use of Investigational Drugs in Treatment. *Journal of the American Medical Association*, 259, 2267–70.

Young, J.H. (1967). *The Medical Messiahs: A Social History of Health Quackery in Twentieth-Century America*, Princeton University Press, Princeton.

Young, J.H. (1972). The Persistence of Medical Quackery in America. *American Scientist*, 60, 318–26.

Young, R.S.K. (1987). Federal Regulation of Laetrile. In Engelhardt, T. and Caplan, A.L. (eds), *Scientific Controversies; Case Studies in the Resolution and Closure of Disputes in Science and Technology*, Cambridge University Press, Cambridge, 333–41.

Yoxen, E. (1983). *The Gene Business*, Pan Books, London and Sydney.

Index